Springer-Verlag Berlin Heidelberg New York
London Paris Tokyo Hong Kong

Peter A. Miescher (Ed.)

Systemic Lupus Erythematosus

With 21 Figures and 24 Tables

Springer

Professor Dr. Peter A. Miescher
Division d'Hématologie
Centre de Transfusion Sanguine
Hôpital Cantonal Universitaire
25, rue Micheli-du-Crest
CH-1211 Geneva 4, Switzerland

ISBN-13: 978-3-642-79624-1 e-ISBN: 978-3-642-79622-7
DOI: 10.1007/978-3-642-79622-7

Softcover reprint of the hardcover 1st Edition 1995

Typesetting: Satztechnik K. Steingraeber, 69126 Heidelberg
SPIN 10497796 27/3136-5 4 3 2 1 0 - Printed on acid-free paper

Contents

Introduction

Peter A. Miescher

Division d'Hématologie, Centre de Transfusion Sanguine, Hôpital Cantonal Universitaire, 25, rue Micheli-du-Crest, CH-1211 Genève 4, Suisse

During the past 50 years, systemic lupus erythematosus (SLE) has been the main subject in the field of immunopathology. Each individual discovery was followed by the discovery of a multitude of related immune phenomena. Thus, the false-positive VDR reaction opened the door to additional antibodies leading to the concept of the anti-phospholipid syndrome. The demonstration of anti-nuclear antibodies led to the discovery of a cascade of antibodies against various constituents of the cell nucleus. Today's concept of a genetic predisposition emerged with the discovery of the H2 system in mice by Snell and subsequently of the immune response genes by Benacerraf and McDevitt.

This book reflects the present status of our understanding of this protean disease. Izui covers the various animal models which clearly show that different gene combinations can lead to the final clinical expression of SLE, with HLA class II genes probably responsible for the targeting of the autoimmune response. Similarly, research on cytokines in SLE patients has shown that SLE is a syndrome depending on different pathways. Handwerger stresses the possible co-involvement of lymphocyte tropic viruses which may lead, depending on the genetic predisposition, to the clinical picture of SLE. Horwitz describes different cytokine constellations depending on whether we are dealing with the initiation or perpetuation of autoimmunity. We, thus, are no longer focusing on single cytokines but rather on the entire cytokine network.

Apoptosis may play an important role in the initiation process. Furthermore, genetically based alterations of cell metabolism may also be of importance, stressing the participation of non-immune parameters in the genetic predisposition to SLE.

Antibodies to cell membrane antigens are a frequent finding in SLE. Autoimmune haemolytic anaemia and severe thrombocytopenia are readily acknowledged as being due to the respective antibodies against cell membrane antigens. More complex are the cold reacting antibodies against CD45 and other lymphocyte membrane antigens, a subject which is well covered by Winfield and associates. Are these antibodies a consequence of SLE or are they directly implicated in the lymphopenia or other pathological events? Or do they represent a physiogenetic attempt by the immune system to restore homeostasis in response to aggressive autoimmune stimulation?

Anti-phospholipid antibodies discussed in the chapters by Roubey and Harris represent another hot subject in lupus research. Do these antibodies cause thrombosis, CNS damage and thrombocytopenia, etc., or are they a consequence of an autoaggression against various endothelial targets? With regard to pregnancy, they certainly appear to be directly involved in miscarriage. Whatever the mechanism, the physician has to offer help to his patients. In the case of serious problems of deep vein thrombosis, life-long anti-coagulation becomes mandatory whether or not antiphospholipid antibodies are present. The same measures are necessary for the treatment of haemorrhagic processes within the brain. Even after one single cerebral vascular accident, anti-coagulation becomes advisable since a second serious accident may occur even years after the first.

Lockshin covers the important subject of lupus pregnancies and neonatal SLE. Again, with or without antiphospholipid antibodies, ASA is probably advisable for all patients with SLE to prevent placental infarction. A more complex problem concerns antibodies to RO-SSA and LA-SSP. Neonatal lupus, a rare condition, appears to be clearly linked to maternal antibodies to these antigenic targets. Rosenberg emphasises that a child with SLE presents a special challenge to the physician. Indeed, the disease activity must be controlled rapidly with as little cortisone as possible. In our experience, cyclosporin is very helpful in this regard if given in association with methotrexate and, if necessary, the more toxic cyclophosphamide.

The remaining papers deal with the treatment of patients with SLE. Gourley speaks of disease management since so many factors have to be taken into consideration in the attempt to control disease activity while permitting a good quality of life. To try to reach this goal, my own group has developed a drug combination therapy. With regard to CNS involvement, Valesini reports on the possibility of offering a local treatment by intrathecal injection of dexamethasone and methotrexate. Knobler gives a short summary of extracorporeal photochemotherapy where one hopes that lymphocytes active in the disease process will preferentially assimilate the photo-sensitive drug 8-methoxypsoralen. It is assumed that subsequent ultraviolet radiation will kill those lymphocytes which then would serve to immunise patients against the idiotypes of the pathogenic lymphocyte clones.

Another experimental approach is discussed by Maini. However, while anti-TNF therapy has been shown to be effective for remission induction in rheumatoid arthritis (RA), conditions in lupus are different. In particular, in RA we are dealing with a real concentration of the cells of the immune system which are ready to attack the putative autoantigen target (collagen II?). In the case of SLE, we do not have such a concentration; Maini, thus, does not expect anti-TNF to be of much use in the treatment of lupus.

Finally, the question of prognosis is discussed by Esdaile. Fortunately, with every passing decade, the prognosis for patients with SLE gets better and better, both with regard to control of disease activity and quality of life.

Mechanisms of genetic control of murine systemic lupus erythematosus

Shozo Izui, Ramón Merino, Masahiro Iwamoto, Liliane Fossati

Department of Pathology, Centre Medical Universitaire, University of Geneva, CH-1211 Geneva 4, Switzerland

Introduction

The pathogenesis of systemic lupus erythematosus (SLE) is a complex process in which many genetic factors apparently play essential roles in determining the incidence, onset and nature of SLE. The involvement of genetic factors in SLE was initially suggested by the fact that there is a familial tendency for SLE. Since a number of different immunopathological manifestations are found in members of the same family, it is likely that the expression of SLE is controlled by multiple genes and a number of secondary factors. Although the conclusion from family studies have to be considered as preliminary, these studies have led to the concept that a special genetic background is necessary for contracting SLE. A sophisticated genetic analysis is only possible by using animal models of SLE with well-defined genetic backgrounds, preferably congenic strains of mice differing at defined genetic loci. The availability of several SLE-prone mice such as (NZB x NZW)F_1, MRL-*lpr/lpr* and BXSB with different genetic backgrounds (reviewed in [112]) offers an invaluable opportunity for elucidating the mechanisms by which genetic factors participate in the pathogenesis of SLE. In this article, we will review the current understanding for the role of various genetic factors and abnormalities involved in different strains of lupus-prone mice.

Multigenic features of murine SLE

Since Helyer and Howie [30] first reported the development of an SLE-like syndrome in the F_1 progeny of the NZB and NZW strains, the genetic basis for SLE in (NZB x NZW)F_1 hybrids (NZB x W) has been investigated in a number of laboratories. Early genetic studies on New Zealand mice have demonstrated that many individual autoimmune traits segregate independently of each other in (NZBxW) x NZW backcross mice [102], in the F_2 generation of NZBxW [40] mice and in the

Correspondence to: S. Izui

Table 1. Possible genetic factors involved in murine systemic lupus erythematosus (SLE)

1. Immunoglobulin variable region genes
2. T cell receptor genes
3. MHC class II genes
4. Genes regulating apoptosis
– the *Fas* apoptosis gene: the *lpr* mutation
– the *gld* gene: the Fas ligand
5. The *Yaa* gene: intercellular adhesion molecule (?)
6. Genes for expression of nephritogenic autoantigens
– genes encoding and/or regulating the expression of serum retroviral gp70 antigen
7. Genes regulating the immunoglobulin class switching
– genes for cytokines and/or their receptors
- the *xid* gene: Bruton's tyrosine kinase (?)

lpr, lymphoproliferation; *gld*, generalized lymphoproliferative disease; *Yaa*, Y chromosome-linked autoimmune acceleration; *xid*, X chromosome-linked immunodeficiency

recombinant inbred strains derived from the NZB strain crossed with normal strains [8, 88]. This suggests that there is no common genetic defect causing overall autoimmune responses, but each of the autoimmune traits is under the control of separate genetic mechanisms, at least in the New Zealand strain. Multiple, unlinked genes are apparently responsible for the production of a variety of autoantibodies and the expression of various disease manifestations.

Since the major features of NZBxW autoimmune disease are not present in the parental strains, genes from each parent most likely act in concert to produce the F_1 phenotype. Although the precise nature and number of genes involved in the development of SLE remain unclear, several genes have been investigated as candidate genes to be implicated in SLE in the last decades (Table 1). They include immunoglobulin (Ig) variable (V) region genes encoding autoantibodies with pathogenic specificity, T cell receptor genes and the major histocompatibility complex (MHC) genes. In addition, in view of the complexity of the immune network, there can be a number of other different kinds of genes, which may play an active role in the regulation of autoimmune responses, such as genes for cytokines or their receptors, genes regulating apoptosis, and genes regulating the expression of nephritogenic autoantigens, etc.

The immunoglobulin variable region genes

In an attempt to gain a better understanding of the genetic origin of autoantibodies characteristic in SLE, the V gene usage in autoantibodies has been extensively analyzed to determine whether lupus autoantibodies are encoded by unique Ig gene segments present in the normal germ-line repertoire, but not expressed in immune responses against exogenous antigens, and whether the autoantibody response is genetically and structurally restricted. Nucleic acid sequence studies on the V regions of various autoantibodies derived from lupus-prone mice have clearly demonstrated that these lupus autoantibodies use the same germ-line repertoire as anti-foreign antibodies (reviewed in [11, 55]). In addition, it has been shown that autoantibody responses in lupus-prone mice are quite heterogeneous in terms of V region gene usage, indicating that a large variety of Ig gene segments are capable of encoding lupus autoantibodies. All these results strongly argue against the idea that spontaneous development of autoantibodies in lupus-prone mice is related to the abnormality in the Ig V region genes.

The T cell receptor genes

Based on the fact that the NZW strain contributes to the switch from IgM autoantibodies (an NZB trait) to IgG autoantibodies in NZBxW mice [56], which is dependent on the presence of $CD4^+$ T cells [99, 121], it is conceivable that the influence of the NZW strain can be on the T cell function. The analysis of the T cell receptor (TCR) gene complex has revealed an unusual TCR β-chain allele in NZW mice, characterized by the deletion of $C_\beta 1$, $D_\beta 2$ and $J_\beta 2$ gene segments [57, 81]. An attractive hypothesis is that a deletion of these elements could result in the unusual joining of $J_\beta 1$ to $C_\beta 2$, which may lead to the generation of a harmful autoreactive T cell repertoire. In fact, studies on (NZBxW) x NZB backcross and TCR congenic NZBxW mice by Shirai and his co-workers [33, 124] have shown a statistically significant association of the NZW TCR β chain allele with autoimmune manifestations characteristic of NZBxW mice. However, two other studies failed to show any association of disease expression with the presence of the NZW allele in (NZBxW) x NZB backcross mice [58] and in NZBxW F_2 mice [82]. This discrepancy can be in part due to the fact that the effect of the NZW TCR allele was incomplete in the study by the former group [33, 124]. Nevertheless, it should be stressed that autoreactive T cells responsible for SLE are apparently well developed in T cells bearing the non-NZW TCR allele in the thymic microenvironment of the appropriate autoimmune genetic background, as observed in NZB mice carrying the $H\text{-}2^{bm12}$ haplotype [13] as well as in two other SLE strains of mice (MRL and BXSB). Apparently, the NZW TCR β-chain deletion is not an indispensable genetic defect for the development of typical murine SLE.

The demonstrations that specific TCR V_β genes are required for responses to certain autoantigens in the case of experimental allergic encephalomyelitis, collagen-induced arthritis and insulin-dependent diabetes (reviewed in [2]) have prompted the exploration of a possible association of particular TCR V_β gene(s) with SLE. Relative over-representation of T cells expressing TCR $V_\beta 8$ family genes has been reported in MRL-*lpr/lpr* mice [28, 98, 103]. Furthermore, it has been claimed that the $V_\beta 8$ T cells may play a critical role in the development of a lupus-like syndrome in MRL-*lpr/lpr* mice, since the selective diminution of $V_\beta 8^+$ T cells by treating them with either staphylococcal enterotoxin B (SEB) or anti-$V_\beta 8$ monoclonal antibody resulted in an inhibition of autoimmune disease in MRL-*lpr/lpr* mice [18, 52]. However, the interpretation of these results should be cautious, since repeated injections of SEB or anti-$V_\beta 8$ monoclonal antibody could lead to a persistent activation of T cells, resulting in a massive production of cytokines such as tumor necrosis factor-α (TNF-α). This would cause a profound effect on the immune system, thereby preventing the excessive stimulation of autoimmune responses. In fact, repeated injections of recombinant TNF-α have been shown to delay the development of SLE in NZBxW mice [45] and of autoimmune diabetes in non-obese diabetic (NOD) mice [48, 95]. Further experiments are awaited to clarify to what extent the $V_\beta 8^+$ T cells indeed contribute to the development of lupus-like autoimmune syndrome in MRL-*lpr/lpr* mice. It should be mentioned, however, that the development of a severe form of SLE in (NZB x BXSB)F_1 hybrid mice despite clonal deletion of $V_\beta 8^+$ T cells due to the expression of endogenous superantigens strongly argues against the idea that $V_\beta 8^+$T cells are an essential element for the development of autoimmune responses in murine SLE.

The MHC-linked genes

The MHC class II I-A genes. The studies on F_1 backcross animals carried out by several groups have shown that the renal disease of NZBxW mice depends on the action of at least three genes or clusters of closely linked genes [54, 58, 62, 63]. Although results from backcross studies have been difficult to interpret in terms of the precise number of genes involved, it has been claimed that one is contributed by the NZB strain and two, unlinked, contributed by the NZW strain. Significantly, one dominant gene from the NZW strain maps within the H-2 (MHC for mouse) region, which was confirmed by the subsequent study on NZB and NZW H-2 congenic mice [31]. Since the genes encoding for MHC molecules participate in both the regulation of the immune response and the selection of T cell specificities from the repertoire, it is conceivable that the NZW MHC class II ($I\text{-}A^z$) genes are one of the major contributors to NZBxW disease. Supporting this are the demonstrations that autoimmune disease manifestations are dependent on the presence of $CD4^+$ T cells [121] and that the development of SLE can be blocked by treatment with anti-I-A^z antibodies [4].

Extensive studies in New Zealand mice using (NZBxW) x NZB backcross, NZBxW F_2 and H-2 congenic NZBxW mice by several groups have consistently demonstrated that the H-$2^{d/z}$ hybrid MHC class II molecules produced in NZBxW mice may act as restriction elements for their autoimmune disease [33, 58, 82]. The role of hybrid class II molecules in the development of murine lupus was also suggested in studies on (NZW x BXSB)F_1 hybrid mice [51] and on F_2 offspring of NZW x SWR crosses [25]. Collectively, it has been proposed that heterozygous pairing of an α chain from one haplotype with a β chain from the other haplotype might produce a mixed haplotype hybrid class II molecule capable of presenting disease-inducing peptides and interacting with the TCR [32, 83].

Other evidence that supports the role of MHC class II molecules in the regulation of murine SLE is the recent description of a new line of NZB mice bearing the H-2^{bm12} haplotype [13]. The introduction of the *bm12* mutation in the I-A_β chain in NZB mice, in contrast to conventional NZB (H-2^d) or NZB.H-2^b congenic mice, results in a dramatic increase of autoantibody production and the rapid development of severe lupus nephritis indistinguishable from that of NZBxW mice. This finding is particularly interesting because the *bm12* mutation differs by only three amino acid residues at positions 67, 70 and 71 of the I-A_β molecule, as compared with that of the wild-type H-2^b haplotype. This suggests that these three amino acid residues located in the peptide-binding groove of the I-A^{bm12} molecules are important for the induction of autoimmunity in the context of an NZB background. However, recent studies by Cohen et al. [16] have shown that there was no significant enhancement of anti-DNA autoantibody production in C57BL/6 (B6)-*lpr/lpr* mice carrying the *bm12* mutation, as compared with conventional B6-*lpr/lpr* (H-2^b) mice. Apparently, an exacerbating effect of the *bm12* mutation on NZB mice cannot be generalizable to all strains of mice. Nevertheless, this is the first direct demonstration that the I-A molecules play a critical role in the development of SLE, since NZB.H-2^{bm12} mice do not express the I-E molecules. It should be mentioned that the production of Coombs' anti-erythrocyte and anti-thymocyte autoantibodies is far lower in NZB.H-2^b mice than NZB (H-2^d) and NZB.H-2^{bm12} mice [78]. This emphasizes the association of the MHC haplotype with individual autoimmune responses characteristic in SLE, supporting the idea that autoimmune responses occurring in lupus-prone mice are under the MHC control, as is the case of immune responses against foreign antigens.

Table 2. Mortality rate of 50% for H-2 congenic BXSB and (NZB x BXSB)F_1 hybrid mice

Mice	H-2	Female	*Yaa* male[a]
BXSB	b/b	> 18 mo	8 mo
	d/b	ND[b]	10 mo
	d/d	ND	> 18 mo
(NZB x BXSB)F_1	b/b	7 mo	5.5 mo
	d/b	9 mo	5.5 mo
	d/d	15 mo	6.5 mo

[a]The development of SLE was markedly delayed in BXSB and (NZB x BXSB)F_1 male mice lacking the *Yaa* gene; mo, months
[b]Not determined

It is now clear that the MHC class II genes provide at least some of the genetic requirements for the predisposition of New Zealand mice to lupus nephritis. However, it was not established whether a unique mixed class II haplotype molecule and/or a mutant class II molecule is crucial for the development of typical murine lupus or whether conventional MHC class II molecules are sufficient in mice with the appropriate autoimmune genetic background. In this regard, it should be mentioned that male BXSB mice bearing the conventional H-2^b haplotype develop a typical lupus [6, 77]. Strikingly, BXSB male mice bearing the H-2^d [68] or H-2^k haplotype (Dixon and McConahey, personal communication) exhibit a far-lower production of autoantibodies and less evidence of lupus nephritis with a marked prolonged survival rate, as compared with mice bearing the wild-type H-2^b haplotype (Table 2).

Since only male BXSB mice develop severe SLE, which results in part from the action of a mutant *Yaa* (Y chromosome-linked autoimmune acceleration) gene (discussed below), it is difficult to determine whether the observed MHC effect on the development of SLE is mediated by acting on the *Yaa* gene or by regulating the development of autoimmune responses, independently of the *Yaa* gene. This question was addressed by studying the effect of the H-2^b and H-2^d haplotypes on the development of SLE in (NZB x BXSB)F_1 hybrid mice [71], whose H-$2^{d/b}$ heterozygous females develop a typical SLE in the absence of the *Yaa* gene [77]. Our results have demonstrated that the development of SLE was markedly delayed in female F_1 hybrid mice homozygous for the H-2^d haplotype, as compared with those bearing the H-2^b haplotype (Table 2). This clearly indicates that the protective effect of the H-2^d is not mediated through the *Yaa* gene action, but is acting directly on the development of autoimmune responses.

It is significant that the conventional H-2^b haplotype exerts an effect sufficient to initiate and promote autoimmune responses responsible for the development of SLE in mice with the appropriate background, while the H-2^d and H-2^k haplotypes are a resistant (or protective) haplotype for SLE. This notion is supported by observations made in H-2^b congenic BXSB and B6-*lpr/lpr* mice, in which the H-2^d and H-2^k, but not H-2^b, inhibit autoantibody production ([16, 68] and Dixon and McConahey, personal communication). In addition, the fact that both the H-$2^{b/b}$ homozygous and H-$2^{d/b}$ heterozygous (NZB x BXSB)F_1 hybrid mice similarly develop SLE, as observed in BXSB mice (Table 2), excludes the implication of hybrid class II molecules in the development of SLE in (NZB x BXSB)F_1 hybrid mice. The dominant effect of the H-2^b haplotype on autoimmune responses was also recognized in H-$2^{b/k}$ heterozygous BXSB mice (Dixon and McConahey, personal communication). However, in studies on B6-*lpr/lpr* mice, the dominant effect of the H-2^b haplotype was less evident: the autoantibody production in $H-2^{d/b}$ B6-*lpr/lpr* mice was substantially lower than that of $H-2^{b/b}$ B6-*lpr/lpr* mice [16]. It is possible that there may exist some gene-dosage effect of the MHC class II molecules on the development of autoimmune responses, as described for immune responses to certain foreign antigens [72]. The MHC class II gene-dosage effect on autoimmune responses can be dependent on other factors in the genetic background of various mouse strains; it may be more apparent in mice whose genetic background is not predisposed to autoimmune diseases, such as B6 mice, than in lupus-prone BXSB and (NZB x BXSB)F_1 mice. Alternatively, the expression of the I-E molecules in $H-2^{d/b}$ heterozygotes (absent in $H-2^{b/b}$ mice because of the deletion of the promoter region of the Eα gene [64]) may exert some inhibitory effect on autoimmune responses, as recently observed in I-Eα^d BXSB transgenic mice [70]. Although the protective effect conferred by the transgene has not been totally elucidated (discussed below), our recent studies on different lupus-prone mice have shown that the protective effect of an E_α^d transgene varies in lupus-prone mice, depending on the severity of the disease developing in mice studied (unpublished observation). Thus, it may not be surprising that the inhibitory effect of the I-E molecules on autoimmune responses can be much greater in B6-*lpr/lpr* mice than in lupus-prone BXSB and (NZB x BXSB)F_1 mice, which develop more severe SLE than B6-*lpr/lpr* mice [42, 77].

It is striking that the *Yaa* gene totally abrogates the MHC effect on the development of SLE occurring in (NZB x BXSB)F_1 mice, since in the presence of the *Yaa* gene, $H-2^{d/d}$ F_1 males developed SLE as severe as $H-2^{b/b}$ F_1 males (Table 2) [71]. It should be noted that the *lpr* gene could similarly overcome the MHC effect in mice, depending on their genetic background, as the presence of the *lpr* mutation markedly accelerates the progression of SLE in MRL mice bearing the $H-2^k$ haplotype, which confers a protection on BXSB mice. Notably, the difficulty of defining MHC association in human SLE may be partly explained by the abolishment of the MHC effect by the presence of powerful accelerating factors, such as the *Yaa* or *lpr* gene.

At present, the precise molecular and cellular mechanisms by which the MHC class II molecules are predisposing to the development of SLE are still unclear. Considering the central role of the MHC molecules in the generation of the T cell repertoire, we favor the idea that the MHC control of the autoimmune syndrome is likely to be a consequence of thymic selection, by the predisposing MHC haplotype, of a harmful autoreactive T cell repertoire. In this regard, a recent study of Forsgren et al. [21] is relevant. They have demonstrated that in allophenic mouse chimeras, constructed by the fusion of B6 and NOD embryos, the development of autoimmune insulitis correlates with the MHC chimerism in thymus cortical regions; only the mice bearing thymus cortical regions expressing the NOD H-2 haplotype develop lymphoid cell infiltration in pancreatic islets. As discussed below, autoreactive T cells can be positively selected even in non-autoimmune mice bearing appropriate MHC haplotypes such as $H-2^b$; but they can be optimally activated only in mice with an autoimmune background.

The MHC class II I-E genes. The inhibition conferred by the $H-2^d$ or $H-2^k$ haplotype on autoimmune responses in BXSB or B6-*lpr/lpr* mice could be in part related to the expression by these mice of MHC class II I-E molecules, absent in BXSB and B6 mice bearing the $H-2^b$ haplotype. In fact, it has been shown that I-E molecules could exhibit a suppressive activity on immune responses [84]. More recently, several groups have reported that the development of spontaneous autoimmune diabetes in NOD mice can be prevented by the expression of I-E molecules through an I-E α-chain transgene [9, 61, 116]. Although the mechanisms by which the I-E molecules protect NOD mice from the development of an autoimmune diabetes are still controversial [9, 19, 87], one possibility is that this protection could be a consequence of the clonal deletion or anergy of I-E-reactive T cells, which potentially contain autoreactive T cells, due to I-E expression in NOD I-E$^+$ transgenic mice [90]. However, such a possibility seems unlikely in the case of lupus-prone mice, since I-E$^+$ H-2$^{b/d}$ BXSB heterozygous male mice exhibit clonal deletion of I-E-reactive T cell populations at an extent comparable to that observed in I-E$^+$ BXSB.H-2^d mice [68], but still develop a typical lupus-like autoimmune disease, as do conventional I-E$^-$ BXSB (H-2^b) male mice. These results strongly argue against the hypothesis that the expression of the I-E molecule and consequent clonal deletion or anergy of potential autoreactive T cells are responsible for the prevention of the lupus-like autoimmune disease in I-E$^+$ BXSB.H-2^d and BXSB.H-2^k mice.

To explore a possible protective effect of the I-E molecules on the development of SLE, we have recently generated I-E_α^d transgenic BXSB mice. The expression of the I-E molecules through an I-E α-chain transgene almost completely prevents autoantibody production and subsequent lupus nephritis in BXSB mice [70]. The development of the autoimmune syndrome in irradiated I-E$^+$ BXSB transgenic mice reconstituted with non-transgenic bone marrow cells rules out the possibility that the E_α^d transgene conferred the protection by the induction of regulatory T cells or clonal deletion of potential autoreactive T cells as a result of I-E expression. It should be mentioned that the lupus-like autoimmune syndrome developing in (NZB x BXSB)F_1 and (NZW x BXSB)F_1 female mice in the absence of the *Yaa* gene is similarly inhibited by the presence of the E_α^d transgene, while the E_α^d transgene exhibits only a partial or little protective effect in (NZB x BXSB)F_1 and (NZW x BXSB)F_1 male mice expressing the *Yaa* gene, which develop a more severe form of SLE than their females (unpublished observation). Thus, the E_α^d transgene is capable of preventing SLE by inhibiting the development of autoimmune responses, but its protective effect apparently depends on the severity of the disease and can be counteracted by the *Yaa* gene.

It is significant that the expression of the I-E molecules at the level provided by the H-2$^{b/d}$ or H-2$^{b/k}$ heterozygous state does not protect BXSB mice from their autoimmune syndrome ([68] and Dixon and McConahey, personal communication). This suggests that the lack of the autoimmune syndrome in the BXSB transgenic mice may be related to the generation of an unusually high level of I-E α chains, probably due to the large copy number of the E_α^d transgene carried by these mice. Of interest, in mice bearing I-A^b and I-E molecules, it has been shown that one of the major self peptides presented by the I-A^b molecules is derived from the I-E α chain [94]. Thus, one may speculate that overexpression of I-E α chains in the transgenic mice could lead to an increased formation of peptides derived from this chain which are presented in the peptide-binding groove of I-A^b molecules. In fact, on B cells from BXSB mice bearing the E_α^d transgene, an increased fraction of the I-A^b molecules contain in their binding groove the I-E α-chain-derived peptide [70]. This raises the possibility that an increased presentation of I-E a chain peptides by the I-A^b molecules might prevent excessive activation of the B cells bearing these peptides, and hence the lack of autoimmune syndrome in the transgenic BXSB mice. In fact, when irradiated BXSB mice were reconstituted with a mixture of bone marrow cells from non-transgenic and transgenic BXSB male mice, I-E$^+$ transgenic B cells produced far less anti-DNA autoantibodies than I-E$^-$ B cells derived from non-transgenic mice [70]. These results support the idea that a lower activation of B cells bearing an I-E α-chain peptide in their I-A^b molecule is the mechanism preventing SLE in the transgenic mice. It should be emphasized that the BXSB transgenic mice by themselves do not show any features of immune deficiency and display normal antibody responses against T cell-dependent antigens. This excludes the possibility that immune deficiency due to overexpression of the transgene product, as observed in mice bearing a high copy number of the A_β^k transgene [26], is a cause of the protection of SLE by the E_α^d transgene.

Based on these results, we propose an entirely novel mechanism by which the E_α^d transgene protects BXSB mice against SLE: overexpression of I-E α chains results in the generation of excessive amounts of a peptide displaying a high affinity to the I-A^b molecule, thereby competing with pathogenic autoantigen-derived peptides for presentation by B cells and preventing their excessive stimulation. Since I-E α-chain-derived peptides apparently have a high affinity for I-A molecules other than the I-A^b [35], this mechanism might also be responsible for the protection against the development of autoimmune diabetes by the expression of an E_α^d transgene in NOD mice. Further understanding of the protective mechanism conferred by the E_α^d transgene may elucidate the molecular and cellular bases central to the development of murine SLE.

The TNF-α gene. One of the intriguing observations is that NZW mice have a unique allele of the *TNF-α* gene, which is located in the H-2 region [75]. In fact, when the ability to produce TNF-α following the stimulation with bacterial lipopolysaccharides was assessed, NZW mice were capable of producing only limited amounts of TNF-α, as compared with NZB mice, and NZBxW mice are an intermediate producer [45]. Interestingly, repeated administrations of recombinant TNF-α caused a significant delay in the development of SLE in NZBxW mice [45]. These results have led to a hypothesis that the *TNF-α* gene of the NZW strain, whose 5' regulatory region sequence is apparently responsible for the reduced levels of TNF-α production [49], contributes to lupus-like autoimmune disease in NZBxW mice by rendering them a lower producer of TNF-α. Accordingly, the apparent MHC association of lupus in New Zealand mice may in part reflect a linkage to the *TNF-α* gene. However, it should be stressed that two other lupus-prone MRL-*lpr/lpr* and BXSB mice produce high levels of TNF-α [49], and that the variability of the ability to produce TNF-α can be similarly seen in patients with SLE, depending on the HLA-DR haplotype [47]. It may be that the different types of MHC-associated genetic predisposition could operate through different mechanisms, involving various genes.

Genes regulating apoptosis

The Fas apoptosis gene: the lpr mutation. Genetic studies on New Zealand mice have failed to demonstrate the presence of a common genetic defect which causes a predisposition to some or all autoimmune traits. However, the clearest example of the influence of a single gene on the development of autoimmunity is the effect of several mutant genes, which have been described to be involved in the development and progression of murine SLE. One of the single mutant genes which has been most extensively studied is the *lpr* (lymphoproliferation) mutation, which was first described in lupus-prone MRL-*lpr/lpr* and CBA/K1Jms-lpr^{cg}/lpr^{cg} mice [6, 65, 76]. The *lpr* mutation provokes a massive enlargement of lymph nodes with the accumulation of a particular subset of T cells that are phenotypically Thy-1^+CD3^+CD4^-CD8^-, but express the B220 antigen characteristic of B cells [65, 74, 122]. In addition, this mutation not only accelerates the progression of autoimmune disease in lupus-prone MRL mice, but also induces the production of a broad spectrum of autoantibodies in mice not predisposed to SLE [6, 42, 53].

The *lpr* gene, mapped to mouse chromosome 19 [119], was recently found to cause defects in the Fas antigen due to the insertion of an endogenous retrovirus in the Fas gene in MRL-*lpr/lpr* mice [3, 14, 123] or due to a point mutation in the intracellular region of the Fas gene in CBA/K1Jms-lpr^{cg}/lpr^{cg} mice [118]. The *Fas* gene is expressed in lymphoid and non-lymphoid cells, and the *Fas* protein is involved in the transduction of apoptotic signals [37, 114, 125]. A more recent study has shown that the Fas protein is highly expressed in $CD4^+CD8^+$ immature thymocytes, the stage at which most thymocytes die by apoptosis, and in activated mature T and B cells in normal mice, but not in MRL-*lpr/lpr* mice [20]. It is conceivable that the abnormal regulation of the apoptotic pathway, due to the lack of functional Fas protein, in mice bearing the *lpr* mutation could result in not only a failure of thymic selection and survival of autoreactive T cells, but also an extension of the functional lifespan and prevention of antigen-induced apoptotic death of autoreactive B cells. This would end up with an induction and/or acceleration of a lupus-like autoimmune syndrome.

The gld gene. The *gld* (generalized lymphoproliferative disease) mutation, first described in the C3H/HeJ strain [93], induces an autoimmune disease and marked lymphoadenopathy phenotypically indistinguishable from those induced by the *lpr* mutation [17]. Results obtained by bone marrow transplantation experiments between *lpr* and *gld* mice or between *gld* and normal mice strongly suggest that the molecule affected by the *gld* gene, mapped to mouse chromosome 1 [93, 100], is an apoptosis-inducing ligand, whose receptor may be the Fas protein [5, 108]. This prediction was recently confirmed: the *gld* mutation affects the ligand for the Fas protein due to a point mutation in the putative binding site [110]. It is worth noting that a recent report described two cases of patients who developed clinical and immunological features resembling those seen in *lpr* and *gld* mice [106].

The bcl-2 and related genes. Studies on mice bearing the *lpr* and *gld* mutations clearly indicate the importance of the genes regulating apoptosis in the development of lupus-like autoimmune disease. Since a number of genes are implicated in the process of apoptosis, one of the genetic defects in other lupus-prone mice such as New Zealand and BXSB mice may be related to those operating in apoptosis. In fact, a recent study has shown the resistance of surface Ig-mediated apoptosis of mature B cells in NZBxW mice [115]. The abnormality in apoptosis in NZBxW B cells would account for the B cell abnormality described in NZB and NZBxW mice, such as increased polyclonal B cell activation [38] and the T cell-independent production of IgG anti-DNA autoantibodies [92]. However, one cannot totally exclude the possibility that the observed resistance of apoptotic death in mature B cells from NZBxW mice is a secondary phenomenon due to an increased polyclonal B cell activation occurring spontaneously early in the life of NZBxW mice: the latter abnormality may be determined by another genetic defect of NZBxW mice.

Nevertheless, it can be speculated that one of the defects in NZBxW mice may be the failure to eliminate efficiently autoreactive B cells upon interaction with autoantigens, which may be an important pathway for a selective expansion of autoreactive B cells, and hence the pathogenesis of SLE. This view is consistent with the finding that overexpression in B-lineage cells of the *bcl-2* transgene, which blocks programmed cell death [117], leads to spontaneous development of an SLE-like autoimmune syndrome in (C57BL/6 x SJL)F_1 mice [109], although it should be noted that the development of autoimmune disease apparently depends on the genetic background of mice to which the *bcl-2* transgene was introduced. In addition, it has been recently shown that the *bcl-2* gene is able to counteract apoptotic cell death of mature autoreactive B cells upon interaction with autoantigens [80]. However, the fact that the expression of *bcl-2* is not enhanced in B cells from NZBxW mice suggests that a *bcl-2* independent mechanism can be responsible for the abnormal resistance to apoptosis of mature B cells in NZBxW mice. Notably, a recent discovery of several *bcl-2*-related genes which inhibit or share the action of *bcl-2* may be highly relevant [10, 85].

The Yaa gene

Another as-yet-unidentified mutant gene present on the Y chromosome of the BXSB strain is the *Yaa* gene, which accelerates the development of autoimmune disease in the BXSB strain [77]. The fact that the *Yaa* gene can accelerate the progression of SLE only in mice predisposed to SLE [34, 44] markedly contrasts with the action of the *lpr* and *gld* genes: the two latters are able to generate autoimmune manifestations even in mice lacking an apparent SLE genetic background [42, 53, 93]. Strikingly, the autoimmune enhancing activity of the *Yaa* gene is selective [34, 43, 66], which differs from the generalized enhancement of autoantibody production in the presence of the *lpr* or *gld* mutation. This strongly suggests that the molecular defect of the *Yaa* gene is likely to differ from those of the *lpr* and *gld* genes.

It is intriguing that the capacity of the *Yaa* gene to promote autoimmune responses depends on the levels of autoantibodies spontaneously produced in different lupus-prone mice in the absence of the *Yaa* gene. Marked enhancement of autoantibody production mediated by the *Yaa* gene is observed only in lupus-prone mice that spontaneously synthesize relatively low amounts of autoantibodies, but not in mice which already produce substantially high titers. This raises an attractive hypothesis that the *Yaa* gene might promote autoimmune responses only if they occur spontaneously at a low level. This is in agreement with our recent observation that the *Yaa* gene is able to potentiate immune responses against foreign antigens only in mice who are genetically (MHC-linked) low responding, but not high responding [22]. In high-responder mice, because of the presence of sufficient antigen-specific T cell help, the *Yaa* gene may not promote any additional help, while in low-responder mice capable of generating a limited antigen-specific T cell help, the *Yaa* gene-mediated helper effect is essential for the enhancement of immune responses. Thus, the *Yaa* gene-related help may play a crucial role for promoting antibody responses against antigens to which mice respond poorly, and not for those to which antigen-specific T cell help is sufficient to activate B cells.

This hypothesis can provide one explanation for the selective autoimmune-enhancing activity of the *Yaa* gene in several lupus-prone mice. Accordingly, the *Yaa* gene effect on spontaneous autoimmune responses in different lupus-prone mice may be related to differences in the capacity of T helper cells specific for autoimmune responses, which are likely to be in part controlled by the MHC class II genes. This can be best illustrated in H-2^b and H-2^d congenic (NZB x BXSB)F_1 hybrid mice [71]. In these hybrid mice, the *Yaa* gene potentiates only slightly autoimmune responses in the F_1 hybrid mice bearing the H-2^b haplotype, which apparently provides sufficient T cell help for lupus autoantibody responses, as documented by high titers of autoantibodies in the absence of the *Yaa* gene. In contrast, the *Yaa* gene prominently enhances autoimmune responses in the F_1 hybrids bearing the H-2^d haplotype, which does not confer a high-responder phenotype for autoimmune responses, resulting in a dramatic acceleration of their SLE.

To further define the cellular mechanism responsible for the *Yaa* gene-mediated acceleration of autoantibody production, experiments were performed for the analysis of anti-DNA autoantibody production occurring spontaneously in autoimmune *Yaa*$^+$ (NZW x B6.*Yaa*)F_1 male and non-autoimmune *Yaa*$^-$ (NZW x B6)F_1 male double bone marrow cell chimeric mice [67]. We have observed that anti-DNA antibodies are selectively produced by B cells from mice bearing the *Yaa* gene. A parallel, selective age-dependent increase in the Ig of the *Yaa*$^+$ origin indicates that B cells from mice bearing the *Yaa* gene are preferentially activated in the *Yaa*$^+$-*Yaa*$^-$ bone marrow cell chimeras to produce anti-DNA autoantibodies and hypergammaglobulinemia. This study strongly suggests that the *Yaa* gene abnormality is most likely to be expressed at least at the level of B cells, which is responsible for the selective activation of *Yaa*$^+$ autoreactive B cells.

If the *Yaa* gene abnormality is related to a defect in the molecules regulating apoptosis, as in the case of the *lpr* mutation, selective autoantibody production by *Yaa*$^+$ B cells in the *Yaa*$^+$-*Yaa*$^-$ bone marrow cell chimeras can be explained. In fact, similar preferential production of autoantibodies by B cells of the *lpr* origin has been noted in different types of *lpr*-non-*lpr* chimeric mice (neonatal, radiation or allophenic chimeras) [50, 79, 86, 107]. However, this possibility appears to be less likely, because of the comparable production of antibodies against foreign antigens by both *Yaa*$^+$-*Yaa*$^-$ B cell populations in *Yaa*$^+$-*Yaa*$^-$ bone marrow cell chimeras following their immunization [67]. In addition, as mentioned above, remarkable differences in the autoimmune potentiating effect between the *Yaa* gene and the *lpr* gene in lupus-prone and non-autoimmune mice further argue that the molecular defect of the *Yaa* gene is likely to be different from that of the *lpr* gene.

We would like to propose the following model (Fig. 1). The *Yaa* gene abnormality may be associated with the expression of a molecule on the surface of B cells, which may be encoded directly by the *Yaa* gene or whose expression may be regulated by the *Yaa* gene. This putative *Yaa*-related molecule could operate as an intercellular adhesion-like molecule, thereby promoting the low-avidity interaction of autoreactive T and B cells. Accordingly, this *Yaa*-mediated help can neither potentiate immune responses in the absence of T cell help nor enhance responses in the presence of sufficient T cell help. In view of our hypothesis, the selective enhancement of immune responses to either self or foreign antigens may be explained by differences in the capacity of T helper cells specific for given antigens, as discussed above. In the presence of sufficient antigen-specific T cell help, the hypothetical *Yaa*-related adhesion molecule may not provide any additional help. Consequently, there are no enhanced immune responses against self or foreign antigens even in the presence of the *Yaa* gene, when mice are genetically high responders to these antigens. In contrast, the *Yaa* gene-mediated helper effect may be essential for the promotion of immune responses against self or foreign antigens in mice that have only a limited activity of T helper cells specific for given antigens.

This model proposed here may be relevant to theoretical considerations on how the *Yaa* gene induces and/or accelerates the development of autoimmune responses in lupus-prone BXSB mice. Recent studies on two different models of transgenic mice

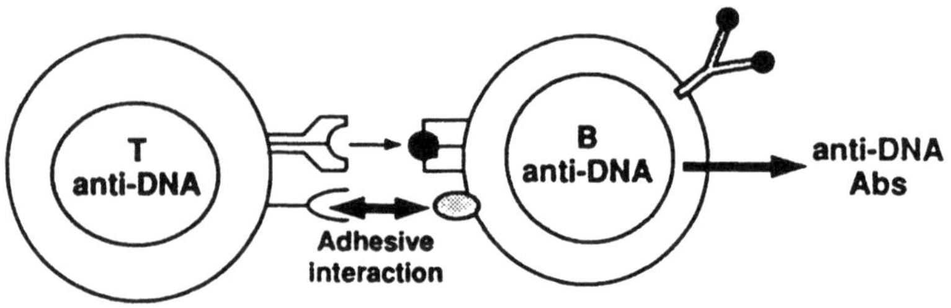

Fig. 1. A hypothetical model of the *Yaa* gene-mediated enhancement of autoantibody production. B cells express a molecule related to the *Yaa* gene on their surface, and this putative *Yaa*-related molecule behaves as an intercellular adhesion-like molecule. Its binding to a specific ligand expressed on T cells is able to potentiate the low-avidity interaction between autoantigen-specific T helper cells and autoreactive Yaa^+ B cells. It is possible that this putative *Yaa*-related adhesion molecule may also be expressed on T cells, and that their homotypic interaction plays a crucial role in the T-B interaction in mice expressing the *Yaa* gene. The lack of autoimmune responses in non-autoimmune B6 and CBA/J mice bearing the *Yaa* gene can be explained by the lack of the expression of the *Yaa*-related molecule and/or its ligand, which requires additional autosomal abnormalities present only in lupus-prone mice. • DNA; *Yaa*-related adhesion molecule; ⊃– ligand for the putative *Yaa*-related molecule

have shown that "autoreactive" T cells specific to the dominant determinants derived from transgene products become tolerant, while "autoreactive" T cells specific to minor ones are able to evade tolerance induction [15, 73]. This is consistent with the fact that the expression of endogenous superantigens or the injection of exogenous superantigens efficiently leads to a clonal deletion of corresponding T cells in I-E^+ lupus-prone mice at an extent comparable to non-autoimmune mice [52, 59, 68, 70, 97], and that T cells specific for the dominant determinant derived from I-E α chains are tolerant in autoimmune BXSB mice expressing the I-E molecules (unpublished observation). Thus, one can postulate that autoreactive T cells with high affinity to self antigens (probably the dominant determinants derived from self antigens) are subject to the clonal deletion even in lupus-prone mice, while T cells with lower affinity to self antigens (probably minor determinants of self antigens) may not be completely deleted during the process of thymic negative selection. The latter autoreactive T cells are not stimulated under normal conditions, because the affinity of T cell receptors to self-peptide-MHC complexes is not high enough to be activated or because such peptides may not be sufficiently presented by antigen-presenting cells. However, in the presence of the *Yaa* mutation, the *Yaa*-linked adhesion molecule could decrease the threshold for antigen receptor-dependent stimulation, leading to the activation of autoreactive T cells capable of recognizing the minor determinants of self antigens presented in the context of the appropriate MHC class II molecules. The absence of autoimmune responses in B6 and CBA/J mice even in the presence of the *Yaa* gene [34, 39] could be explained either by the lack of the expression of the putative *Yaa*-linked adhesion molecule or its ligand, which possibly requires additional autosomal defects present only in lupus-prone mice.

The retroviral gp70 gene

Additional genes which may be involved in the pathogenesis of SLE are those encoding nephritogenic autoantigens or regulating their expression. One of the autoantigens which plays an important role in the development of murine lupus nephritis is the retroviral major envelope glycoprotein, gp70. In support is the documentation that the gp70 antigen, which is secreted by liver cells [29], is found in circulating immune complexes (IC) and glomerular IC deposits within diseased kidneys of lupus mice [6, 39, 126]. gp70-anti-gp70 IC become apparent in the circulation close to the onset of disease, and their concentrations rise with the progression of lupus nephritis [39, 40, 63], constituting good evidence that gp70-anti-gp70 IC are a potential source of renal injury in lupus-prone mice.

It has been clear that not only lupus-prone mice but also many non-autoimmune mice have relatively high concentrations of gp70 in their sera; however, only lupus-prone mice spontaneously develop antibodies directed against this serum retroviral gp70 as a result of their immunological abnormalities [39]. Since it appears that the more gp70 is expressed, the more anti-gp70 antibodies are produced in lupus-prone mice [41], the quantity of gp70 antigen, as a source for antigenic stimulation and for IC formation, can be one of the significant factors in the pathogenesis of murine SLE. This is supported by our preliminary studies that BXSB.gp70 transgenic mice expressing increased amounts of the gp70 antigen rapidly developed lupus nephritis as a result of selective acceleration of anti-gp70 autoimmune responses and an increased formation of gp70-anti-gp70 IC. If this is indeed the case, an abnormal production of certain cytokines, which are able to stimulate the production of acute phase proteins, due to a possible genetic abnormality may be additionally involved in the pathogenesis of murine SLE, since serum retroviral gp70 behaves as an acute phase protein [29].

Genes involved in the pathogenic process of autoantibodies

It should be stressed that while the *lpr* or *gld* mutation is able to induce the formation of various autoantibodies at substantial levels in B6 and C3H/HeJ mice, these mice lacking an apparent SLE background develop only mild glomerular lesions [42, 53, 93]. This indicates that in addition to the *lpr* or *gld* mutation, supplementary genetic abnormalities are necessary to elicit the full manifestations of SLE. In fact, a recent genetic analysis performed on the MRL-*lpr/lpr* strain and its cross with non-autoimmune mice have proposed the presence of two loci on chromosomes 7 and 12, tentatively named *Lrdm-1* and *Lrdm-2* (*lpr* renal disease modifier), which could be involved in the generation of lupus nephritis in MRL-*lpr/lpr* mice [120].

One of the important factors involved in the pathogenetic process of lupus nephritis could be that controlling the quality of autoantibodies with immunopathological consequences. In fact, we have recently shown that spontaneous production of rheumatoid factors with cryoglobulin activity was found prominently in lupus-prone MRL-*lpr/lpr* mice, but rarely in B6 and C3H/HeJ mice bearing the *lpr* or *gld* mutation [101]. Studies on murine monoclonal autoantibodies have demonstrated that murine IgG3 antibodies exhibit a cryoglobulin activity because of their unique physicochemical property of the $\gamma 3$ constant region [1], and that a significant fraction of IgG3 monoclonal autoantibodies derived from lupus-prone mice are highly nephritogenic, generating "wire-loop"-like glomerular lesions characteristic in human lupus nephritis [7, 24, 36, 60, 91, 111]. Thus, the lack of production of cryogenic autoantibodies with immunopathological consequences may partly explain the development of only limited autoimmune pathology in B6 and C3H/HeJ mice bearing the *lpr* or *gld* mutation. This idea was further supported by the fact that the development of lupus nephritis was markedly delayed in a substrain of MRL-*lpr/lpr* mice, designated MRL-*lpr/lpr.ll* (long-lived), which produce autoantibodies at levels comparable to conventional MRL-*lpr/lpr* mice, but only limited amounts of IgG3 cryoglobulins [23].

Although the cellular and molecular basis of the production of IgG3 cryoglobulins has not been fully understood, it is significant that the spontaneous production of IgG3 antibodies is highly dependent on the presence of $CD4^+$ T cells in lupus-prone mice, which is not the case in non-autoimmune mice [69]. Recent studies have shown that one of the T cell cytokines, interferon-γ (IFN-γ), is able to promote the production of IgG3 [105], while another T cell cytokine, interleukin 4 (IL-4) can down-regulate the IgG3 synthesis [104]. Our preliminary studies have suggested that an alteration of a balance between IFN-γ and IL-4 may be responsible for the diminished IgG3 production in the MRL-*lpr/lpr.ll* substrain. Since IFN-γ has been shown to play an important role in the progression of murine SLE [46], one of the accelerating effects ascribed to IFN-γ, in addition to its immune potentiating activity, may be related to the enhanced production of IgG3 autoantibodies with a highly pathogenic potential.

Obviously, the abnormality in the genes regulating the production of IgG3 antibodies could be one of the important genetic factors in the pathogenesis of murine SLE. In this regard, it should be mentioned that the development of lupus nephritis in several lupus-prone mice is markedly retarded by the presence of the *xid* (X chromosome-linked immunodeficiency) gene, which causes a selective defect of IgM and IgG3 production (reviewed in [96]). Recent studies have revealed that a molecular defect of the *xid* mutation may be associated with functional abnormality of Bruton's tyrosine kinase [89, 113], which is implicated in the human X-linked agammaglobulinemia, characterized by a failure to produce B cells. However, in the *xid* mice, B cells are present, but respond abnormally to activating signals [96]. It remains to be elucidated how a single amino acid mutation within the amino-terminal unique region of Bruton's tyrosine kinase found in the *xid* mice leads to a selective effect on the IgM and IgG3 production in mice. Finally, it should be stated that human IgG3 has physicochemical properties similar to those of murine IgG3 [12, 27]. It is of importance that the presence of IgG3 cryoprecipitable autoantibodies should be reassessed in relation to clinical manifestations to determine whether IgG3 cryoprecipitable autoantibodies are useful and predictive markers in patients with SLE and related rheumatic diseases.

Conclusion: multiple distinct genetic pathways for murine SLE

Genetic analysis of SLE in several lupus-prone mice has revealed that multiple, unlinked genes are required for the expression of various autoimmune manifestations, and that several, quite distinct genetic backgrounds are compatible with this disease. It appears that individual lupus-prone strains of mice have quite distinct genetic defects, but end up with the similar immunopathological abnormalities responsible for the development of lupus-like autoimmune disease.

Although the nature of these genetic components has not been fully defined, it is becoming clear that certain genes such as the MHC class II genes and the genes regulating apoptosis apparently play a crucial role in the development of autoimmune responses characteristic in SLE. However, it should be stressed that while immunologically normal B6 mice beating the predisposing MHC haplotype are able to develop significant autoimmune responses in the presence of the *lpr* or *gld* mutation causing the abnormality of apoptotic death, they fail to develop a severe form of lupus nephritis. Since it is highly likely that different genetic components are involved at various levels of the disease process in SLE, the absence of genetic abnormalities at certain levels of the disease process may well explain the lack of the full manifestations of SLE in mice without an appropriate SLE background. These genetic abnormalities can be those for cytokines and their receptors, for intercellular adhesion molecules and their ligands, for intracellular signal transduction molecules, for regulating the IgG class switching, for regulating the expression of nephritogenic autoantigens, etc. Therefore, the variations of the onset, severity and nature of SLE observed among various lupus-prone mice could be interpreted as the result of different assortments of various genetic defects implicated in SLE. Obviously, further identification of the genetic defects present in lupus-prone mice, but lacking in mice with non-autoimmune backgrounds, is of paramount importance for the understanding of the immunopathogenetic mechanism of SLE, and is indeed the subject under an extensive investigation.

Acknowledgements. The studies from the authors' laboratory discussed in this review were supported by a grant from the Swiss National Foundation for Scientific Research.

References

1. Abdelmoula M, Spertini F, Shibata T, Gyotoku Y, Luzuy S. Lambert PH, Izui S (1989) IgG3 is the major source of cryoglobulins in mice. J Immunol 143:526
2. Acha-Orbea H, Steinman L, McDevitt HO (1989) T cell receptors in murine autoimmune diseases. Annu Rev Immunol 7:371
3. Adachi M, Watanabe-Fukunaga R, Nagata S (1993) Aberrant transcription caused by the insertion of an early transposable element in an intron of the Fas antigen gene of *lpr* mice. Proc Natl Acad Sci USA 90:1756
4. Adelman NE, Walling DL, McDevitt HO (1983) Treatment of (NZB x NZW)F_1 disease with anti-I-A monoclonal antibodies. J Exp Med 158:1350
5. Allen RD, Marshall JD, Roths JB, Sidman CL (1990) Differences defined by bone marrow transplantation suggest that *lpr* and *gld* are mutations of genes encoding an interacting pair of molecules. J Exp Med 172:1367
6. Andrews BS, Eisenberg RA, Theofilopoulos AN, Izui S, Wilson CB, McConahey PJ, Murphy ED, Roths JB, Dixon FJ (1978) Spontaneous murine lupus-like syndromes. Clinical and immunopathological manifestations in several strains. J Exp Med 148:1198
7. Berney T, Fulpius T, Shibata T, Reininger L, Van Snick J, Shan H, Weigert M, Marshak-Rothstein A, Izui S (1992) Selective pathogenicity of murine rheumatoid factors of the cryoprecipitable IgG3 subclass. Int Immunol 4:93
8. Bocchieri MH, Cooke A, Smith JB, Weigert M, Riblet RJ (1982) Independent segregation of NZB immune abnormalities in NZB x C58 recombinant inbred mice. Eur J Immunol 12:349
9. Böhme J, Schuhbaur B, Kanagawa O, Benoist C, Mathis D (1990) MHC-linked protection from diabetes dissociated from clonal deletion of T cells. Science 249:293
10. Boise LH, Gonzalez-Garcia M, Postema CE, Ding L, Lindsten T, Turka LA, Mao X, Nunez G, Thompson CB (1993) *bcl-x*, a *bcl-2*-related gene that functions as a dominant regulator of apoptotic cell death. Cell 74:597
11. Bona CA (1988) V genes encoding autoantibodies: molecular and phenotypic characteristics. Annu Rev Immunol 6:327
12. Capra JD, Kunkel HG (1970) Aggregation of γG3 proteins: relevance to the hyperviscosity syndrome. J Clin Invest 49:610
13. Chiang BL, Bearer E, Ansari A, Dorshkind K, Gershwin ME (1990) The *bm12* mutation and autoantibodies to dsDNA in NZB.H-2^{bm12} mice. J Immunol 145:94
14. Chu J-L, Drappa J, Parnassa A, Elkon KB (1993) The defect in Fas mRNA expression in MRL/lpr mice is associated with insertion of the retrotransposon, *ETn*. J Exp Med 178:723
15. Cibotti R, Kanellopoulos JM, Cabaniols JP, Halle-Panenko O, Kosmatopoulos K, Sercarz E, Kourilsky P (1992) Tolerance to a self-protein involves its immunodominant but does not involve its subdominant determinants. Proc Natl Acad Sci USA 89:416

16. Cohen PL, Creech E, Nakul-Aquaronne D, McDaniel R, Ackler S, Rapoport RG, Sobel ES, Eisenberg RA (1993) Antigen nonspecific effect of major histocompatibility complex haplotype on autoantibody levels in systemic lupus erythematosus-prone *lpr* mice. J Clin Invest 91:2761
17. Davidson WF, Dumont FJ, Bedigian HG, Fowlkes BJ, Morse HC III (1986) Phenotypic, functional and molecular genetic comparisons of the abnormal lymphoid cells of C3H-*lpr/lpr* and C3H-*gld/gld* mice. J Immunol 136:4075
18. de Alboran I, Gonzalo JA, Kroemer G, Lconardo E, Marcos MAR, Martinez AC (1992) Attenuation of autoimmune disease and lymphocyte accumulation in MRL/*lpr* mice by treatment with anti-$V_{\beta}8$ antibodies. Eur J Immunol 22:2153
19. Deng H, Apple R, Clare-Salzer M, Trembleau S, Mathis D, Adorini L, Sercarz E (1993) Determinant capture as a possible mechanism of protection afforded by major histocompatibility complex class II molecules in autoimmune disease. J Exp Med 178:1675
20. Drappa J, Brot N, Elkon KB (1993) The Fas protein is expressed at high levels on $CD4^+CD8^+$ thymocytes and activated mature lymphocytes in normal mice but not in the lupus-prone strain, MRL-*lpr/lpr*. Proc Natl Acad Sci USA 90:10 340
21. Forsgren S, Dahl U, Söderström A, Hohnberg D, Matsunaga T (1991) The phenotype of lymphoid cells and thymic epithelium correlates with development of autoimmune insulitis in NOD-C57BL/6 allophenic chimeras. Proc Natl Acad Sci USA 88:9335
22. Fossati L, Merino R, Iwamoto M, Izui S (1994) Selective enhancing effect of the *Yaa* gene on immune responses against self and foreign antigens. Eur J Immunol (in press)
23. Fossati L, Takahashi S, Merino R, Iwamoto M, Aubry JP, Nose M, Spach C, Motta R, Izui S (1993) An MRL/MpJ-*lpr/lpr* substrain with a limited expansion of *lpr* double-negative T cells and a reduced autoimmune syndrome. Int Immunol 5:525
24. Fulpius T, Spertini F, Reininger L, Izui S (1993) Immunoglobulin heavy chain constant region determines the pathogenicity and the antigen-binding activity of rheumatoid factor. Proc Natl Acad Sci USA 90:2345
25. Ghatak S, Sainis K, Owen FL, Datta SK (1987) T-cell-receptor β- and I-Aβ-chain genes of normal SWR mice are linked with the development of lupus nephritis in NZB x SWR crosses. Proc Natl Acad Sci USA 84:6850
26. Gilfillan S, Aiso S, Michie SA, McDevitt HO (1990) Immune deficiency due to high copy number of an A^k_{β} transgene. Proc Natl Acad Sci USA 87:7319
27. Grey HM, Kohler PF, Terry WD, Franklin EC (1968) Human monoclonal γG-cryoglobulins with anti-γ-globulin activity. J Clin Invest 47:1875
28. Groghan TW, Davignon J-L, Evans J, Allison JP, Eisenberg RA, Frelinger JA, Cohen PL (1989) Diminished expression of the T cell receptor on the expanded lymphocyte population in MRL/Mp-*lpr/lpr* mice. Autoimmunity 2:97
29. Hara I, Izui S, Dixon FJ (1982) Murine serum glycoprotein gp70 behaves as an acute phase reactant. J Exp Med 155:345
30. Helyer BJ, Howie JB (1963) Spontaneous auto-immune disease in NZB/Bl mice. Br J Haematol 9:119
31. Hirose S, Nagasawa R, Sekikawa I, Hamaoki M, Ishida Y, Sato H, Shirai T (1983) Enhancing effect of H-2-linked NZW gene(s) on the autoimmune traits of (NZB x NZW)F_1 mice. J Exp Med 158:228
32. Hirose S, Ueda G, Noguchi K, Okada T, Sekigawa I, Sato H, Shirai T (1986) Requirement of H-2 heterozygosity for autoimmunity in (NZB x NZW)F_1 hybrid mice. Eur J Immunol 16:1631
33. Hirose S, Tokushige K, Kinoshita K, Nozawa S, Saito J, Nishimura H, Shirai T (1991) Contribution of the gene linked to the T cell receptor β chain gene complex of NZW mice to the autoimmunity of (NZB x NZW)F_1 mice. Eur J Immunol 21:823
34. Hudgins CC, Sternberg RT, Klinman DM, Reeves MPJ, Steinberg AD (1985) Studies of consomic mice bearing the Y chromosome of the BXSB mouse. J Immunol 134:3849
35. Hunt DF, Michel H, Dickinson TA, Shabanowitz J, Cox AL, Sakaguchi K, Appella E, Grey HM, Sette A (1992) Peptides presented to the immune system by the murine class II major histocompatibility complex molecule I-A^d. Science 256:1817
36. Itoh J, Nose M, Takahashi S, Ono M, Terasaki S, Kondoh E, Kyogoku M (1993) Induction of different types of glomerulonephritis by monoclonal antibodies derived from an MRL/*lpr* lupus mouse. Am J Pathol 143:1436
37. Itoh N, Yonehara S, Ishii A, Yonehara M, Mizushima S-I, Sameshima M, Hase A, Seto Y, Nagata S (1991) The polypeptide encoded by the cDNA for human cell suface antigen Fas can mediate apoptosis. Cell 66:233

38. Izui S, McConahey PJ, Dixon FJ (1978) Increased spontaneous polyclonal activation of B lymphocytes in mice with spontaneous autoimmune disease. J Immunol 121:2213
39. Izui S, McConahey PJ, Theofilopoulos AN, Dixon FJ (1979) Association of circulating retroviral gp70-anti-gp70 immune complexes with murine systemic lupus erythematosus. J Exp Med 149:1099
40. Izui S, McConahey PJ, Clark JP, Hang LM, Hara I, Dixon FJ (1981) Retroviral gp70 immune complexes in NZB x NZW F_2 mice with murine lupus nephritis. J Exp Med 154:517
41. Izui S, Hara 1, Hang LM, Elder JH, McConahey PJ, Dixon FJ (1984) Association of elevated serum glycoprotein gp70 with increased gp70 immune complex formation and accelerated lupus nephritis in autoimmune male BXSB mice. Clin Exp Immunol 56:272
42. Izui S, Kelley VE, Masuda K, Yoshida H, Roths JB, Murphy ED (1984) Induction of various autoantibodies by mutant gene *lpr* in several strains of mice. J Immunol 133:227
43. Izui S, Masuda K, Yoshida H (1984) Acute SLE in F_1 hybrids between SB/Le and NZW mice: prominently enhanced formation of gp70 immune complexes by a Y chromosome-associated factor from SB/Le mice. J Immunol 132:701
44. Izui S, Higaki M, Morrow D, Merino R (1988) The Y chromosome from autoimmune BXSB/MpJ mice induces a lupus-like syndrome in (NZW x C57BL/6)F_1 male mice, but not in C57BL/6 male mice. Eur J Immunol 18:911
45. Jacob CO, McDevitt HO (1988) Tumour necrosis factor-α in murine autoimmune "lupus" nephritis. Nature 331:356
46. Jacob CO, Van Der Meide PH, McDevitt HO (1987) In vivo treatment of (NZB x NZW)F_1 lupus-like nephritis with monoclonal antibody to γ-interferon. J Exp Med 166:798
47. Jacob CO, Fronek Z, Lewis GD, Koo M, Hansen JA, McDevitt HO (1990) Heritable major histocompatibility complex class II-associated differences in production of tumor necrosis factor α: relevance to genetic predisposition to systemic lupus erythematosus. Proc Natl Acad Sci USA 87:1233
48. Jacob CO, Sadakazu A, Michie SA, McDevitt HO, Acha-Orbea H (1990) Prevention of diabetes in nonobese diabetic mice by tumor necrosis factor (TNF): similarities between TNF-α and interleukin 1. Proc Natl Acad Sci USA 87:968
49. Jacob CO, Hwang F, Lewis GD, Stall AM (1991) Tumor necrosis factor alpha in murine systemic lupus erythematosus disease models: implications for genetic predisposition and immune regulation. Cytokine 3:551
50. Katagiri T, Azuma S, Toyoda Y, Mori S, Kano K, Cohen PL, Eisenberg RA (1992) Tetraparental mice reveal complex cellular interactions of the mutant, autoimmunity-inducing *lpr* gene. J Immunol 148:430
51. Kawano H, Abe M, Zhang D, Saikawa T, Fujimori M, Hirose S, Shirai T (1992) Heterozygosity of the major histocompatibility complex controls the autoimmune disease in (NZW x BXSB)F_1 mice. Clin Immunol Immunopathol 65:308
52. Kim C, Siminovitch KA, Ochi A (1991) Reduction of lupus nephritis in MRL/*lpr* mice by a bacterial superantigen treatment. J Exp Med 176:1431
53. Kimura M, Mohri H, Shimada K, Wakabayashi T, Kanai Y, Matsuzawa A (1990) Serological and histological characterization of the new mutant strain of *lpr* mice, CBA/K1Jms-lpr^{cg}/lpr^{cg}. Clin Exp Immunol 79:123
54. Knight JG, Adams DD (1978) Three genes for lupus nephritis in NZB x NZW mice. J Exp Med 147:1653
55. Kofler R, Dixon FJ, Theofilopoulos AN (1987) The genetic origin of autoantibodies. Immunol Today 8:374
56. Kohno A, Yoshida H, Sekita K, Maruyama N, Ozaki S, Hirose S, Shirai T (1983) Genetic regulation of the class conversion of dsDNA-specific antibodies in (NZB x NZW)F_1 hybrid. Immunogenetics 18:513
57. Kotzin BL, Barr VL, Palmer E (1985) A large deletion within the T-cell receptor β-chain gene complex in New Zealand White mice. Science 229:167
58. Kotzin BL, Palmer E (1987) The contribution of NZW genes to lupus-like disease in (NZB x NZW) F_1 mice. J Exp Med 165:1237
59. Kotzin BL, Babcock SK, Herron LR (1988) Deletion of potentially self-reactive T cell receptor specificities in L3T4$^-$, Lyt-2$^-$ T cells of *lpr* mice. J Exp Med 168:2221
60. Lemoine R, Berney T, Shibata T, Fulpius T, Gyotoku Y, Shimida H, Sawada S, Izui S (1992) Induction of "wire-loop" lesions by murine monoclonal IgG3 cryoglobulins. Kidney Int 41:65

61. Lund T, O'Reilly L, Hutchings P, Kanagawa O, Simpson E, Gravely R, Chandler P, Dyson J, Picard JK, Edwards A, Kioussis D, Cooke A (1990) Prevention of insulin-dependent diabetes mellitus in non-obese diabetic mice by transgenes encoding modified I-A β-chain or normal I-E α-chain. Nature 345:727
62. Maruyama N, Ohta K, Hirose S, Shirai T (1980) Genetic studies of autoimmunity in New Zealand mice. Associations among natural thymocytoxic autoantibody (NTA), renal disease, and H-2 complex. Immunol Lett 2:1
63. Maruyama N, Furukawa F, Nakai Y, Sasaki Y, Ohta K, Ozaki S, Hirose S, Shirai T (1983) Genetic studies of autoimmunity in New Zealand mice. IV. Contribution of NZB and NZW genes to the spontaneous occurrence of retroviral gp70 immune complexes in (NZB x NZW)F_1 hybrid and the correlation to renal disease. J Immunol 130:740
64. Mathis DJ, Benoist C, Williams II VE, Kanter M, McDevitt HO (1983) Several mechanisms can account for defective E_α gene expression in different mouse haplotypes. Proc Natl Acad Sci USA 80:273
65. Matsuzawa A, Moriyama T, Kaneko T, Tanaka M, Kimura M, Ikeda H, Katagiri T (1990) A new allele of the *lpr* locus, lpr^{cg}, that complements the *gld* gene in induction of lymphadenopathy in the mouse. J Exp Med 171:519
66. Merino R, Shibata T, de Kossodo S, Izui S (1989) Differential effect of the *lpr* and *Yaa* genes on the acceleration of lupus-like syndrome In MRL/MpJ mice. Eur J Immunol 19:2131
67. Merino R, Fossati L, Lacour M, Izui S (1991) Selective autoantibody production by Yaa^+ B cells in autoimmune Yaa^+-Yaa^- bone marrow chimeric mice. J Exp Med 174:1023
68. Merino R, Fossati L, Lacour M, Lemoine R, Higaki M, Izui S (1992) H-2-linked control of the *Yaa* gene-induced acceleration of lupus-like autoimmune disease in BXSB mice. Eur J Immunol 22:295
69. Merino R, Iwamoto M, Fossati L, Izui S (1993) Polyclonal B cell activation arises from different mechanisms in lupus-prone (NZB x NZW)F_1 and MRL-MpJ-*lpr/lpr* mice. J Immunol 151:6509
70. Merino R, Iwamoto M, Fossati L, Muniesa P, Araki K, Takahashi S, Huarte J, Yamamura K, Vassalli JD, Izui S (1993) Prevention of systemic lupus erythematosus in autoimmune BXSB mice by a transgene encoding I-E α-chain. J Exp Med 178:1189
71. Merino R, Iwamoto M, Gershwin ME, Izui S (1994) The *Yaa* gene abrogates the MHC association of murine lupus in (NZB x BXSB)F_1 hybrid mice. Clin Invest 94:521
72. Milich DR, Hughes JL, Houghten R, McLachlan A, Jones JE (1989) Functional identification of agretopic and epitopic residues within an HBcAg T cell determinant. J Immunol 143:3141
73. Milich DR, McLachlan A, Raney AK, Houghten R, Thomton GB, Maruyama T, Hughes JL, Jones JE (1991) Autoantibody production In hepatitis B e antigen transgenic mice elicited with a self T-cell peptide and inhibited with nonself peptides. Proc Natl Acad Sci USA 88:4348
74. Morse HC III, Davidson VJF, Yetter RA, Murphy ED, Roths JB, Coffman RL (1982) Abnormalities induced by the mutant gene *lpr*: expansion of a unique lymphocyte subset. J Immunol 129:2612
75. Müller U, Jongeneel CV, Nedospasov SA, Lindahl KF, Steinmetz M (1987) Tumour necrosis factor and lymphotoxin genes map close to H-2D in the mouse major histocompatibility complex. Nature 325:265
76. Murphy ED, Roths JB (1979) Autoimmunity and lymphoproliferation: induction by mutant gene *lpr*, and acceleration by a male-associated factor in strain BXSB mice. In: Rose NR, Bigzzi PE, Wemer NL (eds) Genetic control of autoimmune disease. Elsevier North Holland, New York, pp 207-221
77. Murphy ED, Roths JB (1979) A Y chromosome-associated factor in strain BXSB producing accelerated autoimmunity and lymphoproliferation. Arthritis Rheum 22:1188
78. Naiki M, Yoshida SH, Watanabe Y, Izui S, Ansari AA, Gershwin ME (1993) The contribution of I-A^{bm12} to phenotypic and functional alterations among T-cell subsets in NZB mice. J Autoimmun 6:131
79. Nemazee D, Guiet C, Buerki K, Marshak-Rothstein A (1991) B lymphocytes from the autoimmune-prone mouse strain MRL/*lpr* manifest an intrinsic defect in tetraparental MRL/*lpr*-DBA/2 chimeras. J Immunol 147:2536
80. Nisitani S, Tsubata T, Murakami M, Okamoto M, Honjo T (1993) The *bcl-2* gene product inhibits clonal deletion of self-reactive B lymphocytes in the periphery but not in the bone marrow. J Exp Med 178:1247
81. Noonan DJ, Kofler R, Singer PA, Cardenas G, Dixon FJ, Theofilopoulos AN (1986) Delineation of a defect in T cell receptor β genes of NZW mice predisposed to autoimmunity. J Exp Med 163:644

82. Noonan DJ, McConahey PJ, Cardenas GJ (1990) Correlations of autoimmunity with H-2 and T cell receptor β chain genotypes in (NZB x NZW)F_2 mice. Eur J Immunol 20:1105
83. Nygard NR, McCarthy DM, Schiffenbauer J, Schwartz BD (1993) Mixed haplotypes and autoimmunity. Immunol Today 14:53
84. Oliveira DBG, Mitchison NA (1989) Immune suppression genes. Clin Exp Immunol 75:167
85. Oltvai ZN, Milliman CL, Korsmeyer SJ (1993) BCL-2 heterodimerizes in vivo with a conserved homolog, Bax, that accelerates programed cell death. Cell 74:609
86. Perkins DL, Glaser RM, Mahon CA, Michaelson J, Marshak-Rothstein A (1990) Evidence for an intrinsic B cell defect in *lpr/lpr* mice apparent in neonatal chimeras. J Immunol 145:549
87. Podolin PL, Presser A, DeLarato NH, Fischer PA, Peterson LB, Wicker LS (1993) I-E^+ nonobese diabetic mice develop insulitis and diabetes. J Exp Med 178:793
88. Raveche ES, Novotny EA, Hausen CT, njo JH, Steinberg AD (1981) Genetic studies in NZB mice. V. Recombinant inbred lines demonstrate that separate genes control autoimmune phenotype. J Exp Med 153:1187
89. Rawlings DJ, Saffran DC, Tsukuda S, Largaespada DA, Grimaldi JC, Cohen L, Mohr RN, Bazan JF, Howard M, Copeland NG, Jerkins NA, Witte ON (1993) Mutation of unique region of Bruton's tyrosine kinase in immunodeficient XID mice. Science 261:358
90. Reich EP, Sherwin RS, Kanagawa O, Janeway CA Jr (1989) An explanation for the protective effect of the MHC class II I-E molecule in murine diabetes. Nature 341:326
91. Reininger L, Berney T, Shibata T, Spertini F, Merino R, Izui S (1990) Cryoglobulinemia induced by a murine IgG3 rheumatoid factor: skin vasculitis and glomerulonephritis arise from distinct pathogenic mechanisms. Proc Natl Acad Sci USA 87:10038
92. Reininger L, Radaszkiewicz T, Kosco M, Melchers F, Rolink AG (1992) Development of autoimmune disease in SCID mice populated with long-term in vitro proliferating (NZB x NZW)F_1 pre-B cells. J Exp Med 176:1343
93. Roths JB, Murphy ED, Eicher EM (1984) A new mutation, *gld* that produces lymphoproliferation and autoimmunity in C3H/HeJ mice. J Exp Med 159:1
94. Rudensky AY, Preston-Hurlburt P, Hong SC, Barlow A, Janeway CA Jr (1991) Sequence analysis of peptides bound to MHC class II molecules. Nature 353:622
95. Satoh J, Seino H, Abo T, Tanaka S-I, Shintani S, Ohta S, Tamura K, Sawai T, Nobunaga T, Oteki T, Kumagai K, Toyota T (1989) Recombinant human tumor necrosis factor α suppresses autoimmune diabetes in nonobese diabetic mice. J Clin Invest 84:1345
96. Scher I (1982) The CBA/N mouse strain: an experimental model illustrating the influence of the X-chromosome on immunity. Adv Immunol 33:1
97. Scott DE, Kisch WJ, Steinberg AD (1993) Studies of T cell deletion and T cell anergy following in vivo administration of SEB to normal and lupus-prone mice. J Immunol 150:664
98. Seki S, Abo T, Ohteki T, Sugiura K, Kumagai K (1991) Unusual $\alpha\beta$-T cells expanded in autoimmune *lpr* mice are probably a counterpart of normal T cells in the liver. J Immunol 147:1214
99. Sekigawa I, Ishida Y, Hirose S, Sato H, Shirai T (1986) Cellular basis of in vitro anti-DNA antibody production: evidence for T cell dependence of IgG-class anti-DNA antibody synthesis in the (NZB x NZW)F_1 hybrid. J Immunol 136:1247
100. Seldin MF, Morse HC III, Reeves JP, Seribner CL, LeBoeuf RC, Steinberg AD (1988) Genetic analysis of autoimmune *gld* mice. I. Identification of a restriction fragment length polymorphism closely linked to the *gld* mutation within a conserved linkage group. J Exp Med 167:688
101. Shibata T, Spertini F, Berney T, Izui S (1992) Rheumatoid factors (RF) in mice bearing the *lpr* or *gld* mutation: selective production of RF cryoglobulins in MRL-/MpJ-*lpr/lpr* mice. Clin Exp Immunol 87:190
102. Shirai T (1982) The genetic basis of autoimmunity in murine lupus. Immunol Today 3:187
103. Singer PA, Mcevilly RJ, Noonan DJ, Dixon FJ, Theofilopoulos AN (1986) Clonal diversity and T-cell receptor β-chain variable gene expression in enlarged lymph nodes of MRL-*lpr/lpr* lupus mice. Proc Natl Acad Sci USA 83:7018
104. Snapper CM, Paul WE (1987) Interferon-γ and B cell stimulatory factor-1 reciprocally regulate Ig isotype production. Science 236:944
105. Snapper CM, McIntyre TM, Mandler R, Pecanha LMT, Finkelman FD, Lees A, Mond JJ (1992) Induction of IgG3 secretion by interferon γ: a model for T cell-independent class switching in response to T cell-independent type 2 antigens. J Exp Med 175:1367

106. Sneller MC, Straus SE, Jaffe ES, Jaffe JS, Fleisher TA, Stetler-Stevenson M, Strober W (1992) A novel lymphoproliferative/autoimmune syndrome resembling murine *lpr/gld* disease. J Clin Invest 90:334
107. Sobel ES, Katagiri T, Katagiri K, Morris SC, Cohen PL, Eisenberg RA (1991) An intrinsic B cell defect is required for the production of autoantibodies in the *lpr* model of murine systemic autoimmunity. J Exp Med 173:1441
108. Sobel ES, Kakkanaiah VN, Cohen PL, Eisenberg RA (1993) Correction of *gld* autoimmunity by co-infusion of normal bone marrow suggests that *gld* is a mutation of the Fas ligand gene. Int Immunol 5:1275
109. Strasser A, Whittingham S, Vaux DL, Bath ML, Adams JM, Cory S, Harris AW (1991) Enforced *BCL2* expression in B-lymphoid cells prolongs antibody responses and elicits autoimmune disease. Proc Natl Acad Sci USA 88:8661
110. Takahashi T, Tanaka M, Brannan CI, Jenkins NA, Copeland NG, Suda T, Nagata S (1994) Generalized lymphoproliferative disease in mice, caused by a point mutation in the Fas ligand. Cell 76:969
111. Takahashi S, Itch J, Ono M, Yamamoto T, Nose M, Kyogoku M (1993) cDNA sequence analysis of nephritogenic IgG3 monoclonal antibodies derived from an MRL/*lpr* lupus mouse. Mol Immunol 30:177
112. Theofilopoulos AN, Dixon FJ (1985) Murine models of systemic lupus erythematosus. Adv Immunol 37:269
113. Thomas JD, Sideras P, Smith CIE, Vorechovsky I, Chapman V, Paul WE (1993) Colocalization of X-linked agammaglobulinemia and X-linked immunodeficiency genes. Science 261:355
114. Trauth BC, Klas C, Peters AMJ, Matzku S, Möller P, Falk W, Debatin KM, Krammer PH (1989) Monoclonal antibody-mediated tumor regression by induction of apoptosis. Science 245:301
115. Tsubata T, Murakami M, Honjo T (1994) Antigen-receptor cross-linking induces peritoneal B-cell apoptosis in normal but not autoimmunity-prone mice. Curr Biol 4:8
116. Uehira M, Uno M, Kürner T, Kikutani H, Mori K, Inomoto T, Uede T, Miyazaki J, Nishimoto H, Kishimoto T, Yamamura K (1989) Development of autoimmune insulitis is prevented in E_{α}^{d} but not A_{β}^{k} NOD transgenic mice. Int Immunol 1:209
117. Vaux DL, Cory S, Adams JM (1988) *Bcl-2* gene promotes haemopoietic cell survival and cooperates with c-*myc* to immortalize pre-B cells. Nature 335:440
118. Watanabe-Fukunaga R, Brannan CI, Copeland NG, Jerkins NA, Nagata S (1992) Lymphoproliferation disorder in mice explained by defects in Fas antigen that mediates apoptosis. Nature 356:314
119. Watanabe-Fukunaga R, Brannan CI, Itoh N, Yonehara S, Copeland NG, Jerkins NA, Nagata S (1992) The cDNA structure, expression, and chromosomal assignment of the mouse Fas antigen. J Immunol 148:1274
120. Watson ML, Rao JK, Gilkeson GS, Ruiz P, Etcher EM, Pisetsky DS, Matsuzawa A, Rochelle JM, Seldin MF (1992) Genetic analysis of MRL-*lpr* mice: relationship of the Fas apoptosis gene to disease manifestations and renal disease-modifying loci. J Exp Med 176:1645
121. Wofsy D, Seaman WE (1985) Successful treatment of autoimmunity in NZB/NZW F_1 mice with monoclonal antibody to L3T4. J Exp Med 161:378
122. Wofsy D, Hardy RR, Seaman WE (1984) The proliferating cells in autoimmune MRL/*lpr* mice lack L3T4, an antigen on "helper" T cells that is involved in the response to class II major histocompatibility antigens. J Immunol 132:2686
123. Wu J, Zhou T, He J, Mountz JD (1993) Autoimmune disease in mice due to integration of an endogenous retrovirus in an apoptosis gene. J Exp Med 178:461
124. Yanagi Y, Hirose S, Nagasawa R, Shirai T, Mak TW, Tada T (1986) Does the deletion within T cell receptor β-chain gene of NZW mice contribute to autoimmunity in (NZB x NZW)F_1 mice? Eur J Immunol 16:1179
125. Yonehara S, Ishii A, Yonehara M (1989) A cell-killing monoclonal antibody (anti-Fas) to a cell surface antigen co-downregulated with the receptor of tumor necrosis factor. J Exp Med 169:1747
126. Yoshiki T, Mellors RC, Strand M, August JT (1974) The viral envelope glycoprotein of murine leukemia virus and the pathogenesis of immune complex glomerulonephritis of New Zealand mice. J Exp Med 140:1011

The role of cytokines in the immunopathogenesis of lupus

Barry S. Handwerger[1,2,3], **Violeta Rus**[1], **Ludmila da Silva**[1], **Charles S. Via**[1,2,3]

[1]Division of Rheumatology and Clinical Immunology, Department of Medicine and
[2]Department of Microbiology and Immunology, University of Maryland School of Medicine
[3]Department of Veterans Affairs Medical Center, Baltimore, MD 21201, USA

Introduction

Systemic lupus erythematosus is a disease characterized by B cell hyperactivity, autoantibody production and immune complex deposition in vital organs [175]. Increasing evidence indicates a critical role for T cells, particularly $CD4^+$ cells, in driving B cell hyperactivity. For example, work in mice has shown that actions which inhibit T cell function or deplete T cells, particularly $CD4^+$ T cells, improve disease outcome [65, 146, 160, 207]. Many laboratories have presented data which suggest that T cell-derived cytokines may play a critical role in driving B cell differentiation and hyperactivity in lupus (see below). Furthermore, much of the immunopathology in lupus is mediated by IgG autoantibodies [175], a T cell-dependent isotype.

Studies of murine T cell clones has allowed the subdivision of $CD4^+$ helper (Th) cells based on their cytokine secretion profile [115]. Th1 cells produce IL-2 and IFN-γ, but not IL-4, IL-5, IL-6 or IL-10, and mediate delayed-type hypersensitivity (DTH). Th2 cells secrete IL-4, IL-5, IL-6 and IL-10, but not IFN-γ or IL-2, and promote antibody production. Subsequent to the description of Th1 and Th2 cells, there has been a tendency for investigators to denote an in vitro and vivo immune response as either Th1 cell- or Th2 cell-mediated based on whether the response involves primarily cell-mediated immunity (CMI) or humoral immunity, or whether increased amounts of IL-2/IFN-γ or IL-4/IL-5/IL-10 are present in the response. This categorization, however, is overly simplistic. CMI responses are clearly affected by cytokines other than those produced by Th1 cells [131, 167] and humoral responses are promoted by cytokines other than those produced by Th2 cells [49, 122, 158]. Further complicating the matter, many of the cytokines produced by $CD4^+$ Th1 or Th2 cells can also be produced by other cells [1, 13, 38, 48, 51, 82, 120, 130, 149, 212]. Additionally, a single cytokine may affect both CMI and antibody-mediated responses. For example, IFN-γ plays a central role in DTH [115, 167], yet it also serves as a B cell differentiation factor promoting the production of IgG2a antibodies

Correspondence to: B.S. Handwerger, 8-34 MSTF, 10 S. Pine Street, Baltimore, MD 21201-1192, USA

[158]. Moreover, the cytokines produced by Th1 and Th2 cells can cross-regulate each other. For example, IL-4 and IL-10 inhibit Th1 cell responses [131, 167] and IFN-γ inhibits the effects of IL-4 on B cells [19, 133]. This review discusses several cytokines and examines their direct and cross-regulatory effects in the pathogenesis of lupus. The data presented in this review is summarized in Table 1.

Table 1. Cytokines in lupus

Cytokine	Human	Mouse
IL-1		
IL-1 production	↓ or normal	↓, normal, ↑
IL-1 receptor expression	↑ B cells	
IL-1 responsiveness	↓ T cells, ↑ B cells	–
In vivo effects of IL-1	–	IL-1 accelerates disease in NZB and accelerates arthritis in MRL/lpr
IL-2		
IL-2 production	↓ or normal	↓, ↑ during 1st week of GVHD, then ↓
IL-2 receptor expression	↓ β chain ↑ or normal α chain	↓ on MRL/lpr DN T cells and on PN T cells, normal on MRL/lpr B cells
Soluble IL-2 receptors	↑	↑
IL-2 responsiveness	↓ T cells	↓ T cells and B cells induces
In vivo effects of IL-2	–	autoimmunity in neonatally thymectomized or athymic mice inhibits lymphoproliferation and autoimmunity in MRL/llpr; in P → F_1 GVHD model, anti-IL-2 mAb converts acute into chronic GVHD; anti-IL-2R mAb inhibits disease in NZB and NZB/W
IFN-γ		
IFN-γ production	↓	↓ in PN and GVHD
↑ in lpr and gld		
IFN-γ responsiveness	–	normal NZB/W and MRL/lpr B cells, ↓ in NZB B cells
In vivo effects of anti-IFN-γ mAb	–	anti-IFN-γ inhibits autoimmunity in NZB and lymphadenopathy in MRL/lpr; IFN-γ accelerates disease in NZB and NZB/W
IL-3		
IL-3 production	–	↓ in lpr (stimulated in vitro) ↓ or ↑ in lpr (spontaneous)
IL-4		
IL4 production	↑ or normal	↑ in PN, lpr, GVHD normal in BXSB
IL-4 responsiveness	normal or ↓ (B cells)	Normal, ↓, ↑ (B cells)
In vivo effects of anti-IL-4 mAb	–	Anti-IL-4 mAb inhibits IgE production and autoimmunity in GVHD-induced lupus
IL-5		
IL-5 production	–	Normal in PN
IL-5 responsiveness	–	↑ in NZB and NZB/W normal in BXSB, MRL/lpr

Table 1. Continued

IL-6		
IL-6 production	↑	↓
IL-6 receptor expression	↑ B cells	↑ on B cells in MRL/lpr ↓ on $CD4^+$ T cells in MRL/lpr
soluble IL-6 receptors	–	↑ in MRL/lpr, NZB/W, male BXSB
IL-6 responsiveness	↑ B cells	↑ B cells
IL-10		
IL-10 production	–	↑ in PN and GVHD
In vivo effects of anti-IL-10 mAb and IL-10	–	Anti-IL-10 mAb inhibits disease in NZB/W and reverses defect in IFN-γ production in PN and GVHD; IL-10 accelerates autoimmunity in NZB/W
TNF-α		
TNF-α production	–	↑ in MRL/lpr (unstimulated), normal in GVHD (unstimulated) ↓ in NZB/W, NZB (post in vitro stimulation)
In vivo effects of TNF-α and anti-TNF-α	–	High-dose TNF-α inhibits and low-dose TNF-α accelerates autoimmunity in NZB/W; anti-TNF-α inhibits inflammatory pulmonary lesions in MRL/lpr
IL-12		
In vivo effects of IL-12	–	IL-12 converts chronic to acute GVHD in P → F_1 GVHD model
TGF-β		
In vivo effects of TGF-β	–	Possible autoimmune disease in TGF-β_1 knockout mice
M-CSF		
Serum M-CSF	–	↑ in MRL/lpr
Kidney M-CSF	–	↑ in MRL/lpr
GM-CSF		
GM-CSF production	–	↓ in lpr
Eta-1		
Eta-1 production	–	↑ in MRL/lpr
Other B cell stimulatory cytokines		
Serum NZB-SF	–	↑ in NZB
Production of uncharacterized BCGF and/or BCDF	–	↑ lpr
Response to 50- and 12-kDa BCGF	↑	–

IL, interleukin; GVHD, graft-versus-host disease; DN, double-negative; P → F_1. parent-into-F_1; mAb, monoclonal antibody, R, receptor; IFN, interferon; TNF, tumor necrosis factor; TGF, transforming growth factor; M, macrophage; CSF, colony-stimulating factor; G, granulocyte; Eta, early T lymphocyte activation-1; BCG(D)F, B cell growth (differentiation) factor(s)

Interleukin-1

IL-1 production

The exact role of IL-1 in the immunological and pathological alterations that occur in lupus is controversial. Monocytes from some, but not all, lupus patients [8, 14, 20, 118, 206] have a defect in IL-1 production in vitro. Peritoneal and bone marrow-derived macrophages from some strains of lupus mice [17, 39, 42, 96, 102] have also been reported to have a defect in IL-1 production. In MRL mice, the defect in IL-1 production is fully expressed at birth and appears to be due to an intrinsic macrophage abnormality [95, 96]. In contrast, LPS-stimulated IL-1 production by splenic macrophages from older PN mice is variable, with some mice producing normal amounts of IL-1 and others having a mild-to-moderate defect (Handwerger, submitted for publication). Hepatic macrophages from NZB/W mice [46] produce normal amounts of IL-1 following in vitro lipopolysaccharide (LPS) stimulation and glomerular macrophages from MRL/lpr mice express markedly increased levels of IL-1α and IL-1β mRNA [20, 21]. Increased IL-1 mRNA levels also have been detected in the spleens of mice with graft-versus-host disease (GVHD)-induced lupus [10], the renal cortices of NZB/W mice with lupus nephritis [20, 23], and freshly isolated peripheral blood mononuclear cells (PBMC) from patients with active lupus [97, 100]. In addition, high levels of IL-1 production has been observed in unstimulated short-term cultures of purified B cells from lupus patients [172].

IL-1 responsiveness: IL-1 receptor expression

T cells from lupus patients have been reported to have a defect in IL-1 responsiveness [8], while B cells from lupus patients hyperrespond to IL-1 [100, 108, 172]. B cells from lupus patients contain a significantly increased percentage of IL-1 receptor-bearing cells [172].

Effects of in vivo administered IL-1

In vivo administration of low-dose recombinant IL-1α (rIL-1α) to female NZB/W mice accelerates renal injury and mortality when treatment is initiated at 4 months of age, while administration of higher-dose rIL-1α has no effect on proteinuria or survival [23]. In vivo administration of rIL-1β accelerates the onset and progression of spontaneous arthritis in MRL/lpr mice [72].

Interleukin-2

IL-2 production

A defect in IL-2 production following in vitro stimulation of T cells with mitogens or antigens has been demonstrated in most strains of mice that spontaneously develop lupus [11, 29, 64, 142–145, 176, 185, 208, 209] and in mice with GVHD-induced lupus [191, 194] or with lupus induced by immunization with antibodies bearing the pathogenic anti-DNA antibody idiotype 16/6 [16]. In addition, T cells from patients with lupus have been reported to have a significant defect in the production of IL-2 following mitogenic or antigenic stimulation in vitro [3, 7, 34, 71, 98, 99, 113, 116, 147, 154, 155, 166, 197]. This finding, however, has not been universally confirmed [41, 128]. Via et al. [197] have recently demonstrated that lupus patients are heterogeneous with respect to the ability of their T cells to produce IL-2 following in vitro stimulation with influenza A virus (Flu) or allogeneic cells; 35% of patients exhibited a normal IL-2 response to both antigens, 46% of patients demonstrated a defective response to Flu but normal response to allogeneic cells, and 19% of patients showed a defective response to both antigens. In lupus patients, the defect in IL-2 production following in vitro stimulation with allogeneic major histocompatibility complex (MHC) antigens has been reported to be manifested by only $CD4^+$ cells [166] or by both $CD4^+$ and $CD8^+$ T cells [198]. The defect in IL-2 production following in in vitro stimulation with phytohemagglutinin is exhibited by both $CD4^+$ and $CD8^+$ T cells [116]. In PN mice, the defect in IL-2 production following in vitro stimulation with concanavalin A (Con A) is manifested by $CD4^+$ T cells ([64] and Handwerger, manuscript in preparation). Defective IL-2 production by T cells from lupus patients [99, 101] and lupus mice [191, 192] may be related to excessive "suppressor cell" activity. In lupus patients, the suppressor cells are $CD8^+$ $HLA\text{-}DR^+$ and $Leu7^+$ [99, 101]. The exact nature of the "suppressor cell" and the underlying mechanisms of suppression, however, have not been fully elucidated. It is possible that the defect in IL-2 production is related to the overproduction of cytokines, such as IL-4 and IL-10, that are capable of inhibiting immune responses mediated by Th1 cells [131, 167]. Defective monocyte-macrophage or antigen-presenting cell (APC) function also appears to play an important role in the diminished IL-2 production manifested by T cells from lupus patients [197, 208]. The defect in IL-2 production, however, is not due solely to defective IL-1 production by APC, since the exogenous addition of IL-1 to culture does not correct the defect in IL-2 production exhibited by lupus patients [34, 98] or PN mice (Handwerger, submitted for publication).

Defective IL-2 production by lupus T cells can be reversed by costimulating the cells with phorbol myristate acetate (PMA) [30, 143, 144, 155], which suggests that the defect is secondary to an abnormality in intracellular signalling that results in diminished activation of protein kinase C. Defective IL-2 production in vitro also can be reversed by preculturing the T cells in the absence of mitogens [71, 75, 145]. Although the mechanisms responsible for this phenomenon are unclear, the data suggest that the defect in IL-2 production may be related to a reversible. "exhaustion" of T cells, resulting from their continuous in vivo activation [75] or from the secretion of inhibitory factors by activated T cells [71]. Lupus patients have a significant increase in the percentage of activated T cells in their peripheral blood [85, 134, 135, 199, 213] and the percentage of T cells expressing activation markers decreases when the cells are "precultured" prior to in vitro stimulation [71].

The precise role, if any, of defective IL-2 production in the pathogenesis of immunological abnormalities and autoimmunity in lupus is unclear. IL-2 is known to augment natural killer (NK) cell cytotoxic function [91, 180, 200] and to serve as a growth factor for $CD4^+$ helper T cells and $CD8^+$ cytotoxic T cells (CTL) [49, 55, 56, 66, 151, 201, 202]. Exogenous addition of IL-2 to culture can partially or totally correct the defect in NK cell function in lupus patients [163, 182] and totally reverse the defect in the in vitro generation of cytotoxic T lymphocytes (CTL) manifested by lupus patients [182] and autoimmune PN mice (Handwerger, submitted for publication). These data suggest that, to a large extent, diminished NK cell and CTL function in lupus may be secondary to defective IL-2 production. In addition, exogenous IL-2 partially reverses the proliferative defect manifested by peripheral blood mononulear cells (PBMC) from lupus patients in allogeneic [182] or autologous [166, 198] mixed lymphocyte cultures. A defect in IL-2 production alone, however, is not sufficient for the induction of lupus. Approximately half of clinically healthy, consanguineous household and nonhousehold relatives of lupus patients have a defect in IL-2 production similar to the lupus probands [141], suggesting a genetic basis for the defect, independent of the presence of lupus.

IL-2 responsiveness: IL-2 receptor expression

T cells from several strains of lupus mice [11, 208, 209] and some lupus patients [81, 92, 116, 166, 169] have a defect in IL-2 responsiveness. This finding, however, has not been universally confirmed [34, 113]. In lupus patients, the defect involves $CD4^+$ T cells, but not $CD8^+$ T cells [116, 166], and appears to be primarily related to an abnormality in the induction of the p70/75 β chain of the IL-2 receptor [77, 140, 169]. The induction of the p55 IL-2 receptor α chain on activated T cells is also abnormal in some, but not all, lupus patients [77, 92, 116]. Following in vitro stimulation with Con A, the percentage of $CD4^+$ T cells from 10- to 12-month-old, autoimmune PN mice that express the p55 α chain of the IL-2 receptor is significantly decreased compared to either young (3-month-old) PN mice or age- and sex-matched DBA/2 controls. Con A-activated $CD8^+$ T cells from both PN and DBA/2 mice exhibit a mild, comparable, age-related decrease in the percentage of cells that express IL-2 receptor a chain (Handwerger, submitted for publication). Double-negative ($CD4^-$ $CD8^-$) T cells from MRL/lpr mice do not express the α chain of the IL-2 receptor; expression of the β chain on those cells is controversial [61, 139, 170]. Since IL-2 up-regulates the expression of IL-2 receptors [106, 136], the defects in IL-2 receptor expression and IL-2 responsiveness could be due, in part, to diminished IL-2 production [206]. However, the addition of exogenous rIL-2 to culture does not correct the defect in IL-2 receptor expression manifested by T cells from older PN mice (Handwerger, submitted for publication).

Although the percentage of LPS-stimulated B cells that express IL-2 receptors is comparable in MRL/lpr and normal mice, LPS-stimulated B cells from MRL/lpr and NZB/W mice, in contrast to B cells from normal control mice, proliferate in response to IL-2. The IL-2-responsive population consists predominantly of large B cells [94]. Although IL-2 does not induce the proliferation of B cells from patients with lupus [108], it does enhance the proliferative response of lupus B cells to *Staphylococcus aureus* Cowan I (SAC) [184]. An important role of IL-2 receptor-bearing cells in the pathogenesis of lupus nephritis has been suggested by the finding that treatment of female NZB/W mice, beginning at 6 weeks of age, with an anti-IL-2 receptor monoclonal antibody (mAb) significant inhibits the development of immune complex-mediated renal disease [84].

Following activation, T cells release a soluble form of the IL-2 receptor into blood and tissue culture medium. In lupus patients, B cells also may release soluble IL-2 receptors [15]. Lupus patients and lupus mice have elevated serum or plasma levels of soluble IL-2 receptors [15, 26, 76, 150, 174, 205, 210]. Plasma IL-2 receptor levels, which tend to increase prior to and during acute exacerbations of disease activity and fall back toward baseline values following treatment, correlate in lupus patients with the levels of anti-double-stranded DNA antibody and the third and fourth components of complement, but not with a disease activity index [174, 210].

Effect of in vivo administered anti-IL-2 mAb or IL-2

GVHD can be induced in inbred mice by in vivo injection of parental T cells [44, 45, 74]. The injection of C57BL/6 (B6) spleen cells into (C57BL/6 x DBA/2) F_1 mice ($B6D2F_1$) results in acute GVHD, with profound immunodeficiency and early mortality [58, 129, 194]. In contrast, the injection of DBA/2 spleen cells into B6D2F$_1$, mice results in a chronic, immunostimulatory GVHD, characterized by autoantibody production and the induction of a lupus-like disease. Although B6D2F$_1$ mice with acute or chronic GVHD exhibit defective IL-2 production 2 or more weeks after the induction of disease [194], within the first 24–48 h of disease induction, mice with both forms of GVHD exhibit striking elevations in spontaneous IL-2 production in vitro [189] and in splenic IL-2 mRNA expression [53]. The enhanced production of IL-2, which is dependent on donor CD4$^+$ T cells, persists for 7 to 9 days after GVHD induction. Treatment of acute GVHD mice with anti-IL-2 mAb S4B6 for the first 2 weeks of disease alters the nature of the disease process [190]. Anti-IL-2-treated GVHD mice exhibit many features of chronic, immunostimulatory GVHD, including lupus-like autoimmunity. These data demonstrate that, although enhanced IL-2 production early during the course of disease induction may be a feature of some forms of lupus, the subsequent development of B cell hyperactivity and production of autoantibodies may not be IL-2 dependent.

Neonatal thymectomy of normal CBA/H mice results in decreased numbers of splenic and lymph node T cells and a transient increase in T cells in the peritoneal cavity. The peritoneal cavity T cells are predominantly CD4$^-$ and CD8$^-$ (double negative) and selectively overexpress the $V_\beta 11$ family of T cell receptors (TCR) [12]. The percentage of $V_\beta 11^+$ T cells also is increased in the spleens of neonatally thymectomized CBA/H mice. The $V_\beta 11$ gene family encodes an I-E-reactive TCR that is normally deleted in the thymus of I-E$^+$ CBA/H mice. Intraperitoneal (i.p.) injection of an IL-2/vaccinia recombinant virus construct that releases large amounts of human IL-2 into neonatal thymectomized CBA/H mice induces the conversion of the double-negative T cells into CD4$^+$ T cells and CD8$^+$ T cells that proliferate in response to anti-$V_\beta 11$ mAb and induces the production of anti-DNA antibodies, rheumatoid factors and interstitial nephritis. Inoculation of the same construct into young athymic nude mice also induces overt autoimmunity. These data strongly suggest that IL-2 can enhance the autoaggressive activity of T cells that bear self-reactive TCR, which are normally deleted in the thymus. In contrast to these findings, however, when MRL/lpr mice are inoculated with the IL-2/vaccinia recombinant virus construct, the mice exhibit prolonged survival, diminished autoantibody production, decreased renal disease, no development of arthritis, improved thymic differentiation and restoration of normal numbers of mature T cells in peripheral lymphoid organs [62]. Thus, the exact role of IL-2 in the pathogenesis of lupus is still unclear.

Interferon-γ

IFN-γ production

T cells from lupus patients have a diminished ability to produce IFN-γ following in vitro stimulation with mitogen or IL-2 [153, 162, 182, 183], a defect that can be reversed by addition of PMA to culture [154] or by stimulating the cells with the calcium ionophore A23187 plus PMA [162]. T cells from older, autoimmune PN mice ([64] and Handwerger, submitted for publication) and mice with GVHD-induced lupus [37] also exhibit a defect in IFN-γ production. In contrast, Con A-stimulated spleen cells from male BXSB mice produce normal levels of IFN-γ [185], and T cells from lpr and gld mice produce increased amounts of IFN-γ [24, 31, 185]. In lpr mice, the IFN-γ is produced by CD4$^+$ (and probably CD44^{hi}) T cells [24, 31]. The ability of double-negative T cells from lpr mice to produce IFN-γ is controversial [31, 107, 117].

Because patients with lupus and older, autoimmune PN mice manifest a defect in IFN-γ production, while lpr and gld mice produce increased amounts of IFN-γ, the precise role that IFN-γ plays in the induction and maintenance of autoimmunity in lupus is unclear. IFN-γ has pleiotropic effects on immune and non-immune cells [179], including the ability to inhibit the proliferation of Th2 cells [52] and to block the proliferative and immunoglobulin-secretory response of B cells to antigen plus Th2 cells or Th2 cell-derived cytokines, such as IL-4 [19, 133]. Thus, defective IFN-γ production may contribute to the induction and maintenance of autoimmunity in lupus by facilitating increased production of B cell-stimulatory cytokines by Th2 cells and enhancing the responsiveness of B cells to those cytokines. In contrast, several lines of evidence suggest that IFN-γ may have a deleterious effect in lupus. IFN-γ is able to induce or up-regulate MHC class II gene expression [211], an effect which may contribute to the immunopathogenesis of autoimmunity [22]. NZB, NZB/W and MRL/lpr mice all have high serum levels of IgG2a [161, 176], an IFN-γ-induced immunoglobulin isotype [158]. The effects of in vivo-administered IFN-α, IFN-γ and anti-IFN-γ (see below) also suggest that IFN-γ may play a central role in the induction of lupus in some patients and in some strains of lupus mice. Thus, it is possible that, because of its pleiotropic effects, either decreased or increased IFN-γ production may induce immunoregulatory alterations that result in autoantibody production and autoimmune disease.

IFN-γ responsiveness

B cells from NZB/W and MRL/lpr mice respond normally to IFN-γ [89, 112], while B cells from NZB mice exhibited defective IFN-γ responsiveness [89].

Effects of in vivo administered IFN-α, IFN-γ and anti-IFN-γ

In vivo administration of anti-IFN-γ mAb delays the onset of proteinuria and anti-DNA antibody production and prolongs survival in NZB/W mice [68], and reduces lymphadenopathy and the expansion of double-negative T cells in MRL/lpr mice [28], while treatment of NZB or NZB/W mice with IFN-γ accelerates the development of autoantibodies, glomerulonephritis and death [47, 67, 80]. In contrast, neither IFN-γ nor anti-IFN-γ mAb alters the course of disease in GVHD-induced lupus in mice [187], and administration of IFN-γ to normal C57BL/6 mice does not induce autoantibody production [32]. A contributing role for IFN-γ in lupus is also supported by the observation that rIFN-α and rIFN-γ therapy for malignancy or chronic hepatitis has been associated with the induction of autoantibody production [43, 138] and several autoimmune diseases [2, 25, 57, 109, 137, 138, 147], including lupus [43, 203].

Interleukin-3

Santoro et al. [145] have reported that CD4$^+$ T cells from the spleens of MRL/lpr and B6/lpr mice exhibit a defect in Con A-stimulated IL-3 production compared to similar cells from congenic +/+ mice. MacNeil et al. 11031 have reported that splenic T cells from MRL/lpr and MRL/+ mice have a marked defect in their ability to produce IL-3 following in vitro stimulation with pokeweed mitogen (PWM). This defect is due to an abnormality in accessory cell function, since the addition of peritoneal exudate cells from normal, histocompatible CBA mice restores the ability of T cells from MRL/+ and young MRL/lpr mice to produce IL-3. Defective IL-3 production could also be restored by addition of PMA to the cultures or by preincubation of the T cells in tissue culture for 2 days before addition of PWM. Davignon et al. [33] have reported that spleen cells and lymph node cells from MRL/lpr and B6/lpr mice spontaneously produce much less IL-3 in culture than do cells from normal control mice. This defect was due to the lack of IL-3 production by the high proportion of $B220^{+}/CD4^{-}$ $CD8^{-}$ T cells. Following in vitro depletion of that cell population, B6-lpr lymph node cells produced normal amounts of IL-3. Palacios [123], in contrast, has reported that spleen cells from MRL/lpr mice, but not normal control mice, spontaneously secrete IL-3 in vitro. Spontaneous IL-3 production was detected in MLR/lpr mice as young as 6 weeks of age and increased with age. The reasons for these disparate results are unknown.

Interleukin-4

IL-4 production

Elevated levels of IL-4 have been found in the sera of some lupus patients [42]. Purified B cells from lupus patients have been reported to spontaneously produce a soluble factor with IL-4-like activity [171]. In contrast, Tan et al. [168] and Linker-Israeli et al. [100] have reported that peripheral blood lymphocytes from lupus patients do not spontaneously express elevated levels of IL-4 mRNA.

Spleen cells from male BXSB mice produce normal amounts of IL-4 following in vitro Con A stimulation [185], while in vitro-activated lymph node cells from C3H/lpr [31] and MRL/lpr [24] mice and hepatic lymphocytes from MRL/lpr mice [105] produce significantly more IL-4 than lymphocytes from control mice. The cells responsible for the increase in IL-4 production following in vitro stimulation of MRL/lpr lymph node cells are $CD4^{+}$ (and probably $CD4^{hi}$) T cells and not the double-negative T cells that accumulate in the lymphoid organs of lpr mice [24]. Umland et al. [185], in contrast, have reported that Con A-stimulated spleen cells from 6-to 7-month-old MRL/lpr mice produce significantly less IL-4 mRNA and IL-4 protein than controls. Spleen cells from PN mice have a significant, age-related increase in their ability to produce IL-4 following in vitro stimulation with Con A ([64] and Handwerger, submitted for publication). $CD4^{+}$ T cells are responsible for the increased IL-4 production. In the DBA/2-into-B6D2F_1 model of GVHD-induced lupus, increased splenic expression of IL-4 mRNA is seen as early as 2 to 4 days after injection of parental cells ([53, 195] and Rus and Via, manuscript in preparation) and increased production of IL-4 by donor $CD4^{+}$ cells is observed beginning 2–3 weeks after the injection of donor T cells [10, 37].

IL-4 responsiveness

Anti-μ- or anti-IgM-stimulated B cells from lupus patients proliferate normally when rIL-4 is added to culture on day 0, [50, 86]; however, in a restimulation assay, where B cells are preincubated for 3 days with anti-IgM, the proliferative response of B cells from lupus patients to IL-4 was significantly decreased compared to normal controls [86]. rIL-4 augments the proliferation of SAC-stimulated B cells from lupus patients and enhances the IgG plaque-forming cell response of B cells from lupus patients that have been stimulated in vitro with SAC plus rIL-1 and/or rIL-6 [171].

IL-4 augments the proliferative response of anti-μ-stimulated B cells from PN mice (da Silva and Handwerger, unpublished observation). Older PN mice exhibit a marked hypergammaglobulinemia, characterized primarily by an increase in the concentration of serum IgG1 (da Silva and Handwerger, manuscript in preparation); mice with GVHD-induced lupus have significantly increased serum IgG1 and IgE concentrations [40, 187]. These data suggest that IL-4 plays an important role in the B cell hyperactivity of these mice, since IgG1 and IgE are IL-4-dependent immunoglobulin isotypes [157]. The percentage of splenic B cells secreting IgG1 following in vitro stimulation with LPS plus IL-4 is normal in MRL/lpr and NZB/W mice, but markedly reduced in NZB mice [89]. In contrast, Minoda et al. [112] have reported that small, resting B cells from older NZB/W mice hyperproliferate in response to LPS plus IL-4.

Effect of in vivo administered anti-IL-4 mAb

A critical role of IL-4 in the induction of B cell hyperactivity and disease in mice with GVHD-induced lupus has been suggested by the observation that treatment of the mice with anti-IL-4 mAb prevents the increase in IgE production [40] and delays the onset of proteinuria and significantly prolongs survival [187].

Interleukin-5

The possible role of IL-5 in the pathogenesis of lupus has not been extensively evaluated. Tominaga et al. [178] have reported that transgenic mice carrying the mouse IL-5 gene have high serum levels of IL-5, IgM and IgA and produce polyreactive IgM autoantibodies reactive with single-stranded DNA (ssDNA), double-stranded DNA (dsDNA) and cardiolipin. The production of IL-5 by T cells from lupus patients or lupus mice has not been extensively studied. In contrast to 3-month-old PN mice, spleen cells from approximately one-half of autoimmune, 10- to 12-month-old PN mice produce increased amounts of IL-5 following in vitro Con A stimulation; however, this increase appears to be a normal age-related phenomenon, since an equivalent increase is observed in age-and sex-matched normal controls (Handwerger, submitted for publication). IL-5, however, may play a role in the B cell hyperactivity of PN mice, since older PN mice exhibit a two- to threefold increase in serum IgA concentration compared to normal controls (da Silva and Handwerger, manuscript in preparation) and they produce IgA anti-dsDNA and anti-ssDNA antibodies ([63] and Handwerger, submitted for publication). IgA is an IL-5-dependent immunoglobulin isotype [18, 27]. B cells from NZB and NZB/W mice [4, 68, 186], but not BXSB or MRL/lpr mice [186], hyperrespond to IL-5 or a combination of IL-4 and IL-5.

Interleukin-6

IL-6 production

Increasing evidence suggests an important role of IL-6 in the B cell hyperactivity and immunopathology of lupus. Older, autoimmune, MRL/lpr mice [164] and patients with active lupus, but not those inactive lupus patients, have increased serum IL-6 levels [3, 97, 100, 110, 159, 165]. In lupus patients, increased levels of IL-6 correlate with disease activity, but not with anti-DNA antibody concentrations [159]. Elevated levels of IL-6 are present in the cerebrospinal fluid of lupus patients with central nervous system (CNS) involvement [9, 69] and in the urine and renal glomeruli of patients with lupus nephritis [60, 73]. With successful treatment of CNS lupus, cerebrospinal fluid IL-6 levels decrease significantly [69]. Urinary IL-6 levels correlate with the renal pathology score [73].

T cells, B cells and monocyte-macrophages from lupus patients produce increased amounts of IL-6 [3, 70, 86–88, 100, 119, 127, 165, 171]; however, T cells produce much less IL-6 than do B cells [87, 88]. Following in vitro mitogenic stimulation, lymph node cells from MRL/lpr [173], C3H/lpr [31] and C3H/gld mice [31], but not NZB/W mice [173], produce increased amounts of IL-6. Increased macrophage production of IL-6 has been demonstrated in mice with host-versus-graft disease (HVGD)-induced lupus [188]. Allen et al. [10] have reported that 2 weeks after induction of disease, mice with GVHD-induced lupus express normal splenic IL-6 mRNA levels. In contrast, we have observed that splenic IL-6 mRNA levels are increased in mice with GVHD-induced lupus (Rus and Via, unpublished observation). The reasons for this discrepancy are unclear.

IL-6 responsiveness: IL-6 receptor expression

In contrast to B cells from normal individuals, which do not spontaneously express IL-6 receptors, the majority of B cells from lupus patients do spontaneously express IL-6 receptors [119]. Furthermore, B cells from lupus patients have been reported to respond well to IL-6 [86–88, 100, 171]. The enhanced response of B cells from patients with active lupus may be related to a defect in a suppressor cell population that normally inhibits IL-6-induced IgG production [204].

MRL/lpr mice, in contrast to normal control mice, overexpress IL-6 receptors on splenic B cells and lack IL-6 receptor expression on peripheral $CD4^+$ T cells [90]. Older MRL/lpr, NZB/W and male BXSB mice have high serum levels of soluble IL-6 receptor (sIL-6R), suggesting that elevated sIL-6R levels in aged mice may be a common phenomenon in lupus-prone mice [164].

IL-6 may play an important role in the induction of anti-DNA antibodies in lupus patients and lupus mice. Immunoglobulin and anti-DNA antibody production in vitro by B cells from lupus patients is promoted by IL-6 and inhibited by anti-IL-6 or anti-IL-6 receptor antibodies [86–88, 100, 119]. IL-6 induces B cells from old NZB/W mice, but not young NZB/W or BALB/c mice, to produce IgG and IgG anti-DNA antibodies [5, 6, 111], and enhances IgG (particularly IgG1) production by B cells from mice with HVGD-induced lupus [188]. Anti-IL-6 mAb inhibits the in vitro production of anti-DNA antibodies by old NZB/W spleen cells [5] and anti-IL-6 receptor mAb markedly reduces the spontaneous in vitro hyperproduction of IgG1 by spleen cells from mice with HVGD-induced lupus [188]. The production of IL-6 and IgG anti-DNA antibody in vitro by spleen cells from old NZB/W mice is macrophage dependent [6].

Interleukin-10

IL-10 mRNA expression is increased in the spleens of mice 2–3 weeks after the induction of GVHD-induced lupus ([10, 37, 53] and Rus and Via, unpublished observation). Spleen cells from older, autoimmune PN mice also spontaneously express increased levels of IL-10 mRNA ([64] and Handwerger, Svetic and Gause, manuscript in preparation), and following in vitro stimulation with Con A or anti-CD3 mAb, $CD4^+$ T cells from older autoimmune PN mice secrete increased amounts of IL-10 ([64] and Handwerger, submitted for publication).

Several lines of evidence suggest that IL-10 may play a role in the pathogenesis of immunoregulatory abnormalities and in the initiation and/or maintenance of autoimmune disease in lupus. DeWit et al. [37] have reported that the addition of neutralizing anti-IL-10 mAb to culture can partially reverse the defect that is exhibited in IFN-γ production by anti-CD3 mAb-stimulated spleen cells from mice with GVHD-induced lupus. Similarly, in preliminary experiments, we have found that the defect in Con A-induced IFN-γ production by $CD4^+$ T cells from older, autoimmune PN mice can be reversed by the exogenous addition to culture of anti-IL-10 mAb (Handwerger, unpublished observations). Ishida et al. [78] have reported that the continuous in vivo administration of neutralizing anti-IL-10 mAb to NZB/W mice delays the onset of proteinuria, glomerulonephritis and anti-dsDNA antibody production and decreases mortality, while the continuous administration of rIL-10 accelerates the onset of autoimmunity. The protective effect of anti-IL-10 mAb appears to be due to the up-regulation of tumor necrosis factor-α (TNF-α) production, since treatment of anti-IL-10 mAb-protected mice with neutralizing anti-TNF-α mAb resulted in the rapid development of autoimmunity.

Tumor necrosis factor-α

Kupffer cells [104], splenic macrophages [104], whole lung preparations [35], and renal cortices [20] from MRL/lpr mice express increased levels of TNF-α mRNA. Infiltrating mononuclear cells appear to be responsible for the increased TNF-α mRNA expression in MRL/lpr lungs [35], while glomerular macrophages, which are prominent only in MRL/lpr mice with active renal disease, appear to be the source of the increased renal expression of TNF-α mRNA [20]. In contrast, following in vitro stimulation with LPS or LPS plus IFN-γ, peritoneal macrophages from NZW and NZB/W mice produce significantly less TNF-α then do macrophages from normal control mice [79] and, 2 weeks after the injection of DBA/2 cells into $B6D2F_1$ mice, splenic TNF-α mRNA levels are normal in mice with GVHD-induced lupus [10].

In vivo treatment of NZB/W mice with 10 μg of rTNF-α, i.p., three times per week, beginning at either 4 months or 6 months of age, improves survival and delays, but does not prevent, the progression of renal disease [59, 79]. Anti-dsDNA antibody titers, however, were unaffected by the TNF-α treatment [59]. In contrast, administration of 2 μg of rTNF-α, i.p., three times per week, beginning at 4 months of age, to NZB/W mice does not affect survival, and administration of 0.2 μg of rTNF-α, i.p., three times per week accelerates renal disease and mortality rate [23]. Thus, the effects of rTNF-α on the progression of lupus in NZB/W mice appear to be dose dependent, with low-dose TNF-α accelerating and high-dose TNF-α inhibiting disease progression. Deguchi and Kishimoto [35] have reported that in vivo treatment of MRL/lpr mice with anti-TNF-α antibodies inhibits the development of inflammatory pulmonary lesions.

Interleukin-12

Via et al. ([196] and J Immunol, in press) have demonstrated that the in vivo administration of IL-12 on days 0–5 after injection of DBA/2 spleen cells into B6D2F$_1$ mice stimulates the development of acute GVHD in mice that otherwise would have developed chronic, autoimmune GVHD. This effect apparently is not due to the ability of IL-12 to induce increased IFN-γ production, since the concomitant administration of neutrlizing anti-IFN-γ mAb does not affect the ability of IL-12 to convert chronic GVHD to acute GVHD.

Tansforming growth factor-β

Shull et al. [152] have reported that during the first 17–34 days of life TGF-β1 knockout mice develop a rapidly fatal wasting syndrome, associated with the presence of inflammatory cell infiltrates and tissue necrosis in multiple organs. The etiopathogenesis of the syndrome, which resembles to some extent polymyositis and Sjogren's syndrome, is unknown – it may be secondary to an infectious agent and/or an autoimmune process. The potential relevance of this model to lupus is as yet unclear.

Macrophage-colony-stimulating factor (CSF) and granulocyte-macrophage CSF

Yui et al. [214] have demonstrated that MRL/lpr mice have an increased serum level of M-CSF, which is detectable in mice as young as 1 week of age. Serum M-CSF levels in MRL/lpr mice decrease between 2 months and 4 months of age and then steadily increase thereafter. MRL/+, B6/lpr, C3H/lpr, NZB/W and normal control mice, in contrast, do not express detectable serum levels of M-CSF. The source of the M-CSF In the sera of MRL/lpr mice has not been clearly defined. The kidneys of MRL/lpr mice express significantly elevated levels of M-CSF mRNA, while steady-state M-CSF mRNA levels in lymph nodes, spleen, liver, lung and bone marrow of MRL/lpr are similar to those in control mice.

Lymph node cells and spleen cells from MRL/lpr and B6/lpr mice spontaneously produce significantly less GM-CSF in culture than do lymphoid cells from control mice [33]. This defect appears to be due to the accumulation of double-negative T cells, which are immunologically nonfunctional and do not produce GM-CSF, in the lymphoid organs of lpr mice. The in vitro production of GM-CSF by B6/lpr lymph node cells that have been depleted of double-negative T cells is normal.

Early T lymphocyte activation-1

Lymph node cells, splenocytes, thymocytes and the lungs of MRL/lpr mice spontaneously express very high levels of mRNA for T cell cytokine early T lymphocyte activation-1 (Eta-1) [125]. Eta-1 has been shown to bind to macrophages through an RGD motif and alter their mobility and activation state [124, 156], and to stimulate IgM and IgG production by mixtures of macrophages and B cells [93].

Increased Eta-1 mRNA expression, which occurs in double-negative T cells, but not CD4$^+$ T cells or CD8$^+$ T cells, begins with the onset of autoimmune disease and continues throughout the course of the disease [125]. Both the lpr gene and MRL background genes contribute to the maximal expression of Eta-1 mRNA in MRL/lpr mice. The increased expression of Eta-1 mRNA by lymphoid cells from MRL/lpr mice and the ability of Eta-1 to stimulate IgM and IgG production suggest that Eta-1 may play a role in the induction of autoimmune disease in these mice. The possible role of Eta-1 in the induction or maintenance of lupus-like disease in other murine models of lupus or in patients with lupus has not as yet been reported.

Other B cell stimulatory cytokines

Several laboratories have reported that T cells from patients with lupus secrete increased amounts of an uncharacterized B cell growth factor(s) (BCGF) and a B cell differentiation factor(s) (BCDF) [70, 108, 132]. The finding of increased BCGF production, however, has not been universally confirmed [54, 70, 121]. This discrepancy may be secondary to increased in vitro consumption of BCGF by lupus B cells [121]. B cells from lupus patients also secrete B cell stimulatory cytokines [126, 171]. The B cell stimulatory factors spontaneously secreted by lupus B cells possess IL-1, IL-4 and IL-6 activity [171].

T cells from MRL/lpr and B6/lpr mice spontaneous produce high levels of an uncharacterized BCDF that induces IgM and IgG production by LPS-activated B cells [132, 177]. Increased BCDF production is apparent in MRL/lpr mice as early as 1 week of age and increases with age and the appearance of lymphoproliferation [132]. Serum from young NZB mice contains increased amounts of a 66-kDa factor (NZB-SF), which is produced by spleen cells and enhances the proliferation and differentiation of pre-B cells in bone marrow [83].

B cells from patients with lupus hyperrespond in the absence of other in vitro stimulation to a purified 50-kDa BCGF [36] and to recombinant 12-kDa BCGF [50].

Cytokines in lupus – a synthesis

A long-standing debate has been whether B cell hyperactivity and autoantibody production in lupus result from too much T cell help or not enough T cell-mediated suppression. Recent advances in our understanding of cytokine regulation of immune responses have refined our concepts of help and suppression, such that the question now becomes whether B cell hyperactivity in lupus results from excessive production of B cell stimulatory cytokines, from a lack of inhibitory cytokines, or both. An excess of B cell stimulatory cytokines would act to drive antibody production by B cells, including autoreactive B cells, that have bound relevant antigens to their antigen receptors. The lack of inhibitory cytokines, such as IFN-γ, would be important because of their ability to inhibit Th cell production of B cell stimulatory cytokines (e.g., IL-4) and/or to down-regulate the response of B cells to stimulatory cytokines, such as IL-4.

Murine models of spontaneous lupus and models of induced lupus, such as the parent-into-F_1 ($P \rightarrow F_1$) model of GVHD, have been useful in elucidating the importance of cytokines and cell-cell interactions in the pathogenesis of lupus. In the ($P \rightarrow F_1$) GVHD model, depending on the parent and F_1 strain combinations used, mice develop either an acute GVHD, with T cell activation patterns similar to those reported in allograft rejection, or a chronic, lupus-like GVHD, with anti-DNA antibody production and deposition of immune complexes in skin and glomeruli [58, 194]. Because mice are immunologically normal prior to the induction of GVHD, it is possible to determine the sequence of events with respect to cytokines production by which normal mice develop autoimmunity. By comparing results obtained in chronic GVHD mice to those obtained in acute GVHD mice, events that are specific for the induction of humoral autoimmunity can be more clearly delineated.

Although acute and chronic GVHD are clearly distinct entities by 2 weeks of disease, they share several features early on. Initially, in both forms of GVHD, donor $CD4^+$ T cells become activated in response to allogeneic MHC class II molecules on the F_1 host cells [58, 191], which results in a burst of increased IL-2 production by the donor cells during days 1–3 of disease [53, 189]. Subsequently, beginning at approximately days 2–4 [53, 197], increased donor T cell production of B cell stimulatory cytokines is noted, resulting in B cell activation (MHC class II antigen up-regulation) and autoantibody secretion in both forms of GVHD [193]. At 1 week of disease, acute and chronic GVHD begin to diverge. In acute GVHD. donor T cells produce increased amounts of IFN-γ and IL-2, cytokines important in CMI and CTL generation, and reduced amounts of IL-4, IL-10 and IL-6 ([195] and Rus and Via, unpublished observations). As a result, donor $CD8^+$ T cells become activated and develop into mature CTL specific for host MHC class I antigens [194]. Host lymphocytes, including autoantibody-secreting B cells, are eliminated and the profound immunodeficiency that characterizes acute GVHD ensues.

In contrast, chronic GVHD mice do not exhibit the increased production of IFN-γ or IL-2 that is typical of acute GVHD ([37, 195] and Rus and Via, unpublished observations). However, the increased production of B cell stimulatory cytokines (IL-4, IL-10 and possibly IL-6), observed during the 1st week of GVHD, continues in chronic GVHD mice [37, 53, 187]. Due to a reduced number of anti-host precursor CTL in the donor inoculum, significant numbers of donor anti-host CTL do not develop and host MHC class I-bearing cells are not eliminated [191, 194]. Instead, only donor $CD4^+$, allogeneic MHC class II ($H\text{-}2^b$)-reactive, T cells appear to be activated, resulting in the delivery of help to host allogeneic MHC class II-bearing B cells, including autoreactive B cells [114], with the subsequent production of autoantibodies and the development of a lupus-like disease. Increasing data suggest that similar alterations in cytokine production occur in several murine models that spontaneously develop lupus, especially PN mice, and in humans with lupus (see Table 1).

In the $P \rightarrow F_1$ model of GVHD, Via et al. ([190] and unpublished observations) have recently observed that acute and chronic GVHD outcomes can be altered by manipulation of cytokines in vivo. Blocking the early increase in donor T cell IL-2 production with anti-IL-2 mAb treatment in vivo inhibits the development of donor $CD8^+$ anti-host CTL and converts acute GVHD to chronic, autoimmune GVHD [190]. Conversely, chronic GVHD can be converted to acute GVHD if IL-12, a cytokine that promotes IFN-γ production and CTL development [148], is given at disease initiation ([196] and Via et al., J Immunol, in press). These observations indicate that lupus-like disease can result in a setting where the generation of a CTL response to a cell surface antigen (allogeneic MHC molecules in the case of GVHD) is prevented and the secretion of B cell stimulatory cytokines is enhanced, leading to heightened antibody-mediated responses. Conversely, enhancement of CTL and IFN-γ production in this setting blocks lupus- like disease by the elimination of activated autoreactive B cells.

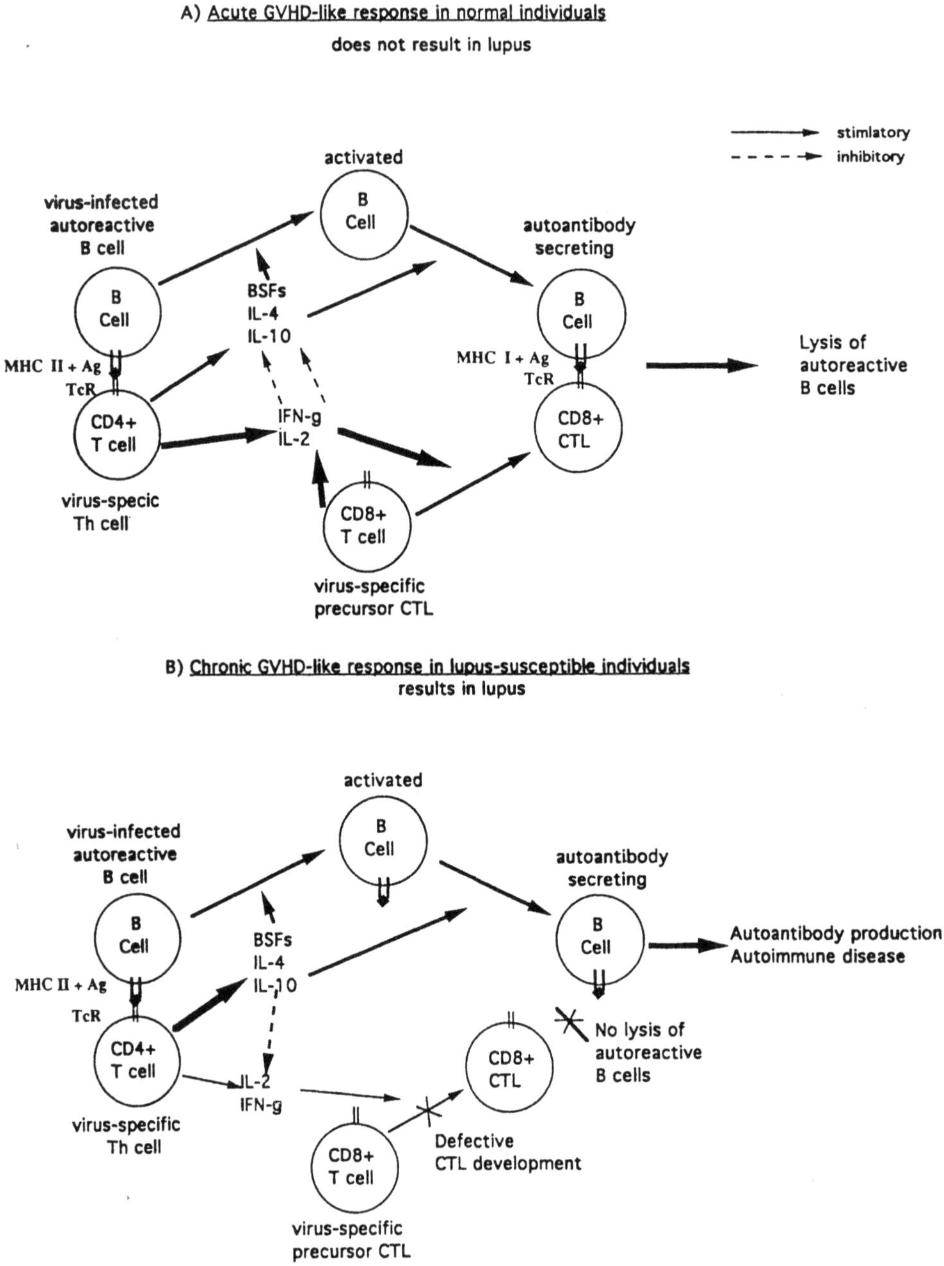

Fig. 1A,B. Autoimmunity resulting from immune response to a B cell tropic virus

These data suggest several possible models which may explain the immunopathogenesis of lupus. In the P $\rightarrow$ F_1 model of GVHD, acute GVHD serves as a model for an immune response that does not result in lupus and chronic GVHD models an immune response to the same antigens that results in lupus (Fig. 1). We postulate that in human and murine lupus, a B cell tropic virus may infect B cells in a non-clonally

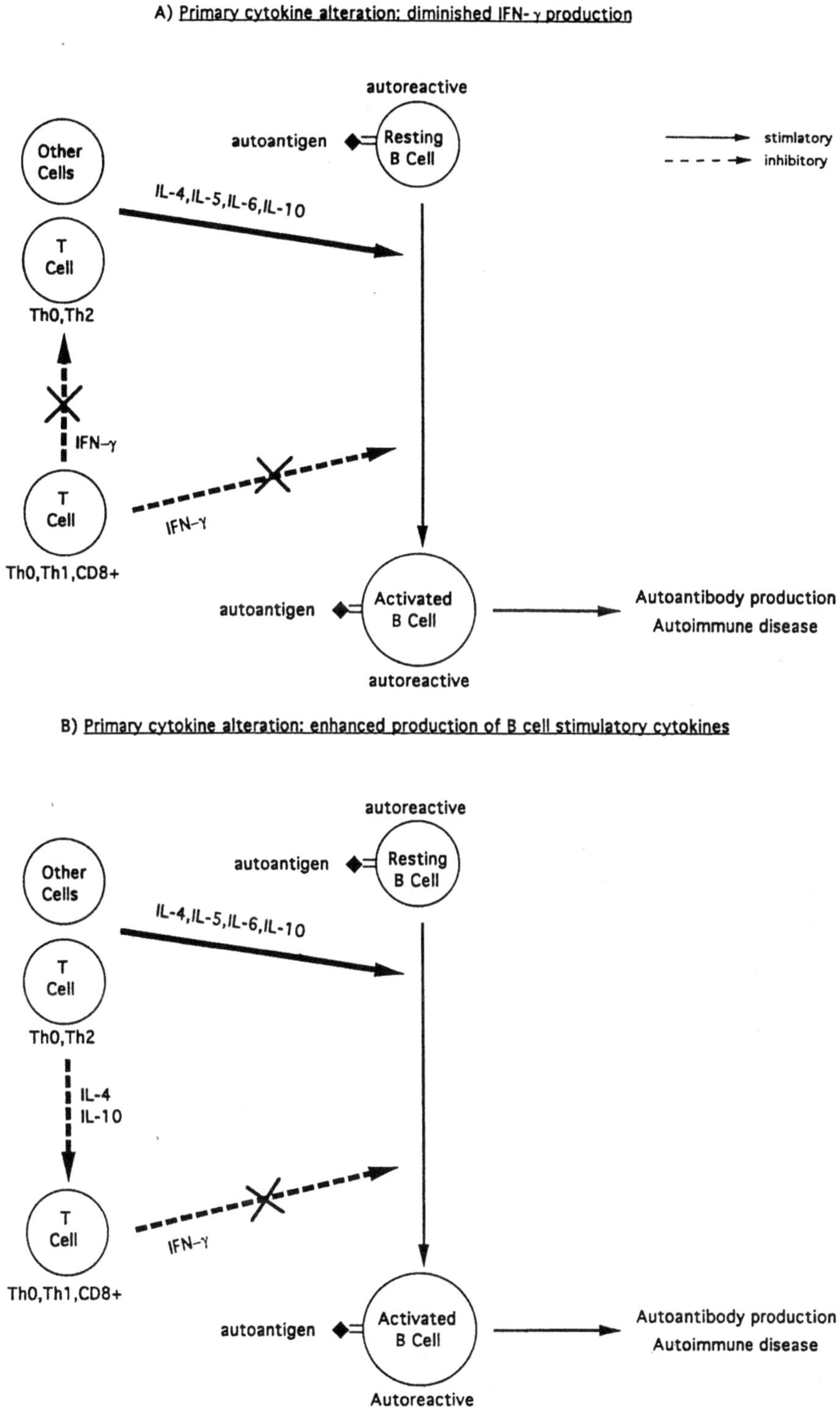

Fig. 2A,B. Autoimmunity resulting from a primary alteration in cytokine production

distributed fashion, which results in activation of virus-specific CD4⁺ T cells and the production of both T cell and B cell stimulatory cytokines. B cells become polyclonally activated and autoreactive B cells which bind relevant autoantigen secrete autoantibodies. In normal individuals (acute GVHD-like responses; Fig. 1A). the development of virus-specific CTL terminates autoantibody production by eliminating virus-infected cells, including autoantibody-secreting B cells. In addition, the continued production of IFN-γ may down-regulate the production of B cell stimulatory cytokines, such as IL-4. In patients who are genetically susceptible to lupus (chronic GVHD-like responses; Fig. 1B), we postulate that lupus may result when the development of virus-specific CTL is defective, either due to reduced numbers of precursor CTL or defective production of IL-2/IFN-γ, which prevents effective CTL maturation. Lack of virus elimination by CTL allows continued presentation of antigen by B cells to virus-specific T helper cells. This results in the provision of polyclonal help (signal 2), in the form of cognate help and/or in the form of IL-4, IL-6 and IL-10, to virus-infected B cells, including autoreactive B cells, which, in turn, leads to autoantibody production. Thus, some instances of lupus may occur when an IL-4/IL-10 response to a foreign antigen is favored over an IL-2/IFN-γ/CTL response.

Alternatively, lupus may develop as a result of an acquired or a genetic defect in T cell activation that results in diminished production of IL-2 and IFN-γ (Fig. 2A). The loss of IFN-γ production would lead to enhanced proliferation of Th2 cells, increased production of Th2 cell-derived B cell stimulatory cytokines, and hyperresponsiveness of B cells to those cytokines, especially IL-4. Autoreactive B cells that have bound autoantigen to their antigen receptors would be driven to differentiate into autoantibody-secreting plasma cells, with the subsequent development of humoral autoimmunity. Conversely, the primary abnormality in lupus may be at the level of excessive production of IL-4, IL-10 and other B cell stimulatory cytokines (Fig. 2B). The excessive production of these cytokines could result from an acquired or genetic defect or from chronic exposure to antigen(s) that preferentially stimulate an IL-4/IL-10 response. The enhanced production of IL-4, IL-10 and other B cell stimulatory cytokines would result in down-regulation of CMI, including IFN-γ production, and would provide signal 2 to autoreactive B cells that had bound autoantigens in vivo, leading to autoantibody production. Genetic or acquired abnormalities that result in a marked enhancement of IFN-γ production or chronic exposure to an antigen that preferentially stimulates high levels of IFN-γ production may also result in the induction of a lupus-like illness, mediated by the ability of IFN-γ to stimulate the production of IgG2a autoantibodies by autoreactive B cells that have bound autoantigens in vivo. The lupus-like illnesses that occurs in MRL/lpr mice and in some patients treated in vivo with IFN-α or IFN-γ may be examples of this pathological mechanism.

Conclusions

Increasing data suggest that human and murine lupus are heterogeneous diseases and that, in genetically susceptible individuals, lupus may be the final common pathway of a number of etiological agents and/or immunological processes. This review has discussed a number of cytokines which appear to be involved in lupus pathogenesis. The models that we have put forward illustrate several possible mechanisms which may lead to lupus. During the next several years, the exact role of these cytokine in the pathogenesis of lupus should become more fully elucidated. Hopefully, this knowledge will provide the framework for newer, highly specific immunotherapeutic approaches to the treatment of this fascinating, complex, and potentially devastating disease.

Acknowledgement. The authors thank Cathy Storrer and Phuong Nguyen for excellent technical assistance and Shirley Harrington for superb secretarial help. This work was supported by NIH grants AI 27885 (B.S.H.) and AI 33882 (C.S.V.), V.A. Merit Review grants (B.S.H. and C.V.S.), research grants from the Maryland Chapters of the Arthritis Foundation and Lupus Foundation (C.S.V.), a V.A. Research Associate Career Development Award (C.S.V.) and research fellowship grant support from the Maryland Chapter of the Arthritis Foundation (V.R. and L. daS.).

References

1. Aarden LA, De Groot ER, Schaap OL, Lansdorp PM (1987) Production of hybridoma growth factor by human monocytes. Eur J Immunol 17:1411
2. Akard LP, Hoffman R, Elias L, Saiers JH (1994) Alpha-interferon and immune hemolytic anemia. Ann Intern Med 105:306
3. Al-Janadi M, Al-Balia S, Al-Dalaan A, Raziuddidn S (1993) Cytokines profile in systemic lupus erythematosus, rheumatoid arthritis, and other rheumatic disease. J Clin Immunol 13:58
4. Alarcon-Riquelme ME, Moller G, Fernandez C (1991) The effects of interleukin 4 and 5 on the differentiation of B cells from (NZB x NZW)F_1 mice. Scand J Immunol 33:119
5. Alarcon-Riquelme ME, Moller G, Fernandez C (1992) Age-dependent responsiveness to interleukin-6 in B lymphocytes from a systemic lupus erythematosus-prone (NZB X NZW)F_1 hybrid. Clin Immunol Immunopathol 62:264
6. Alarcon-Riquelme ME, Moller G, Fernandez C (1993) Macrophage depletion decreases IgG anti-DNA in cultures from (NZB X NZW)F_1 spleen cells by eliminating the main source of IL-6. Clin Exp Immunol 91:220
7. Alcocer-Varela J. Alarcon-Segovia D (1982) Decreased production of and response to interleukin-2 by cultured lymphocytes from patients with systemic lupus erythematosus. J Clin Invest 69:1388
8. Alcocer-Varela J, Laffon A, Alarcon-Segovia D (1983) Defective monocyte production of, and T lymphocyte response to, interleukin-1 in the peripheral blood of patients with systemic lupus erythematosus. Clin Exp Immunol 54:125
9. Alcocer-Varela J, Aleman-Hoey D, Alarcon-Segovia D (1992) Interleukin-1 and interleukin-6 activities are increased in the cerbrospinal fluid of patienta with CNS lupus erythematosus and correlate with local late T-cell activation markers. Lupus 1:111
10. Allen RD, Staley TA, Sidman CL (1993) Differential cytokine expression in acute and chronic murine graft-versus-host disease. Eur J Immunol 23:333
11. Altman A, Theofilipoulos AN, Weiner R, Katz DH, Dixon FJ (1981) Analysis of T cell function in autoimmune murine strains: defects in production of and responsiveness to interleukin 2. J Exp Med 154:791
12. Andreu-Sanchez JL, Moreno de Alboran I, Marcos MAR, Sanchez-Movilla A, Marinez-A C, Kroemer G (1991) Interleukin 2 abrogates the nonresponsive state of T cell expressing a forbidden T cell receptor repertoire and induces autoimmune disease in neonatally thymectomized mice. J Exp Med 173:1323
13. Andrus L, Prowse SJ, Lafferty KL (1981) Interleukin 2 production by both $Ly2^+$ and $Ly2^-$ T-cell subsets. Scand J Immunol 13:297
14. Aotosuka S, Nakamura K, Nakano T, Kawakami M, Goto M, Okawa-Takatsuji M, Kinoshita M, Yokohari R (1991) Production of intracellular and extracellular interleukin-1β and interleukin-1β by peripheral blood monocytes from patients with connective tissue diseases. Ann Rheum Dis 50:27
15. Balderas RS, Josimovic-Alasevic O, Diamantatein T, Dixon FJ, Theofilopoulos AN (1987) Elevated titers of cell-free interleukin 2 receptors in serum of lupus mice. J Immunol 139:1496
16. Blank M, Sredni B, Mozes E, Shoenfeid Y (1990) The effect of the immunomodulator agent AS101 on interleukin-2 production in systemic lupus erythematosus (SLE) induced in mice by a pathogenic anti-DNA antibody. Clin Exp Immunol 79:443

17. Bocchieri MH, Knittweis L, Seaton DS (1984) Cytokine production by NZB, C58, and NZBXC58 recombinant inbred mice. Cell Immunol 88:453
18. Bond MW, Shrader B, Mosmann TR, Coffman RL (1987) A mouse T cell product that preferentially enhances IgA production II. Physicochemical characterization. J Immunol 139:3691
19. Boom WH, Liano D, Abbas AK (1988) Heterogeneity of helper/inducer T lymphocytes. II Effects of interleukin 4- and interleukin 2-producing T cell clones on resting B lymphocytes. J Exp Med 167:1350
20. Boswell JM, Yui MA, Burt DW, Kelley VE (1988) Increased tumor necrosis factor and IL-1β gene expression in the kidneys of mice with lupus nephritis. J Immunol 141:3050
21. Boswell JM, Yui MA, Endres S, Burt DW, Kelley VE (1988) Novel and enhanced IL-1 gene expression in autoimmune mice with lupus. J Immunol 141:118
22. Bottazzo GF, Pujoi-Borrell R, Hanafusa T, Feldmann M (1983) Role of aberrant HLA-DR expression and antigen presentation in induction of endocrine autoimmunity. Lancet II:1115
23. Brennan DC, Yui MA, Wuthrich RP, Kelley VE (1989) Tumor necrosis factor and IL-1 in New Zealand Black/White mice. Enchanced gene expression and acceleration of renal injury. J Immunol 143:3470
24. Budd RC, Schumacher JH, Winslow G, Mosmann TR (1991) Elevated production of interferon-γ and interleukin-4 by mature T cells from autoimmune lpr mice correlates with Pgp-1 (CD44) expression. Eur J Immunol 21:1081
25. Burman P, Totterman TH, Oberg K, Karisson FA (1986) Thyroid autoimmunity in patients on long term therapy with leukocyte-derived interferon. J Clin Endocrinol Metab 63:1086
26. Campen DH, Horwitz DA, Quishmorio FPJr, Ehresmann GR, Martin WJ (1988) Serum levels of interleukin-2 receptor and activity of rheumatic diseases characterized by immune system activation. Arthritis Rheum 31:1358
27. Coffman RL, Shrader B, Carty J, Mosmann TR, Bond MW (1987) A mouse T cell product that preferentially enhances IgA production: I. Biologic characterization. J Immunol 139:3685
28. Cohen PL, Rapoport RG, Eisenberg RA, Finkelman FD (1989) Effects of anti-IFN-γ on MRL/MP-*lpr/lpr* mice. Arthritis Rheum 32:S52
29. Dauphinee MJ, Kipper SB, Wofsy D, Talai N (1981) Interleukin 2 deficiency is a common feature of autoimmune mice. J Immunol 127:2483
30. Davidson WF, Roths JB, Holmes KL, Rudikoff E, Morse HC III (1984) Dissociation of severe lupus-like disease from polyclonal B cell activation and IL 2 deficiency in C3H-*lpr/lpr* mice. J Immunol 133:1048
31. Davidson WF, Catkins C, Hugin A, Giese T, Holmes KL (1991) Cytokines secretion by C3H-*lpr* and -*gld* T cells: Hypersecretion of IFN-γ and tumor necrosis factor-α by stimulated $CD4^+$ T cells. J Immunol 146:4138
32. Davignon J-L, Cohen PL, Eisenberg RA (1990) Immunological effects of recombinant interferon-gamma in vivo in normal mice: failure to induce autoantibodies. Int J Immunopharmacol 12:691
33. Davignon J-L, Kimoto M, Kindier V, De Kossodo S, Vassalli P, lzui S (1988) Selective production of interleukin 3 (IL3) and granuiocyte-macrophaqe colony-stimulating factor (GM-CSF)., in vitro by murine $L3T4^+$ T cells: lack of spontaneous IL-3 and GM-CSF production by $Ly\text{-}2^-/L3T4^-$ *lpr* subset. Eur J Immunol 18:1367
34. de Faucal P, Godard A, Peyrat MA, Moreau JF, Soulillou JP (1984) Impaired IL-2 production by lymphocytes of patients with systemic lupus erythrmatosus. Ann Immunol 135 D:161
35. Deguchi Y, Kishimoto S (1991) Tumour necrosis factor/cachectin plays a key role in autoimmune pulmonary inflammation in lupus-prone mice. Clin Exp Immunol 85:392
36. Delfraissy J-F, Wallon C, Vazquez A, Dugas B, Dormont J, Galanaud P (1986) B cell hyperacitivity in systemic lupus erythematosus: selectively enhanced responsiveness to a high molecular weight B cell growth factor. Eur J Immunol 16:1251
37. De Wit D, Van Mechelen M, Zanin C, Doutrelepont J, M, Velu T, Gerard C, Abramowicz D, Scheerlinck J-P, De Baetselier P, Urbain J, Leo O, Goldman M, Moser M (1993) Preferential activation of Th2 cells in chronic graft-versus-host reaction. J Immunol 150:361
38. Djeu JY, Heinbaugh JA, Holden HT, Herberman RB (1979) Augmentation of mouse natural killer cell activity by interferon and interferon inducers. J Immunol 122:175
39. Donnelly RP, Levine J, Hartwell DW, Frendi G, Fenton MJ, Beller DI (1990) Aberrant regulation of IL-1 expression in macrophages from young autoimmune-prone mice. J Immunol 145:3231

40. Doutrelepont JM, Moser M, Leo O, Abramowicz D, Vanderhaegen ML, Urbain J, Goldman M (1991) Hyper IgE in stimulatory graft-versus-host disease: role of interleukin-4. Clin Exp Immunol 83:133
41. Draeger AM, Van Der Brink HG, Aarden LA (1986) T cell function in systemic lupus erythematosus: normal production of and responsiveness to interleukin 2. Clin Exp Immunol 64:80
42. Dueymers M, Barrier J, Besancenot JF, Cledes J, Conri C, Dien G, Drosos AA, Dueymes JM, Galanaud P, Gribois B, Guillevin L, Hatron PY, lsenberg DA, Jorgensen C, Jouguan J, Lamour A, Le Gaff P, Longy.-Boursier M, Maron R, Massot C, Meyer O, Mottier D, Mountsopouios HM, Philippe P, Piette JC, Sany J, Series C, Shoenfeld Y, Youinou P (1993) Relationship of interleukin-4 to isotypic distribution of anti-double-stranded DNA antibodies in systemic lupus erythematosus. Int Arch Allergy Immunol 101:408
43. Ehrenstein MR, McSweeney E, Swana M, Worman CP, Goldstone AH, Isenberg DA (1993) Appearance of anti-DNA antibodies in patients treated with interferon-α. Arthritis Rheum 36:279
44. Elie R, Lapp WS (1976) Graft-versus-host induced immunosuppression: decreased T cell helper function in vitro. Cell Immunol 21:31
45. Elkins WL (1971) Cellular immunology and the pathogenesis of graft-versus-host reactions. Prog Allergy 15:78
46. Emmendorffer A, Muller M, Wedekind D, Hartung K, Lohmann-Matthes M-L (1993) Expansion of the liver-associated macrophage system in systemic lupus erythematosus-prone NZB/W mice. J Leukoc Biol 53:294
47. Engleman EG, Sonnenfeld G, Dauphinee M, Greenspan JS, Talai N, McDevitt HO, Merigan TC (1981) Treatment of NZB/NZW F_1 hybrid mice with *Mycobacterium bovis* BCG or type 11 interferon preparations accelerates autoimmune disease. Arthritis Rheum 24:1396
48. Enk AH, Katz SI (1992) Identification and induction of keratinocyte-derived IL-10. J Immunol 149:92
49. Farrar JJ, Benjamin WR, Hilfiker ML, Howard M, Fasrrar WL, Fuller-Farrar J (1982) The biochemistry, biology, and role of interleukin 2 in the induction of cytotoxic T cell and antibody-forming B cell response. Immunol Rev 63:129
50. Flescher E, Fossum D, Ballester A, Maizel A, Sharma S, Talai N (1990) Characterization of B cell, growth in systemic lupus erythematosus. Effects of recombinant 12-kDa B cell growth factor, interleukin-4 and transforming growth factor-β. Eur J Immunol 20:2425
51. Fultz MJ, Barber SA, Dieffenbach CW, Vogel SN (1993) Induction of IFN-γ in macrophages by lipopolysaccharide. Int Immunol 5:1383
52. Gajewski TF, Fitch FW (1988) Anti-proliferative effects of IFN-γ in immune regulation. 1. IFN-γ inhibits the proliferation of Th2 but not Th1 murine helper T lymphocytes clones. J Immunol 140:4245
53. Garlisi CG, Pennline KJ, Smith SR, Siegel MI, Umland SP (1993) Cytokine gene expression in mice undergoing chronic graft-versus-host disease. Mol Immunol 30:699
54. Gaspar ML, Alvarez-Mon M, Gutierrez C (1988) The B-cell activation pathways in human systemic lupus erythematosus: Imbalanced in vitro production of lymphokines and association with serum analytical findings. J Clin Immunol 8:266
55. Gillis S, Mochizuki DY, Conion PJ, Hefeneider SH, Ramthun CA, Gillis AE, Frank MB, Henney CS, Watson JD (1982) Molecular characterization of interleukin 2. Immunol Rev 63:167
56. Gillis S, Gillis AE, Henney CS (1983) Monocional antibody directed against interleukin 2. 1. Inhibition of T lymophocyte mitogenesis and the in vitro differentiation of alloreactive cytolytic T cells. J Exp Med 154:983
57. Gisslinger H, Gilly B, Woloszuczuk W, Mayr WR, Havelec L, Linkesch W (1992) Thyroid autoimmunity and hypothyroidism during long-term treatment with recombinant interferon-alpha. Clin Exp Immunol 90:363
58. Gleichmann E, Pals ST, Rolink AG, Radaszkiewicz T, Gleichmann H (1984) Graft-vs-host reactions: clues to the etiology of a spectrum of immunological disease. Immunol Today 5:324
59. Gordon C, Ranges GE, Greenspan JS, Wofsy D (1989) Chronic therapy with recombinant tumor necrosis factor-α in autoimmune NZB/NZWF_1 mice. Clin Immunol Immunopathol 52:421
60. Gordon C, Richards N, Howie AJ, Richardson K, Michael J, Adu D, Emery P (1991) Urinary IL-6: a marker for mesangial proliferation glomerulonephritis? Clin Exp Immunol 6:145
61. Gutierrez-Ramos JC, Pezzi L, Palacios R, Martinez-A C (1989) Expression of the p75 interleukin 2-binding protein on $CD3^{+}4^{-}8^{-}$ Tac^{-} cells from autoimmune MR/MP-*lpr/lpr* mice. Eur J Immunol 19:201, 63.

62. Gutierrez-Ramos JC, Andreu JL, Revilla Y, Vincela E, Martinez-A C (1990) Recovery from autoimmunity of MRL/lpr mice after infection with an interleukin-2/vaccinia recombinant virus. Nature 346:271.
63. Handwerger B, Wasson CS, Movafagh F, Reichlin M (1994) Palmerston North mice produce antibodies to U_1RNP and Sm particles. Clin Res 42:315
64. Handwerger BS, Svetic A, Gause WC (1994) Lupus-like disease in Palmerston North (PN) mice is associated with loss of "naive" $CD4^+$ T cells and excessive expression of B cell stimulatory cytokines. Clin Res 42:138
65. Hang L, Theofilopoulos AN, Balderas RS, Francis SJ, Dixon FJ (1984) The effect of thymectomy on lupus-prone mice. J Immunol 132:1809
66. Hefeneider SH, Conion PJ, Henney CS, Gillis S (1983) In vivo interleukin 2 administration augments the generation of alloreactive cytolytic T lymphocytes and resident natural killer cells. J Immunol 130:222
67. Heremans H, Billiau A, Colombatti A, Hllgers J, De Somer P (1978) Interferon treatment of NZB mice: accelerated progression of autoimmune disease. Infect Immun 21:925
68. Herron LR, Coffman RL, Bond MW, Kotzin BL (1988) Increased autoantibody production by NZB/NZW B cells in response to IL-5. J Immunol 141:842
69. Hirohata S, Miyamoto T (1990) Elevated levels of interleukin-6 in cerbrospinal fluid from patients with systemic lupus erythematosus and central nervous system involvement. Arthritis Rheum 33:644
70. Hirose T, Hara M, Kitani A, Norioks K, Kawagoe M, Nakamura H (1985) Abnormal production of and response to B-cell growth factor and B-cell differentiation factor in patients with sytemic lupus erythematosus. Scand J Immunol 21:141
71. Hishikawa T, Tokano Y, Sekigawa I, Ando S, Takasaki Y, Hashimoto Y, Hirose H, Okumura K, Abe M, Shirai T (1994) HLA-DP^+ T cells and deficient interleukin-2 production in patients with systemic lupus erythematosus. Clin Immunol Immunopathol 55:285
72. Hom JT, Cote H, Bendele AM (1990) Interleukin 1 enchances the development of spontaneous arthritis in MRL/*lpr* mice. Clin Immunol Immunopathol 55:109
73. Horn Y, Iwano M, Hirata E, Shiiki H, Fujii Y, Doni K, Ishikawa H (1993) Role of interleukin-6 in the progressive of mesangial proliferative glomerulonephritis. Kidney Int 43:S71
74. Howard JG, Woodruff MFA (1961) Effects of the graft-versus-host reaction on the immunological responsiveness of the mouse. Proc R Soc Lond Biol Sci 154:532
75. Huang YP, Miescher PA, Zubler RH (1986) The interleukin 2 secretion defect in vitro systemic lupus erythematosus is reversible in rested cultured T cells. J Immunol 137:3515
76. Huang Y-P, Perrin LH, Miescher PA, Zubler RH (1988) Correlation of T and B cell activaties in vitro and serum IL-2 levels in systemic lupus erythematosus. J Immunol 141:827
77. Ishida H, Kumagai S, Umehara H, Sano H, Tagaya Y, Yodoi J, Imura H (1987) Impaired expression of high affinity interleukin 2 receptor on activated lymphocytes from patients with systemic lupus erythematosus. J Immunol 139:1070
78. Ishida H, Muchamuel T, Sakaguchi S, Andrade S, Menon S, Howard M (1994) Continuous administration of anti-interleukin 10 antibodies delays onset of autoimmunity in NZB/W F_1 mice. J Exp Med 179:305
79. Jacob CO, McDevitt HO (1988) Tumour necrosis factor-α in murine autoimmune 'lupus' nephritis. Nature 331:356
80. Jacob CO, van der Meide PH, McDevitt HO (1987) In vivo treatment of (NZB X NZW) F_1 lupus-like nephritis with monoclonal antibody to γ-interferon. J Exp Med 166:798
81. Jira M, Strejcek J, Zavadil Z, Antosova E, Rejholec V (1990) Interleukin-2 activated cells from peripheral blood of patients with systemic lupus erythematosus. Z Rheumatol 49:30
82. Jirik FR, Podor TJ, Hirano, T, Kishimoto T, Loskutoff DJ, Carson DA, Lotz M (1989) Bacterial lipopolysaccharide and inflammatory mediators augment IL-6 secretion by human endothelial cells. J Immunol 142:144
83. Jyonouchi H, Voss RM, Good RA (1991) NZB serum factor (NZB-SF): B cell precursor cell maturation factor identified in murine lupus. Cell Immunol 132:223
84. Kelley VE, Gaulton GN, Hattori M, Ikegami H, Eisenbarth G, Strom TB (1988) Anti-interleukin 2 receptor antibody suppresses murine diabetic insulitis and lupus nephritis. J Immunol 140:59
85. Kitani A, Hara M, Hirose T, Norioka K, Hirose W, Kawagoe M, Nakamura H (1986) Kinetic analysis of 1a expression on T cells in patients with systemic lupus erythematosus. J Clin Lab Immunol 19:59

86. Kitani A, Hara M, Hirose T, Norioka K, Harigai M, Hirose W, Suzuki K, Kawakami M, Kawagoe M, Nakamura H (1989) Heterogeneity of B cell responsiveness to interleukin 4, interleukin 6 and low molecular weight B cell growth factor in discrete stages of B cell activation in patients with systemic lupus erythematosus. Clin Exp Immunol 77:31
87. Kitani A, Hara M, Hirose T, Harigai M, Suzuki K, Kawakami M, Kawaguchi Y, Hidaka T, Kawagoe M, Nakakmura H (1992) Autostimulatory effects of IL-6 on excessive B cell differentiation in patients with systemic lupus erythematosus: analysis of IL-6 production and IL-6R expression. Clin Exp Immunol 88:75
88. Klashman DJ, Martin RA, Martinez-Maza O, Stevens RH (1991) In vitro regulation of B cell differentiation by interleukin-6 and soluble CD23 in systemic lupus erythematosus B cell subpopulations and antigen-induced normal B cells. Arthritis Rheum 34:276
89. Klinman DM (1990) IgG1 and IgG2a production by autoimmune B cells treated in vitro with IL-4 and IFN-γ. J Immunol 144:2529
90. Kobayashi I, Matsuda T, Saito T, Yasukawa K, Kikutani H, Hirano T, Taga T, Kishimoto T (1992) Abnormal distribution of IL-6 receptor in aged MRL/lpr mice: elevated expression on B cell and absence on $CD4^+$ cells. Int Immunol 4:1407
91. Kuribayashi K, Gillis S, Kern DE, Henny CH (1981) Murine NK cell cultures: effects of interleukin-2 and interferon on cell growth and cytotoxic reactivity. J Immunol 126:2321
92. Lakhanpal S, Handwerger BS (1987) Interleukin 2 receptors and responsiveness to recombinant human interluekin 2 in patients with systemic lupus erythematosus. Mayo Clin Proc 62:3
93. Lampe MA, Patarca R, Iregui MV, Cantor H (1991) Polyclonal B cell activation by the Eta-l cytokine and the development of systemic autoimmune disease. J Immunol 147:2902
94. Lehmann KR, Kotzin BL, Portanova JP, Santoro TJ (1986) Interleukin 2 is a proliferative signal for B cells from autoimmune mice. Eur J Immunol 16:1105
95. Levine J, Hartwell D, Beller DI (1991) Imbalanced cytokine production by macrophages from autoimmune-prone mice. Immunol Lett 30:183
96. Levine JS, Pugh BJ, Hartwell D, Fitzpatrick JM, Marshak-Rothstein A, Beller DI (1993) Interleukin-1 dysregulation in an intrinsic defect in macrophages from MRL autoimmune-prone mice. Eur J Immunol 23:2951
97. Linker-Israeli M (1992) Cytokine abnormalities in human lupus. Clin Immunol Immunopathol 63:10
98. Linker-Israeli M, Bakke AC, Kitridou RC, Gendier S, Gillis S, Horwitz DA (1983) Defective production of interleukin 1 and interleukin 2 in patients with systemic lupus erythematosus (SLE). J Immunol 130:2651
99. Linker-Israeli M, Bakke AC, Quismorio FP Jr Horwitz DA (1985) Correction of interleukin-2 production in patients with systemic lupus erythematosus by removal of spontaneously activated suppressor cells. J Clin Invest 75:762
100. Linker-Israeli M, Deans RJ, Wallace DJ, Prehn J, Ozeri-Chen T, Klinenberg JR (1991) Elevated levels of endogenous IL-6 in systemic lupus erythematosus: a putative role in pathogenesis. J Immunol 147:117
101. Linker-Israeli M, Gray JD, Quismorio FP Jr, Horwitz DA (1994) Characterization of lymphocytes that suppress IL-2 production in systemic lupus erythematosus. Clin Exp Immunol 73:236
102. Lu CY, Unanue ER (1982) Spontaneous T-cell lymphokine production and enhanced macrophage la expression and tumoricidal activity in MRL-*lpr* mice. Clin Immunol Immunopathol 25:213
103. MacNeil D, Krystal G, Fairhurst M, Waterfield JD (1986) Correction of defective IL-3 responses to T lymphocytes from autoimmune mice. J Immunol 137:3464
104. Magilavy DB, Rothstein JL (1988) Spontaneous production of tumor necrosis factor α by Kupffer cells of MRL/lpr mice. J Exp Med 168:789
105. Magilavy DB, Foys KM, Gajewski TF (1992) Liver of MRL/lpr mice contain interleukin-4-producing lymphocytes and accessory cells that support the proliferation of Th2 helper T lymphocytes clones. Eur J Immunol 22:2359
106. Malek TR, Ashwell JD (1985) Interleukin-2 upregulates expression of its receptor on a T cell clone. J Exp Med 161:1575
107. Manolios N, Schrieber L, Nelson M, Geczy CL (1989) Enhanced interferon-gamma (IFN) production by lymph node cells from autoimmune (MRL/l, MRL/n) mice. Clin Exp Immunol 76:599
108. Martinez-Cordero E, Alcocer-Varela J, Alarcon-Segovia D (1986) Stimulating and differentiation factors for human B lymphocyte in systemic lupus erythematosus. Clin Exp Immunol 65:598

109. McLaughlin P, Talpaz M, Quesada JR, Saleem A, Barlogie B, Gutterman JU (1985) Immune thrombodcytopenia following α-interferon therapy in patient with cancer. J Am Med Assoc 254:1353
110. Metsarinne KP, Nordstrom DC, Konttinen YT, Teppo AM, Fyhrquist FY (1992) Plasma interleukin-6 and renin substrate in reactive arthritis, rheumatoid arthritis, and systemic lupus erythematosus. Rheumatol Int 12:93
111. Mihara M, Fukui H, Koishihara Y, Saito M, Ohsugi Y (1990) Immunologic abnormality in NZB/W Fl mice. Thymus-independent expansion of B cells responding to Interleukin-6. Clin Exp Immunol 82:533
112. Minoda M, Ohno M, Hamada K, Tomioka Y, Funauchi M, Horiuchi A (1991) Interferon-γ inhibition of interleukin 4-induced hyperproliferation of resting B cell from NZB/NZW F_1 mice. J Clin Lab Immunol 35:57
113. Miyasaka N, Nakumura T, Russell IJ, Talai N (1984) Interleukin 2 deficiencies in rheumatoid arthritis and systemic lupus erythematosus.Clin Immunol Immunopathol 31:109
114. Morris SC, Cheek RL, Cohen PL, Eisenberg RA (1990) Autoantibodies in chronic graft versus host result from cognate T-B Interactions. J Exp Med 171:503
115. Mosmann TR, Coffman RL (1989) TH1 and TH2 cells: different patterns of lymphokine secretion lead to different functional properties. Annu Rev Immunol 7:145
116. Murakawa Y, Takada S, Ueda Y, Suzuki N, Hoshino T, Sakane T (1985) Characterization of T lymphocytes subpopulations responsible for deficient interleukin 2 activity in patients with systemic lupus erythematosus. J Immunol 134:187
117. Murray L, Martens C (1989) The abnormal T lymphocytes in *lpr* mice transcribe interferon-γ and tumor necrosis factor-α genes spontaneously in vivo. Eur J Immunol 19:563
118. Muzes G, Vien CV, Gonzalez-Cabello R, Feher J, Gergely P (1989) Defective production of Interleukin-1 and tumor necrosis factor-alpha by stimulated monocytes from patients with systemic lupus erythematosus. Acta Med Hung 46:245
119. Nagafuchi H, Suzuki N, Mizushima Y, Sakane T (1993) Constitutive expression of IL-6 receptors and their role in the excessice B cell function in patients with systemic lupus erythematosus. J Immunol 151:6525
120. O'Garra A, Chang R, Go N, Hastings R, Haughton G, Howard M (1992) Ly-1 B cells are the main source of B cell-derived interleukin-10. Eur J Immunol 22:711
121. Ogawa N, Itoh M, Goto Y (1992) Abnormal production of B cell growth factor in patients with systemic lupus erythematosus. Clin Exp Immunol 89:26
122. Paetkau V, Shaw J, Mills G, Caplan B (1980) Cellular origins and targets of costimulator (IL 2). Immunol Rev 51:157
123. Palacios R (1994) Spontaneous production of interleukin-3 by T lymphocytes from autoimmune MRL/Mp-*lpr/lpr* mice. Eur J Immunol 14:599
124. Patarca R, Freeman GJ, Singh RP, Wei F-Y, Durfee WT, Blattner F, Regnier DC, Kozak CA, Mock BA, Morse HC Jerrelis TR, Cantor H (1989) Structural and functional studies of the early T lymphocyte activation 1 (*eta-1*) gene: definition of a novel T cell-dependent response associated with genetic resistance to bacterial infection. J Exp Med 170:145
125. Patarca R, Wei F-Y, Singh P, Morasso MI, Cantor H (1990) Dysregulated expression of the T cell cytokine *Eta-1* in $CD4^-8^-$ lymphocytes during the development of murine autoimmune disease. J Exp Med 172:1177
126. Peiton BK, Denman AM (1987) Spontanous production of B cell growth factors by SLE lymphocytes. Clin Exp Immunol 67:159
127. Pelton BK, Hylton W, Denman AM (1992) Activation of IL-6 by UV irradiation of blood mononuclear cells from patients with sytemic lupus erythematosus. Clin Exp Immunol 89:251
128. Perl A, Gonzaler-Cabello R, Onody K, Bodom 1, Gergely P (1986) Independence of depressed lectin-dependent cell-mediated cytotoxicity from Interleukin-2 production. Clin Exp Immunol 65:286
129. Picket K, Hoffmann MK (1977) Suppressor T cells arising in mice undergoing a graft-versus-host response. J Immunol 118:653
130. Plaut M, Pierce JH, Watson CJ, Hanley-Hyde J, Nordan RP, Paul WE (1989) Mast cell lines produce lymphokines in response to cross-linkage of FcεRI or to calcium ionophores. Nature 339:64
131. Powrie F, Menon S, Coffman RL (1993) Interleukin-4 and interleukin-10 synergize to inhibit call-mediated immunity in vivo Eur J Immunol 23:3043

132. Prud'homme GJ, Park CL, Fieser TM, Kofler R, Dixon FJ, Theofilopoulos AN (1983) Identification of a B cell differentiation factor(s) spontaneously produced by proliferating T cells in murine lupus strains of the *lpr/lpr* genotype. J Exp Med 157:730
133. Rabin EM, Mond JJ, Ohara J, Paul W (1986) Interferon-γ inhibits the action of B cell stimulatory factor (BSF)-1 on resting B cells. J Immunol 137:1573
134. Raziuddin S, Danial HB, Kelley M (1988) OKT4$^+$ T cell abnormality in patients with active systemic lupus erythematosus: HLA-DR antigen expression. Clin Immunol Immunopathol 48:42
135. Raziuddin S, Ma N, Al-Wabel AA (1990) Increased circulating HLA-DR$^+$ CD4$^+$ T cells in systemic lupus erythematosus: alterations associated with prednisolone therapy. Scand J Immunol 31:139
136. Reem GH, Yeh NH, Urdal DL, Killian PL, Farrar JJ (1985) Induction and upregulation by interleukin 2 of high-affinity interleukin-2 receptor on thymocytes and T cells. Proc Nati Acad Sci USA 82:8663
137. Ronnblom LE, Alm GV, Oberg KE (1990) Possible induction of systemic lupus erythematosus by interferon-α treatment in patients with a malignant carcinoid tumor. J Immunol Methods 227:207
138. Ronnblom LE, Alm GV, Oberg KE (1991) Autoimmunity after alpha-Interferon therapy for malignant carcinoid tumor. Ann Intern Med 115:178
139. Rosenberg YJ, Nurse F, Begley CG (1989) IL-2 receptor expression in autoimmune MRl-*lpr/lpr* mice: The expanded L3T4$^-$, Lyt-2$^-$ population does not express p75 and cannot generate functional high-affinity IL-2 receptors. J Immunol 143:2216
140. Saiki O, Tanaka T, Kishimoto S (1990) Defective expression of p70/75 interleukin 2 receptor in T cells from patients with systemic lupus erythematosus: a possible defect in the process of increased Intracellular calcium leading to p70/75 expression. J Rheumatol 17:1303
141. Sakane T, Murakawa Y, Suzuki N, Ueda Y, Tsuchida T, Takada S, Yamauchi Y, Tsunematsu T (1989) Familial occurrence of impaired interleukin-2 activity and increased peripheral blood B cells actively secreting immunogiobulins in systemic lupus erythematisis. Am J Med 86:385
142. Santoro TJ, Benjamin WR, Oppenheim JJ, Steinberg AD (1983) The cellular basis for immune Interferon production in autoimmune MRL/-*lpr/lpr* mice. J Immunol 131:265
143. Santoro TJ, Luger TA, Raveche ES, Smolen JS, Oppeheim JJ, Steomberg JJ (1983) In vitro correction of the interleukin 2 defects of autoimmune mice. Eur J Immunol 13:601
144. Santoro TJ, Malek TR, Rosenberg YJ, Morse HC III, Steinberg AD (1984) Signals required for activation and growth of autoimmune T lymphocytes. J Mol Cell Immunol 1:347
145. Santoro TJ, Lehmann KR, Batt RA, Kotzin BL (1987) The role of L3T4$^+$ cells in the pathogenesis of lupus in *lpr*-bearing mice I. Defects in the production on interleukins 2 and 3. Eur J Immunol 17:1131
146. Santoro TJ, Portanova JP, Kotzin BL (1988) The contribution of L3T4$^+$ T cells to lymphoproliferation and autoantibody production in MRL-*lpr/lpr* mice. J Exp Med 167:1713
147. Schilling PJ, Kurzrock R, Kantarjian H, Gutterman JU, Talpaz M (1994) Development of systemic lupus erythematosus after interferon therapy for chronic myelogenous leukemia. Clin Res 42:1536
148. Scott P (1993) IL-12: initiation cytokine for cell-mediated immunity. Science 260:496
149. Seder RA, Boulay Y-L, Finkelman F, Barbier S, Ben-Sasson SZ, Le Gros G, Paul WE (1992) CD8$^+$ T cells can be primed in vitro to produce IL-4. J Immunol 148:1652
150. Semenzato G, Bambara LM, Biasi D, Frigo A, Vinante F, Zuppini B, Trentin L, Feruglio C, Chilosi M, Pizzoio G (1988) Increased serum levels of soluble interleukin-2 receptor in patients with systemie lupus erythematosus and rheumatoid arthritis. J Clin Invest 8:447
151. Shaw J, Caplan B, Paetkau V, Pilarski LM, Delovitch TL, McKenzie IFC (1980) Cellular origins of co-stimulator (IL-2) and its activity in cytotoxic T lymphocyte responses. J Immunol 124:2231
152. Shull MM, Ormsby I, Kier AB, Pawlowski S, Diebold RJ, Yin M, Alien R, Sidman C, Proetzel G, Calvin D, Annunziate N, Doetschman T (1992) Targeted disruption of the mouse transforming growth factor-βl gene results in multifocal inflammatory disease, Nature 359:693
153. Sibbitt WL Jr, Liker L, Spellman CW, Bankhurst AD (1983) Impaired natural killer cell function in systemic lupus erythematosus: Relationship to interleukin-2 production. Arthritis Rheum 26:1316
154. Sibbitt WL Jr, Kenny C, Spellman CW, Led KD, Bankhurst AD (1984) Lymphokines in autoimmunity: relationship between interleukin-2 and interferon-γ production in systemic lupus erythematosus. Clin Immunol Immunopathol 32:166
155. Sierakowski S, Kucharz EJ, Lightfoot RW, Goodwin JS (1989) Impaired T-cell activation in patients with systemic lupus erythematosus. J Clin Invest 9:469

156. Singh RP, Patarca R, Schwartz J, Singh P, Cantor H (1990) Definition of a specific interaction between the early T lymphocyte activation 1 (Eta-1) protein and murine macrophages in vitro and its effects upon macrophages in vivo. J Exp Med 171:1931
157. Snapper CM, Finkelman FD, Paul WE (1988) Differential regulation of IgGl and IgE synthesis by interleukin 4. J Exp Med 167:183
158. Snapper CM, Percher C, Paul WE (1988) IFN-γ stimulated IgG2a secretion by murine B cells stimulated with bacterial lipopolysaccharide. J Immunol 140:2121
159. Spronk PE, Ter Borg EJ, Limburg PC, Kallenberg CGM (1992) Plasma concentration of IL-6 in sytemic lupus erythematosus, an indicator of disease activity? Clin Exp Immunol 90:106
160. Steinberg AD, Roths JB, Murphy ED, Steinberg RT, Raveche ES (1980) Effects of thymectomy or andogen adminstration upon the autoimmune disease of MRL/MP-*lpr/lpr* mice. J Immunol 125:871
161. Steward MW, Hay FC (1976) Changes in immunoglobulin class and subclass of anti-DNA antibodies with increasing age in NZB/W F_1 hybrid mice. Clin Exp Immunol 26:363
162. Stolzenburg T, Binz H, Fontana A, Felder M, Wagenhaeuser F-J (1988) Impaired mitogen-induced interferon-γ production in rheumatoid arthritis and related diseases. Scand J Immunol 27:73
163. Struyf NJ, Snoeck HW, Bridts CH, De Clerck LS, Stevens WJ (1990) Natural killer cell activity in Sjorgren's syndrome and systemic lupus erythematosus: stimulation with interferons and interleukin-2 and correlation with immune complexes. Ann Rheum Dis 49:690
164. Suzuki H, Yasukawa K, Saito T, Narazaki M, Hasegawa A, Taga T, Kishimoto T (1993) Serum soluble interleukin-6 receptor in MRL/lpr mice is elevated with age and mediates the interleukin-6 signal. Eur J Immunol 23:1078
165. Swank AJG, van Rooyen A, Raziuddin S (1989) Interleukin-6 (IL-6) and acute phase proteins in the disease course of patients with sytemic lupus erythematosus. Rheumatol Int 18:263
166. Takada S, Ueda Y, Suzuki N, Murakawa Y, Hoshino Y, Green I, Steinberg AD, Sakane T (1985) Abnormalities in autologous mixed lymphocyte reaction-activated immunologic processes in systemic lupus erythematosus and their possible correction by interleukin 2. Eur J Immunol 15:262
167. Takashima T, Ohnishi K, Tsuyuguchi I, Kishimoto S (1993) Differential regulation of formation of multinucleated gaint cells from concanavalin A-stimulated human blood monocyted by IFN-γ and IL-4. J Immunol 150:3002
168. Tan PL, Blumenstein M, Yeoman S, Watson JD (1989) B cell lymphokines in human systemic lupus erythematosus. Ann Rheum Dis 44:941
169. Tanaka T, Saiki O, Negoro S, Igarashi T, Kuritani T, Hara H, Suemura M, Kishimoto S (1989) Decreased expression of interleukin-2 binding molecules (p70/75) in T cells from patients with systemic lupus erthematosus. Arthritis Rheum 32:552
170. Tanaka T, Nagasaka Y, Kitamurea F (1993) The role on the interleukin-2 (IL-2)/IL-2 receptor pathways in MRL/lpr lymphadenopathy: the expanded $CD4^-8^-$ T cell subset completely lacks functional IL-2 receptors. Eur J Immunol 23:1378
171. Tanaka Y, Saito K, Shirakawa F, Ota T, Suzuki H, Eto S, Yamashita U (1988) Production of B cell-stimulating factors by B cells in patients with systemic lupus erythematosus. J Immunol 141:3043
172. Tanaka Y, Saito K, Suzuki H, Eto S, Yamashita U (1989) Inhibitory effect of anti-class II antibody on the spontaneous activation of B cells in patients with systemic lupus erythematosus: Analysis with IL-1 production and IL-1 receptor expression. J Immunol 143:1584
173. Tang B, Matsuda T, Akira S, Nagata N, Ikehara S, Hirano T, Kishimoto T (1991) Age-associated increase in interleukin-6 in MRL/lpr mice. Int Immunol 3:273
174. Ter Borg EJ, Horst G, Limburg PC, Kallenberg CGM (1990) Changes in plasma levels of interleukin-2 receptor in relation to disease exacerbation and levels of anti-dsDNA and complement in systemic lupus erythematosus. Clin Exp Immunol 82:21
175. Theofilopoulos AN, Dixon FJ (1981) Etiopathogenesis of murine SLE. Immunol Rev 55:179
176. Theofilopoulos AN, Dixon FJ (1985) Murine models of systemic lupus erythematosus. Adv Immunol 37:269
177. Theofilopoulos AN, Prud'homme GJ, Fieser TM, Dixon FJ (1983) B-cell hyperactivity in murine lupus. II Defects in response to and production of accessory signals in lupus-prone mice. Immunol Today 4:317
178. Tominaga A, Takaki S, Koyama N, Katoh S, Matsumoto R, Migita M, Hitoshi Y, Hosoya Y, Yamauchi S, Kanai Y, Miyazaki J, Usuku G, Yamamura K, Takatsu K (1991) Transgenic mice expressing a B cell growth and differentiation factor gene (interleukin 5) develop eosinophilia and autoantibody production. J Exp Med 173:429

179. Trichieri G, Perussia B (1985) Immune interferon: a pleiotrophic lymphocine with multiple effects. Immunol Today 6:131
180. Trinchieri G, Matsumoto-Kobayashi M, Clark SC, Seehra J, London L, Perussia B (1984) Response of resting human peripheral blood natural killer cells to interleukin 2. J Exp Med 160:1147
181. Tsokos GC, Rook AH, Djeu JY, Balow JE (1982) Natural killer cells and interferon responses in patinets with systemic lupus erythematosus. Clin Exp Immunol 50:239
182. Tsokos GC, Smith PL, Christian CB, Lipnick RN, Balow JE, Djeu JY (1985) Interleukin-2 restores the depressed allogeneic cell-mediated lympholysis and natural killer cell activity in patients with systemic lupus erythematosus. Clin Immunol Immunophatol 34:379
183. Tsokos GC, Boumpas DT, Smith PL, Djeu JE, Balow JE, Rook AH (1986) Deficient γ-interferon production in patients with systemic lupus erythematosus. Arthritis Rheum 29:1210
184. Ueda Y, Sakane T, Tsunematsu T (1989) Hyperreactivity of activated B cells to B cell growth factor in patients with systemic lupus erythematosus. J Immunol 143:3988
185. Umland S, Lee R, Howard M, Martens C (1989) Expression of lymphokine genes in splenic lymphocytes of autoimmune mice. Mol Immunol 26:649
186. Umland SP, Go NF, Cupp JE, Howard M (1989) Responsese of B cells from autoimmune mice to IL-5. J Immunol 142:1528
187. Umland SP, Razac S, Nahrebne DK, Seymour B (1992) Effects of in vivo administration of interferon (IFN)-γ, anti-IFN-γ or anti-interleukin-4 monocional antibodies in chronic autoimmune graft-versus-host disease. Clin Immunol Immunopathol 63:66
188. Vandenabeele P, Abramowicz D, Berus D, Van Der Heyden J, Grooten J, Donckier V, Hooghe-Peters EL, Goldman M, Fiers W (1993) Increased IL-6 production and IL-6-mediated lg secretion in murine host-vs-graft disease. J Immunol 150:4179
189. Via CS (1990) Kinetics of T cell activation in acute and chronic forms of murine graft-versus-host disease. J Immunol 146:2603
190. Via CS, Finkelman FD (1993) Critical role of interleukin-2 in the development of acute graft-versus-host disease. Int Immunol 5:565
191. Via CS, Shearer GM (1988) T-cell interaction in autoimmunity: insights from a murine model of graft-verus-host disease. Immunol Today 9:207
192. Via CS, Shearer GM (1988) Functional heterogeneity of L3T4$^+$ T cells in MRL-*lpr/lpr* mice: L3T4$^+$ T cells suppress major histocompatibility complex-self restricted L3T4$^+$ helper cell function in association with autoimmunity. J Exp Med 168:2165
193. Via CS, Shearer GM (1988) Murine graft-versus-host disease as a model for the development of autoimmunity: relevance of cytotoxic T lymphocytes. Ann NY Acad Sci 532:44
194. Via CS, Sharrow SO, Shearer GM (1987) Role of cytotoxic T lymphocytes in the prevention of lupus-like disease occurring in a murine model of graft-vs-host disease. J Immunol 139:1840
195. Via CS, Svetic A, Finkelman FD, Gause WC (1992) Early cytokine production in a murine model of lupus. FASEB J 6:A1447
196. Via CS, Rus V, Gately M, Finkelman FD (1993) IL-12 prevents autoimmunity in a murine model of SLE. Arthritis Rheum 36:S63
197. Via CS, Tsokos GC, Bermas B, Clerici M, Shearer GM (1993) T cell-antigen-presenting cell interactions in human systemic lupus erythematosuse. Evidence for heterogeneous expression of multiple defects. J Immunol 151:3914
198. Volk HD, Diamantstein T (1986) IL-2 normalizes defective suppressor T cell function of patients with systemic lupus erythematosus in vitro. Clin Exp Immunol 66:525
199. Volk HD, Kopp J, Korner IJ, Jahn S, Grunow R, Bartheimes H, Fiebig H (1986) Correlation between the phenotype and the functional capacity of activated T cells in patients with active systemic lupus erythematosus. Scand J Immunol 24:109
200. Vose BM, Bonnard GD (1983) Limiting dilution analysis of the frequency of human T cell and large granular lymphocytes proliferating in response to interleukin 2. I. The effect of lectin on the proliferative frequency and cytotoxic activity of cultured lymphoid cells. J Immunol 130:687
201. Wagner H, Hardt C, Heeg K, Pfizenmaier K, Solbach W, Bartlett R, Stockinger H, Rollinghoff M (1980) T-T cell interactions during cytotoxic T lymphocyte (CTL) responses: T call-derived helper factor (interleukin 2) as a probe to anaiyze CTL responsiveness and thymic maturation of CTL progenitors. Immunol Rev 51:215

202. Wagner H, Hardt C, Rouse BT, Rollinghoff M, Scheurich P, Pfizenmaier K (1982) Dissection of the proliferative and differentiative signals controlling murine cytotoxic T lymphocyte response. J Exp Med 155:1876
203. Wandl UB, Nagel-Hienke M, May D, Kreuzfelder E (1992) Lupus-like autoimmune disease induced by interferon therapy for. myeloproliferative disorders. Clin Immunol Immunopathol 65:70
204. Warrington RJ, Rutherford WJ (1990) Normal mitogen-induced suppression of the interlerukin-6 (IL-6) response and its deficiency in systemic lupus erythematosus. J Clin Invest 10:52
205. Warrington RJ, Sauder PJ, Homik J, Ofosu-Appiah W (1989) Reversible interleukin-2 response defects in systemic lupus erythematosus. Clin Exp Immunol 77:163
206. Whicher JT, Gilbert AMI, Westcott C, Hutton C, Dieppe PA (1986) Defective production of leucocytic endogenous mediator (interleukin 1) by peripheral blood leucocytes of patients with systemic sclerosis, systemic lupus erythematosus, rheumatoid arthritis and mixed connective tissue disease. Clin Exp Immunol 65:80
207. Wofsy D, Seaman WE (1985) Successful treatment of autoimmunity in NZB/NZW F_1 mice with monocional antibody to L3T4. J Exp Med 161:378
208. Wofsy D, Dauphinee MJ, Kipper SB, Talai N (1981) Interleukin-2 deficiency in murine systemic lupus erythematosus. Trans Assoc Am Physicians 194:341
209. Wofsy D, Murphy ED, Roths JB, Dauphinee MJ, Kipper SB, Talai N (1981) Deficient interleukin 2 activity in MRL/Mp and C57BL6J mice bearing the *lpr* gene. J Exp Med 154:1671
210. Wolf RE, Brelsford WG (1988) Soluble interleukin-2 receptors in systemic lupus erythematosus. Arthritis Rheum 31:729
211. Wong GHW, Clark-Lewis I, McKimm-Breschkin JL, Harris A, Schrader JW (1983) Interferon-γ induces enhanced expression of Ia and H-2 antigens on B lymphoid, macrophage and myeloid cell lines. J Immunol 131:788
212. Yoshimoto T, Paul WE (1994) $CD4^+$, $NK1.1^+$ T cells promptly produce interleukin 4 in response to in vivo challenge with anti-CD3. J Exp Med 179:1285
213. Yu D, Winchester RJ, Fu SM, Gibofsky A, Ko HS, Kunkel HG (1980) Peripheral blood 1a-positive T cells: increase in certain diseases and after immunization. J Exp Med 157:91
214. Yui MA, Brissette WH, Brennan DC, Wuthrich RP, Rubin-Kelley VE (1991) Increased macrophage colony-stimulating factor in neonatal and adult autoimmune MRL-*lpr* mice. Am J Pathol 139:255

The cytokine network in the pathogenesis of systemic lupus erythematosus and possible therapeutic implications

David A. Horwitz, Chaim O. Jacob

Division of Rheumatology and Immunology, Department of Medicine, University of Southern California School of Medicine, Los Angeles, CA, USA

Introduction

Systemic lupus erythematosus (SLE) is considered to be the prototype of human autoimmune diseases. It is a disorder of generalized autoimmunity characterized by multisystem organ involvement and autoantibodies against nuclear, cytoplasmic, and cell surface antigens. The mechanisms responsible for the breakdown of tolerance against these self antigens are unknown. Abnormalities of T cells, B cells and antigen-presenting cells result in immune dysregulation, especially in patients with active disease. There is B cell hyperactivity with polyclonal B cell activation and autoantibody formation. By contrast, there is decreased cellular immunity with impaired T cell and natural killer (NK) cell effector functions leading to decreased host defense [50]. For many years investigators have searched for primary abnormalities of T cells which are important in pathogenesis. Most of the T cell abnormalities, however, appear to reflect dysregulation as a consequence of the disease.

To explain the mechanisms responsible for immune dysregulation in SLE, cytokines have received increasing attention. Cytokines are hormone-like low molecular weight proteins, produced by a wide variety of cells, that have profound effects on the immune system. Cytokines mediate a large variety of functions and exert remarkably diverse effects. The number of known cytokines continues to increase and some have been known to have redundant functional properties.

A key question today is not only which cytokines are potentially involved in the pathophysiology of an immune response or disease, but when do these cytokines function and which of their many activities are relevant in vivo. Complexity derives from the fact that the expression of a given cytokine is invariably influenced by other cytokines forming networks of cytokine cascades. Such cascades may represent important features of cytokine action in the programmed growth, differentiation and function of cells. Furthermore, complexity also derives from the large range of cellular

Correspondence to: D.A. Horwitz, USC School of Medicine, 2011 Zonal Avenue, HMR 711, Los Angeles, CA 90033, USA

interactions required for normal immunological function and for tolerance. Thus, the control or modulation of these interactions can occur at several levels and at any or all of these levels then might result in reactivity to self and induce an autoimmune response.

In considering the pathogenesis of SLE, one must distinguish the mechanisms which are responsible for the initiation of this disorder from those involved in perpetuation. Genetic factors are especially important in disease susceptibility and one particular cytokine, tumor necrosis factor-alpha (TNF-α) appears to have an important protective role, possibly at the level of antigen presentation. In both the initiation and perpetuation of disease, cytokines also have well-defined functions in regulating lymphocyte effector functions. Thus, the clinical course of mouse SLE can be significantly altered by several cytokines. This information may be used to predict whether up-regulation or down-regulation of certain cytokines can affect the course of human SLE. Each of these topics will be reviewed. Mouse models of SLE have been especially useful in elucidating genetic factors important in the initiation of SLE while the study of human SLE has provided important clues to understanding the role of cytokines in perpetuation.

Cytokines and the genetic predisposition to SLE

Class II major histocompatibility complex genes regulate TNF-α production

The TNF genes are unique in that they are the only known cytokines located within the major histocompatibility complex, both in mice and human [21, 97, 113]. A striking association between different MHC alleles, especially class II alleles, and various autoimmune diseases has been well established [61]. SLE is a complex autoimmune disease associated with MHC class II DR2, DQw1 and/or DR3 alleles. Despite this clear association, the role of MHC class II molecules in SLE remains largely unknown. It is even questionable whether the MHC genes are indeed the predisposing genes to the disease or rather just markers for other closely linked gene(s). Because the TNF genes are located within the MHC the possibility of the involvement of TNF in autoimmunity is an attractive hypothesis [64].

The production of TNF by peritoneal macrophages activated with lipopolysaccharide (LPS) and interferon (IFN-γ), obtained from various mouse strains revealed a significant variation in the production of this cytokine among the different strains [60, 65]. This variability seemed not to be random but rather MHC associated. For example, Ia^d mice (BALB/c, NZB and DBA/2) produce similar intermediate levels of TNF-α while Ia^q mice (SWR, DBA/1 and B10.Q) produce very high levels of TNF-α.

To extend these studies to humans, the production of TNF by activated peripheral blood lymphocytes or enriched monocyte populations of HLA-A, -B, -C, -DR and -DQ serotyped normal donors was assayed [63]. As in mice, major differences in the level of TNF-α production was found to be associated with MHC class II genotype. DR2- and DQw1-positive individuals were found to produce significantly lower levels of TNF than donors not possessing these specificities. By contrast, normal donors positive for DR3 or DR4 were almost always high producers of the cytokine.

Three lines of evidence strongly suggest that the differences in TNF-α production are stable, inter-individual variations rather than different overall sensitivities of lymphocytes from the different donors to the particular stimulation condition used. First, various methods were used to induce TNF production in vitro including LPS, IFN-γ, concanavalin A (Con A), phorbol myristate acetate (PMA) and phytohemagglutinin (PHA) at various doses and combinations. Although activation by Con A plus PMA gave the highest level of inducibility of both TNF-α and TNF-β, the inter-individual differences were evident in all methods of activation [63]. Second, the levels of TNF-α production in the same subject were highly reproducible in repeated tests, suggesting that these inter-individual variations are stable. Third, there was no correlation between the proliferative responses of lymphocytes to mitogens and, thus, their capability to produce TNF-α levels are not due to individual variation in responsiveness to these mitogens, nor to a qualitative difference in kinetic responses to these mitogens, but are rather due to heritable, stable inter-individual variations.

Class II MHC regulation by IFN-γ and TNF-α

IFN-γ is widely accepted as the principal lymphokine involved in the induction of MHC class II molecules which is a key element in the process of antigen presentation. A significant decrease in MHC class II Ia expression on macrophages in the peritoneum of TNF-α-treated (NZB $\times$ NZW)F1 mice was noted [65, 143]. The observation that class II MHC expression is not up-regulated but actually down-regulated by TNF-α treatment may at least resolve the apparent paradoxical in vivo effects of TNF-α and IFN-γ in (NZB $\times$ NZW)F1 mice. Inappropriate expression of MHC class II molecules by IFN-γ has been suggested to play a role in the initiation of autoimmune processes [13]. Thus, the apparent opposite effects of TNF-α and IFN-γ in regulation of class II MHC molecules in this in vivo system may imply that regulation of la expression is the mechanism by which TNF-α or IFN-γ affect the development of lupus nephritis in the (NZB $\times$ NZW)F1 mice. TNF-α has been shown both to synergize with IFN-γ and also to antagonize IFN-γ regarding regulation of class II MHC expression [17, 49, 111]. Watanabe and Jacob [143] have proposed that depending on the stage of differentiation and maturation of the target cell, TNF-α might synergize or antagonize IFN-γ-induced regulation of MHC class II antigens. In immature cells like HL-60 or THP-1, TNF-α enhances IFN-γ induction of MHC class II antigens, while in differentiated cells like skin fibroblasts or activated macrophages TNF-α down-regulates the IFN-γ-induced class II expression. In bone marrow cells induced to differentiate, in vitro, TNF-α decreased the IFN-γ-induced MHC class II expression in a maturation-dependent fashion [143].

The capability to present antigen is a property of mature, differentiated and activated cells [25] rather than primitive or immature cells. Therefore, the down-regulation of MHC class II expression by TNF-α shown on mature macrophages might be much more relevant biologically than the up-regulatory effect seen on undifferentiated cells.

Cytokines and the initiation of SLE

TNF and IFN-γ in mouse lupus models and human SLE

The (NZB × NZW)F1 hybrid mouse develops a severe autoimmune disease similar to systemic lupus erythematosus (SLE) in humans [137]. Both the human and mouse form of the disease show a strong association with specific alleles of MHC gene products. Although the NZW parental strain is phenotypically normal, most F1 females develop severe glomerulonephritis. The NZW parent, thus, makes a major genetic contribution to the development of nephritis in F1 mice. Backcross studies have shown that the major genetic contribution from NZW mice maps within the H-2 regions [9, 74].

The hypothesis that lymphokines may play a critical role in the pathogenesis of this autoimmune disease by activating the immune system and up-regulating the MHC class II molecules was tested. Since IFN-γ is widely accepted as the principal inducer of class II MHC molecules, the in vivo effects of this lymphokine were tested. Indeed, it was found that IFN-γ-treated (NZB × NZW)F1 mice have an accelerated development of lupus nephritis, while blocking the effect of IFN-γ with monoclonal antibody against mouse IFN-γ caused a significant delay in disease development [62]. Because TNF-α has been shown in vitro to possess similar or additive effects to IFN-γ [17, 108, 145], the in vivo effects of this cytokine were evaluated in comparison to IFN-γ. In contrast to IFN-γ, therapy with recombinant TNF-α induced a very significant diminution in the development of lupus nephritis in the (NZB × NZW)F1 mouse [60]. Furthermore, peritoneal macrophages from NZW parental strain were found to produce very low levels of TNF-α.

To account for the mechanism of low TNF-α production, a restriction fragment length polymorphism of the TNF gene [60] and more recently a polymorphism in a dinucleotide tandem repeat within the 5′ regulatory region of TNF-α gene [65, 67] was found to correlate with the reduced levels of TNF-α prodution seen in NZW mice. Jacob et al. [60] have, therefore, suggested that the NZW parent may contribute to the F1 disease a TNF-α gene capable of only low level of TNF production. Thus, recombinant TNF-α may possibly act as replacement therapy to supplement the low endogenous TNF production.

Additional complexity is demonstrated when some other lupus model systems were tested. Administration of IFN-γ or monoclonal antibody against IFN-γ had no significant effect on disease development in the MRL-lpr/lpr mice (C.O. Jacob, unpublished). Furthermore, TNF-α significantly delays the development of nephritis in (NZB × NZW)F1 and also in the MRL-lpr/lpr model, but it has no protective effect in BXSB mice [65]. The BXSB model is believed to have a totally different genetic basis [99], which may account for the lack of TNF-α effect on disease development in this strain of mice.

An inverse correlation has been found between the level of TNF-α inducibility in peritoneal macrophages in vitro and the effect of TNF-α administration in vivo [65]. Based on these results, it is possible to predict that TNF-α treatment might be beneficial only in situations where TNF-α inducibility is low.

The protective effect of TNF-α in the (NZB × NZW)F1 has been confirmed independently by Gordon et al. [36]. On the other hand, two publications argue that rather than a beneficial effect, TNF-α may have a deleterious effect in mouse lupus. Boswell et al. [12] have found increased mRNA expression of IL-1 and TNF-α

locally in the kidneys of MRL-lpr/lpr mice, suggesting that intra-renal production of these cytokines is responsible for a cascade of events leading to lupus nephritis. Brennan et al. [14] report on enhanced TNF-α and IL-β expression in the kidneys of (NZB $\times$ NZW)F1 mice. The basic concept of the potential role of TNF in autoimmune lupus nephritis is clearly different between these investigators. However, the data of the studies themselves are not necessarily contradictory. Jacob et al. [59, 60, 65] tested TNF-α protein production by stimulated peritoneal macrophages, while others assayed TNF-α mRNA levels locally in the kidneys. It should be noted that there can be a significant discrepancy between the amount of TNF-α mRNA and the amount of TNF-α protein translated. Thus, in certain instances, TNF-α mRNA may be expressed in considerable abundance, while the protein is not expressed or is expressed at a very low level [10, 116].

In addition, the age of mice and different dose of TNF-α given may affect the outcome of this cytokine. Brennan et al. [14] show an accelerating effect only with a very low dose of TNF-α and only if treatment is started after 4 months of age and continued until 8 months of age. It is perhaps possible that this deleterious effect seen with treatment between the age of 4–8 months is related to the observation of Jacob et al. [65] that treatment between 3–9.5 months is less effective than treatment between 3–6 months. This study shows that the earlier TNF-α is given the more effective is its protective effect [61]. A reasonable hypothesis is that TNF-α is involved in a protective model only in the early induction phases of the autoimmune process, rather than in the late effector arm of the disease process. Further investigation will be required to understand the basis of differential dose response to TNF-α.

Searching for mechanisms of TNF-α effect in autoimmune disease

In an attempt to determine the mechanisin(s) by which TNF-α suppresses autoimmunity, different immune cell populations were characterized by flow cytometry on TNF-α-treated and PBS-treated age-matched (NZB $\times$ NZW)F1 mice at 2- to 3-week intervals during and after treatment. TNF-α treatment appeared to have no discernible effects on the frequency or phenotype of B, T, or monocyte cell population in cells from the peritoneal cavity, spleen, lymph node and thymus [65]. There was, however, a slight increase in the number of macrophages and a decrease in Ly-1 + B cells in the peritoneum, especially during the first few weeks of treatment [59, 65]. In contrast to other immune intervention methods applied to the (NZB $\times$ NZW)F1 model system (anti-L3T4 antibody; anti-Ia antibody; TLI; cyclosporine treatment), TNF-α administration seems to have the least overall effect. In previous studies, increased Ly-1 B cell frequencies in NZB mice were interpreted as reflecting polyclonal expansion and activation of an autoantibody producing Ly-1 B cell population [43]. Recently, it was shown that these increases in Ly-1 B cell frequencies actually represent expansion of individual Ly-1 B clones [128], which do not appear to be responsible for the increased autoantibody production observed in these strains. Thus, it is not possible, at this point, to evaluate the significance of the reduction in the frequencies of Ly-1 B cells in TNF-α-treated mice.

Treatment of lupus prone mice with TNF-α does not reduce autoantibody production [65]. These data support previous genetic studies with respect to inheritance of autoantibody production and nephritis development as not being the result of a single gene but rather, result from faulty regulation of independently segregating genes [73, 114, 137].

Furthermore, these data are consistent with findings that TNF-α does not suppress humoral immunity in normal or lupus mice [35, 36]. These observations imply that TNF-α may affect autoimmune disease not through effects on humoral immunity, but via an as yet unidentified mechanism. Indeed, it was suggested that long-term administration of TNF may lead to a suppression of cell-mediated immunity [36], possibly by a systemic macrophage activation, which might inhibit the development of the autoimmune response before the effector stage.

IL-10 and mouse lupus

IL-10 is a cytokine produced by activated TH2 and B lymphocyte subsets as well as macrophages. As many other cytokines, IL-10 mediates a variety of both immunostimulatory and immunosuppressive activities in vitro. Normal BALB/c mice treated continuously from birth until 8 weeks of age with neutralizing anti-IL-10 antibodies show elevated levels of endogenous IFN-γ and TNF-α [56, 57]. Furthermore, the elevated IFN-γ leads to depletion of Ly-1 B lymphocytes, a numerically small subset of B cells, but one from which many autoantibodies are derived in the mouse [56]. These studies in the normal mouse suggested that neutralization of IL-10 may result in some desirable consequences in lupus prone mice (elavation of TNF-α and reduction of autoantibody production). On the other hand, it may induce some undesirable effects as well (elevation of endogenous IFN-γ).

To evaluate these possibilities in vivo, Ishida et al. [58] have treated lupus prone NZB $\times$ NZW mice with neutralizing anti-IL-10 antibodies continuously from birth until 8–10 months of age. The anti-IL-10 treatment substantially delayed onset of autoimmunity in the lupus prone mice as monitored either by overall survival, or by development of proteinuria or overt glomerulonephritis and autoantibody titers in the serum of the mice. Most interestingly, the anti IL-10 protective effect was due to the endogenous up-regulation of TNF-α, since anti-IL-10-protected lupus mice rapidly developed autoimmunity when neutralizing anti-TNF-α antibodies were introduced, even at 30 weeks of age, along with the anti-IL-10 treatment. Consistent with the protective role of anti-IL-10, continuous administration of IL-10 to these lupus prone mice accelerated the onset of autoimmunity. It is noteworthy that the same amount IL-10 administered to non-autoimmune BALB/c mice had no toxic effect and did not induce any autoimmune symptoms. The mechanism of anti-IL-10-mediated protection of lupus prone NZB $\times$ NZW mice strongly supports the protective role for TNF-α in this disease.

Cytokines and the perpetuation of SLE

Cytokine production and responsiveness

The data in this area is inadequate to address the critical issues concerning the role of cytokines in the perpetuation of human SLE. In patients with active SLE, information is available concerning the spontaneous and induced production of some cytokines by their peripheral blood mononuclear cells (PBMC). Some information on serum levels is also available. What is lacking is information about the production of cytokines and the response to these cytokines in the microenvironment where autoimmunity is actually taking place. Table 1 summarizes information currently available.

Table 1. Cytokine production in patients with active SLE

Cytokine	Serum level	Spontaneous release	After stimulation of PBMC in vitro
IL-1	Not detectable	High	Decreased
IL-2	Increased	Low	Decreased
IL-4	Usually not detectable	Low	Low
IL-6	Increased	High	–
IL-10	Normal or high	Normal or high	Normal
TNF-α	Not detectable or ? increased	Variable	Decreased
IFN-γ	Increased	Low	Decreased

SLE, Systemic lupus erythematosus; IL, interleukin; TNF, tumor necrosis factor; IFN, interferon; PBMC, peripheral blood mononuclear cells

An example of the complexity of this issue is information concerning IL-2 production. IL-2 production by stimulated peripheral blood T cells is decreased in SLE [3, 77, 92, 98], but the significance of this finding has been questioned. Initially, it was reported in human SLE that there was an intrinsic defect in the capacity of $CD4^+$ T cells to produce this cytokine [98]. Subsequently, others reported that in most patients, this defect can be explained by $CD8^+$ suppressor cells [78], or because the SLE T cells are already activated and cannot respond to further stimulation [53]. In addition, autoantibodies in SLE serum can inhibit IL-2 production by normal cells [91]. Evidence suggesting ongoing production of IL-2 in vivo includes the finding of increased serum levels of this cytokine [54], and increased IL-2 gene expression in freshly obtained $CD4^+$ T cells from patients with active disease [51]. Although the production of IL-2 is decreased in response to mitogenic stimulation in vitro, this result may not reflect the response to endogenous antigens in vivo.

Not only is the production of IL-2 decreased in SLE, but the response of lymphocytes to IL-2 is also decreased. This has been explained by decreased IL-2 receptor expression [55, 133]. At present, there is little information available about the response of lupus T cells to other cytokines. As described above, TNF-α inducibility is low in (NZB $\times$ NZW)F1 mice and this trait correlates positively with SLE. In human SLE, one group has reported normal TNF-α by mitogen-stimulated lymphocytes, but when phorbol ester was added the amount of TNF-α was significantly decreased [84]. When MHC typing was performed, DR2, DQw1-positive SLE patients show low levels of TNF-α production [63] and this genotype is also associated with an increased incidence of lupus nephritis [27, 60]. Thus, similar to the B/W mouse model of SLE, decreased TNF-α production correlated with nephritis. However, a substantial portion of SLE patients are DR3 associated and these patients do not have a low TNF-α production, similar to MRL-lpr/lpr and BXSB mice which also show moderate to high levels of TNF-α production [65]. Taken together, these studies Suggest that SLE is not a single condition, but rather one that can be subdivided from a genetic point of view into two or more subsets [61, 64]. These data also emphasize that the MHC-associated genetic predisposition may actually proceed through different mechanisms involving different genes in different subsets of the disease.

Cytokines in the development of CD4⁺ T cell effector functions

Certain cytokines fall into two categories based on their effects on T cell effector function. IL-12 and IFN-γ condition T cells to provide help for cytotoxic effector cells and enhance macrophage microbicidal activity. By contrast, IL-4 conditions T cells to become helpers of B cell differentiation [94]. $CD4^+$ T cells that support cell-mediated immunity are called TH1 cells and those that provide B cell help are called TH2 cells. Once T cells have become TH1 cells, they produce IFN-γ upon antigenic stimulation. Similarly, in mice stimulated TH2 cells produce high levels of IL-4 and IL-10. In humans, however, TH1 and TH2 clones both produce IL-10 [147] and other mononuclear populations can produce this cytokine. Importantly, high levels of IFN-γ inhibit IL-4 production and vice versa. Therefore, TH2 cells not only support antibody-secreting B cells, but suppress cell-mediated immunity. Since SLE is characterized by each of these features, one might expect an increased production of IL-4, IL-5 and possibly IL-10 with a corresponding decrease in IFN-γ and IL-12. SLE, however, appears to conform to only part of this model.

Even in mice where this paradigm was first described, the TH1/TH2 dichotomy between humoral and cell-mediated immunity is not complete. TH1 cells also provide B cell help for complement-fixing Ig2a antibodies in mice or IgG1 antibodies in humans. By contrast, IL-4 conditions T cells to provide B cell help for non-complement fixing IgG antibodies [117]. Moreover, one of the principal effects of IL-4 is class switching to IgE. In SLE, pathogenic anti-DNA antibodies are of complement-fixing phenotype and IgE is not increased. In mouse SLE, there is scanty evidence that production of IL-4 is increased in models of SLE with female predominance and even less evidence has been found in human SLE. Stimulated $CD4^+$ T cells from older male BXSB mice produce increased amounts of IL-4 and IFN-γ [18]. The best evidence in mice is that cloned T cells from the NZB/bm-12 strain, which provide help for anti-DNA antibody, produce IL-4, but not IL-2 or IFN-γ [102].

In humans, where it is difficult to study lymphoid organs, the best correlate of cytokine production in vivo would be the spontaneous activity of freshly obtained PBMC. In human SLE, T cell expression of IL-4 mRNA transcripts is decreased and serum levels of IL-4 were not increased [29, 51].

Although IL-4 production does not appear to be increased in human SLE, our laboratory does have preliminary evidence for elevated IL-10 levels. In a study in progress, we have observed markedly increased spontaneous production of IL-10 in several newly diagnosed, untreated SLE patients, but not controls. Moreover, elevated levels of this cytokine were found in the serum of almost all of these patients, but not in the serum of healthy subjects. This preliminary finding of increased IL-10 synthesis in human SLE is of significant interest since: (1) IL-10 inhibits cell-mediated immunity, one of the characteristic features of SLE; and (2) as described above, continuous administration of anti-IL-10 delays the onset of mouse SLE [58]. One other group has also reported high levels of IL-10 in SLE [80a].

Turning now to TH1 cytokines, we have investigated production of 6 different cytokines by unstimulated and mitogen-stimulated lymphocyte subsets and monocytes in studies performed in collaboration with Dr. Giorgio Trinchieri (Wistar Institute, Philadelphia, PA). To date we have studied 10 patients with newly diagnosed, untreated SLE and have found decreased production of IL-12 by Staph A stimulated monocytes that approached statistical significance ($P = 0.06$). Lymphocyte production of IL-12 was not statistically different. Other noteworthy unpublished observations include significantly decreased production of TNFα by lymphocytes and monocytes, and decreased IFNγ production by lymphocytes (see below). Others have found decreased mitogen-induced production of IFN-γ in SLE is decreased [131, 138] and this finding correlates with decreased natural killer cell activity [139]. This issue is not completely settled since information is lacking regarding IFN-jγ production in vivo and serum levels of the cytokine are increased (see below). Apparently, high levels of interferons may be detrimental to humans as in mice since the administration of recombinant IFN to humans can induce an SLE-like syndrome (see below).

In summary, the mouse TH1 and TH2 cytokine paradigm only partially explains the dichotomy between humoral and cellular immunity in human SLE. There is no convincing evidence of increased IL-4 production in SLE and while IFN-γ production may, possibly, be decreased, this cytokine appears to provoke rather than to prevent SLE. The role of IL-10 and IL-12 in human SLE remains to be defined.

Cytokines in the development of CD8⁺ T cell effector functions

$CD8^+$ T cells normally develop the capacity to become cytotoxic effector cells, or to become suppressor cells. Both of these functions are abnormal in SLE. Lupus T cells proliferate normally to anti-CD3 and IL-2, but their cytotoxic capacity was markedly reduced in comparison to normal controls, even after long-term culture with IL-2 [130]. Previously, this laboratory described a pathological circuit in SLE involving $CD8^+$ cells. These T cells inhibit IL-2 production by $CD4^+$ cells and, paradoxically, provide B cell help [79]. $CD8^+$ T cells from patients with active SLE secrete a soluble inhibitor of IL-2 production which has not been characterized [78].

The mechanisms which enable $CD8^+$ cells to become non-specific suppressors of antibody production are poorly understood. Cytokines, however, appear to play an important role. $CD8^+$ cells were responsible for the defects in IFNγ and TNFα production which we recently observed (see above). After depletion of $CD8^+$ cells, the values for these cytokines in the SLE and controls were similar. This was because of a sharp decrease in the control group (unpublished observations). Moreover, TGFβ appears to be important in the *generation* of suppression. Besides using conventional methods to assess T cell dependent antibody production, we have described a monocyte-independent method [47]. Here we can directly assess the effects of well-defined regulatory populations. With this model, we have found that the addition of $CD8^+$ cells to $CD4^+$ T cells and B cells generally has only modest to moderate inhibitory effects on IgM and IgG production. While the addition of NK cells to $CD4^+$ T cells and B cells does not suppress antibody production, the combination of $CD8^+$ cells and NK cells results in marked suppression. This is because of an interaction between $CD8^+$ T cells and NK cells which induces NK cells to produce transforming growth factor-β (TGF-β). This cytokine, in low concentrations, induces $CD8^+$ cells to become suppressor cells. Thus, in addition to the well-known suppressive properties of TGF-β on T cell and NK cell effector functions [85, 103, 132], this cytokine appears to be involved in the generation of suppressor cell activity [40].

The issue of TGF-β in SLE is likely to be complex. While this cytokine in low concentrations may be involved in the generation of suppressor-effectors of antibody production, in high concentrations TGF-β inhibits T cell effector cell functions [106, 132]. These activities are ultimately determined not only by the local concentration of TGF-β, but also by the composition of the cells in the microenvironment which are responsible for the local cytokine cascade. It must also be emphasized that TGF-β is usually detected as a high molecular mass, latent molecule. Biologic activity occurs after conversion to the 25 kDa mature form.

The administration of TGF-β to mice inhibits TH1 cells more than TH2 cells [122], although in vitro studies with human T cells the opposite effect appears to be the case [26]. TGF-β decreased macrophage MHC class II expression [81] and inhibits the T cell response to antigens [69]. These are abnormalities described in SLE and it is likely that increased amounts of TGF-β will be found in response to the chronic inflammatory state. There is one preliminary report suggesting that TGF-β contributes to impaired T cell function in vitro in some lupus patients [20].

Cytokine production and effects on B cells and other antigen-presenting cells

Monocytes/macrophages and B cells produce a large variety of cytokines which include IL-1, IL-6, IL-12, TNF-α, and TGF-β. Each of these cytokines affect B cell function. Spontaneous production of IL-1 [8, 48, 66, 125, 134, 135] and IL-6 [72, 80] by mononuclear cells is increased in SLE. These cytokines contribute to polyclonal B cell activation and autoantibody formation in SLE. Although some workers have reported that sustained antibody production by B cells requires help from other lymphocyte populations [11, 32, 93], there is also evidence of autocrine circuits. Some workers report that IL-1 and IL-6 are spontaneously released by high density B cells and these cytokines then sustain antibody production by low-density B cells [109, 134, 135]. These B cells are extremely sensitive to the effects of IL-6. In contrast to low density B cells from healthy donors, SLE B cells respond to IL-6 to produce IgG and anti-single-stranded (ss)DNA antibody [71]. IL-6 receptors are constitutively expressed on SLE B cells [100]. By blocking these receptors with anti IL-6 receptor antibodies blocked spontaneous Ig production and anti-ssDNA antibody synthesis [71, 100]. There is also one report that normal T cell suppression of B cell responses to IL-6 is lacking [142].

IL-6 production could result from autoimmunity. Nucleosomes are an important source of nuclear autoantigens. These structures are released into the extracellular milieu by cells which undergo apoptosis. In SLE, one group has reported that exposure of lupus PBMC to UV light induces IL-6 production [110]. Another group has reported that, UV light induces keratinocytes in the skin to undergo apoptosis and release nucleosomes [16]. A third group has documented that nucleosomes can induce the spleen cells of lupus mice to produce IL-6 [44]. Taken together, IL-6 may be the consequence of the release and presentation of nucleosomal autoantigens to autoreactive lymphocytes in SLE. It is well established that sunlight exposure can precipitate or exacerbate SLE.

Autoantibodies can also induce IL-6 production. It has been reported that immunization of normal mice with a monoclonal anti-DNA antibody induced an anti-idiotypic antibody which mimicked the effects of DNA and induced spleen cells to produce IL-6 [45].

In addition to the effects of IL-6, SLE B cells produce excessive levels of Ig in response to IFN-γ [28, 33]. This cytokine can either enhance or inhibit B cell function depending upon the cytokine cascade or other regulatory cells present. On one hand, IFN-γ enhances IgG production by purified B cells induced by IL-2 or other soluble T cell factors in both normal controls and SLE. On the other hand, IFN-γ down-regulates the proliferative response of high density B cells to IL-4 in normal subjects. This inhibition, however, is absent in SLE [28].

There has been an increasing attention given to antigen-presenting cells in the pathogenesis and perpetuation of SLE. Lupus patients have well-known defects in their proliferative response to recall antigens [38] and these defects have been localized to monocytes/macrophages [140]. The mechanism responsible for these defects have not been characterized. Lupus monocytes expression of MHC class II antigens is decreased [101, 124] and stimulation of these cells to produce IL-1 is decreased [5, 77]. The explanation for decreased MHC class II is not known. TGF-β can have this effect [31]. The effects of TNF-α and IFN-γ on class II MHC expression has been discussed above.

Correlation between serum or plasma cytokine or cytokine receptor levels and clinical activity of disease

The serum levels of several cytokines is elevated in SLE. IL-2 [54], acid-labile IFN-α [112], IFN-γ [6, 28] and IL-6 [6] are increased and it has been reported that TNF-α may be normal or increased [6, 34, 88]. Serum levels of IFN-α correlate with active disease [70, 87, 141]. Serum IFN-γ is also elevated with evidence of activity [6]. Several groups have reported high levels of serum IL-6 associated with active disease [30, 80, 127] there are exceptions [37, 90]. IL-6 acts on the liver to increase C-reactive protein (CRP) and amyloid A antigen. Nonetheless, although serum levels of IL-6 are elevated, the CRP does not increase as expected in many cases of active SLE. This problem has been reviewed recently, but the explanation remains obscure [34]. One group has found elevated levels of TNF-α in patients with active disease [34], another group found TNF-α levels to be variably elevated [89], another to correlate with thrombocytopenia [6]. Jacob et al. (unpublished data), however, has not found elevated TNF-α in the serum of SLE patients. Certain cytokines have been detected in the cerebral spinal fluid (CSF) of patients with lupus central nervous system disease. These include IL-1 and IL-6 [4, 46]. Another group found increased IFN-α in the CSF of patients with lupus psychosis [123].

One of the reasons serum cytokine levels are difficult to interpret is because cytokine receptors are also shed by activated cells and the cytokine levels may reflect both bound and free cytokine. Shed receptors include: IL-1 [126], IL-2 [104], IL-6 [82, 95, 96], TNF-α [24, 120], IFN-α [105] and many others. The length of this list suggests that the presence of these receptors in serum or plasma is a general phenomenon.

Serum or plasma levels of soluble cytokine receptors also can correlate with active disease. Serum-soluble IL-2 receptors (CD25 or IL-2Rα) are increased in SLE [15, 86, 121, 136, 144] and the levels correlate with disease activity, and may predict exacerbations [15, 136]. Serum IL-2R levels have also been reported to correlate with activity of lupus nephritis [75]. Serum levels of soluble TNF-α receptors are also increased in SLE and correlate with disease activity. Both Type I (p55) and Type II (p75) levels are increased [2]. In our group, increased levels of soluble TNF receptors has been observed in the CSF of patients with lupus central nervous system disease (unpublished observations).

The biological function of soluble cytokine receptors is not well understood. At high concentrations in serum, they can antagonize biological effects. This has been demonstrated for TNF-α and for IL-4 [19, 22]. At lower concentrations soluble cytokine receptors may function as transport proteins for their ligands, protecting them from proteolysis and acting as a reservoir for active or potentially active factors. Soluble TNF receptors have this activity [1]. The binding of soluble IL-6 receptors to IL-6 appears to increase the activity of IL-6 [146].

Therapeutic possibilities

Because of the imbalance between the cellular and humoral divisions of the immune response, cytokines that down-regulate B cell function and up-regulate T cell effector functions should offer the most promise. According to the mouse TH1/TH2 paradigm, up-regulation of IFN-γ or IL-12 and down-regulation of IL-4 and IL-10 would ameliorate this imbalance. As described in this review, however, even in the mouse, TH1 cytokines can provide B cell help and the TH2 cytokine, IL-4, does not appear to be elevated in human SLE. If further studies should reveal increased IL-10 production in human SLE, then attempts to down-regulate this cytokine might be investigated. As described above, continuous administration of anti-IL-10 to B/W mice delayed the onset of SLE and this was achieved by up-regulating TNF-α. Anti-IL-10 and/or TNF-α might be given to the subset of human SLE patients known to have decreased production of TNF-α, those who are HLA-DR2 or HLA-DQw1 positive. The mechanism of action of anti-IL-10 was to up-regulate TNF-α production and the administration of TNF-α to (NZB $\times$ NZW)F1 mice also delayed the onset of SLE (see above). In addition to counteracting the effects of IFN-γ in up-regulating MHC class II expression on antigen-presenting cells, TNF-α has also been reported to suppress autoreactive T cell proliferation.

Table 2. The role of cytokines in modifying the course of SLE

Cytokines
Treatment of NZB/W mice with IL-2 did not have any effect
IFN and IFN inducers accelerate the onset of disease
The administration of anti-IFN-γ antibodies slows the progression of renal disease in NZB/W F1 mice
In humans treatment of patients with IFNα and IFN-γ can induce a lupus-like disease
Administration of TNF-α to NZB/W mice delayed the onset of autoimmune disease
Administration of anti-IL-10 delayed the onset of autoimmunity in NZB/W F1 mice
Anti-IL-6 receptor antibody blocked autoantibody sythesis in vitro
Cytokine genes
Treatment of MRL-lpr/lpr with vaccinia virus genetically engineered to produce recombinant IL-2 lead to improvment of SLE
Transforming growth factor-β genes injected into the skeletal muscle of MRL-lpr/lpr mice decreased autoantibody production

TNF-α in combination with IL-1 has also been reported to up-regulate IL-6 production and this cytokine may be intimately involved in supporting B cell hyperactivity. Blocking IL-6 receptors may be another strategy to down-regulate antibody production in SLE. As stated above, there is little reason to down-regulate IL-4 production in human SLE.

It is unlikely that up-regulating TH1 cytokines will be of therapeutic benefit. Treatment of a patient with presumed rheumatoid arthritis with IFN-γ induced SLE [39, 83] and administration of IFN-α to patients with hematological malignancies has led to the appearance of autoantibodies and even clinical SLE [118, 119]. In fact, blocking rather than administering IFN-γ appears to be a more promising approach. Antibodies to IFN-γ slowed the progression of renal disease in NZB/NZW F1 mice [62]. Clearly, IFN and IFN inducers cannot repair the suppressor cell circuits in SLE and these agents will accelerate disease [23, 129] until the functional properties of $CD8^+$ T cells and NK cells are restored to normal. It is also unlikely that administration of IL-12 will have therapeutic effects. In this laboratory, recombinant IL-12 markedly increased rather than decreased antibody synthesis by SLE B cells in vitro (unpublished studies). It is important to emphasize that most of the positive effects of cytokines documented in mouse SLE have been to delay the onset of disease, rather than to alter the course of fully developed disease.

Since IL-2 production is decreased in both human and mouse SLE, this cytokine has been given to mice as a potential therapeutic agent. Injection of MRL-lpr/lpr mice every 14 days with live vaccinia viruses genetically engineered to produce recombinant IL-2 lead to improvement of SLE [41, 42]. The administration of IL-2 also corrected a T cell activation defect in NZB and MRL-lpr/lpr mice [52]. However, long-term treatment of NZB/NZW F1 mice with IL-2 did not lead to improvement [107]. Because of differing genetic backgrounds of these mice, it is not surprising that the outcomes of different experimental models of SLE would be different. Because of the diverse genetic backgrounds of patients with SLE, one also might expect different responses to a specific cytokine.

As stated above, TGF-β is a strongly suppressive cytokine in high concentrations and induces suppressor cell activity in low concentrations. TGF-β genes injected into the skeletal muscle of MRL-lpr/lpr mice decreased autoantibody production [115]. Because this cytokine appears to be an important co-factor in the generation of suppressor cells in addition to its immunosuppressive effects, it is conceivable that a strategy involving TGF-β could have therapeutic benefit. Because of the complexity of its production, considerably more information about the production and the response of lupus mononuclear cells to this cytokine is needed before this strategy could be implemented.

Acknowledgement. This work was supported in part by NIH grant AR 29 846 and the Southern California Chapter of the Arthritis Foundation (DAH) and by the Arthritis National Research Foundation.

References

1. Aderka D, Engelmann H, Maor Y, Brakebusch C, Wallach D (1992) Stabilization of the bioactivity of tumor necrosis factor by its soluble receptors. J Exp Med 175:323
2. Aderka D, Wysenbeek A, Engelmann H, et al (1993) Correlation between serum levels of soluble tumor necrosis factor receptor and disease activity in systemic lupus erythematosus. Arthritis Rheum 36:1111
3. Alcocer-Varela J, Alarcon-Segovia D (1982) Decreased production of and response to interleukin-2 by cultured lymphocytes from patients with systemic lupus erythematosus. J Clin Invest 69:1388
4. Alcocer-Varela J, Aleman-Hoey D, Alarcon-Segovia D (1992) Interleukin-I and interleukin-6 activities are increased in the cerebrospinal fluid of patients with CNS lupus erythematosus and correlate with local late T-cell activation markers. Lupus 1:111
5. Alcocer-Varela J, Laffon A, Alarcon-Segovia D (1983) Defective monocyte production of, and T lymphocyte response to, interleukin-1 in the peripheral blood of patients with systemic lupus erythematosus. Clin Exp Immunol 54:125

6. al Janadi M, al-Balla S, al-Dalaan A, Raziuddin S (1983) Cytokine profile in systemic lupus erythematousus, rheumtoid arthritis, and other rheumatic diseases. J Clin Immunol 13:58
7. Alleva DG, Burger CJ, Elgert KD (1993) Tumor-induced macrophage tumor necrosis factor-alpha production suppresses autoreactive T cell proliferation. Immunobiology 188:430
8. Aotsuka S, Nakamura K, Nakano T, Kawakami M, Goto M, Okawa-Takatsuji M, Kinoshita M, Yokohari R (1991) Production of intracellular and extracellular interleukin-1 alpha and interleukin-1 beta by peripheral blood monocytes from patients with connective tissue diseases. Ann Rheum Dis 50:27
9. Babcock SK, Appel VB, Schiff M, Palmer E, Kotzin BL (1989) Genetic analysis of the imperfect association of H-2 haplotype with lupus-like autoimmune disease. Proc Natl Acad Sci USA 86:7552
10. Beutler B, Krochin N, Milsark IW, Luedke C, Cerami A (1986) Control of cachectin (tumor necrosis factor) synthesis: mechanisms of endotoxin resistance. Science 232:977
11. Bizar-Scheebaum A, O'Dell JR, Kotzin BL (1987) Anti-histone antibody production by peripheral blood cells in SLE. Arthritis Rheum 30:511
12. Boswell JM, Yui MA, Burt DW, Kelley VE (1988) Increased tumor necrosis factor and IL-1β gene expression in the kidneys of mice with lupus nephritis. J Immunol 141:3050
13. Bottazzo GF, Pujol. Borrel R, Hanafusa T (1983) Role of aberrant HLA-DR expression and antigen presentation in induction of endocrine autoimmunity. Lancet II:1115
14. Brennan DC, Yui MA, Wuthrich RP, Kelley VE (1989) Tumor necrosis factor and IL-1 in New Zealand black/white mice. J Immunol 143:3470
15. Campen DH, Horwitz DA, Quismorio FQ Jr, Ehresmann GR, Martin WJ (1988) Serum levels of interleukin-2 receptor and activity of rheumatic disease characterized by immune system activation. Arthritis Rheum 31:1358
16. Casciola-Rosen LA, Anhalt G, Rosen A (1994) Autoantigens targeted in systemic lupus erythematosus are clustered in two populations of surface structures on apoptotic keratinocytes. J Exp Med 179:1317
17. Chang RJ, Lee SH (1986) Effects of interferon-γ and tumor necrosis factor-α on the expression of an Ia antigen on a murine macrophage cell line. J Immunol 137:2853
18. Chu EB, Ernst DN, Hobbs MV, Weigle WO (1994) Maturational changes in $CD4^+$ cell subsets and lymphokine production in BXSB mice. J Immunol 152:4129
19. Cosman D (1993) The hematopoietin receptor superfamily. Cytokine 5:95
20. Del Guidice G, Crow MK (1993) Role of transforming growth factor beta in systemic autoimmunity. Lupus 2:213
21. Dunham I, Sargent CA, Trowsdale J, Campbell DR (1987) Molecular mapping of the human major histocompatibility complex by pulse field gel electrophoresis. Proc Natl Acad Sci USA 84:7237
22. Ehlers MR, Riordan JF (1991) Membrande proteins with soluble counterparts: role of proteolysis in the release of transmembrane proteins. Biochem 30:10065
23. Engelman EG, Sonnenfeld G, Dauphinee M, Greenspan JS, Talal N, McDevitt HO, Merigan TC (1981) Treatment of NZB/NZW F1 mice with *Mycobacterium Bovis* strain BCG or type II interferon preparations accelerates autoimmune disease. Arthritis Rheum 24:1396
24. Engelmann H, Holtmann H, Brakebusch C, Avni YS, Sarov I, Nophar Y, Hadas E, Leitner O, Wallach D (1990) Antibodies to a soluble form of a tumor necrosis factor (TNF) receptor have TNF-like activity. J Biol Chem 265:14497
25. Falk LA, Wahl LM, Vogel SN (1988) Analysis of Ia antigen expression in macrophages derived from bone marrow cells cultured in granulocyte-macrophages colony-stimulating factor or macrophage colony-stimulating factor. J Immunol 140:2652
26. Fargeas C, Wu CY, Nakajima T, Cox D, Nutman T, Delespesse G (1992) Differential effect of transforming growth factor beta on the synthesis of Th1- and Th2-like lymphokines by human T lymphocytes. Eur J Immunol 22:2173
27. Fronek Z, Timmerman LA, Alper CA, Hahn BH, Kalunian K, Peterlin BM, McDevitt HO (1990) Major histocompatibility complex genes and susceptibility to systemic lupus erythematosus. Arthritis Rheum 33:1542
28. Funacuchi M, Sugishima H, Minoda M, Horiuchi A (1991) Effect of interferon-gamma on B lymphocyte of patients with systemic lupus erythematosus. J Rheumatol 18:368
29. Funauchi M, Minoda M, Horiuchi A (1991) Qualitative difference of anti-DNA antibody-producing cell precursors in the pre-immune B cell repertoire between normal and lupus-prone mice. Clin Exp Immunol 86:106

30. Gabay C, Roux-Lombard P, de Moerloose P, Dayer JM, Vischer T, Guerne PA (1993) Absence of correlation between interleukin 6 and C-reactive protein blood levels in systemic lupus erythematousus compared with rheumatoid arthritis. J Rheumatol 20:815
31. Geiser AG, Letterio JJ, Kulkarni AB, Karlsson S, Roberts AB, Sporn MB (1993) Transforming growth factor-beta 1 (TGF-beta 1) controls expression of major histocompatibility genes in the postnatal mouse: aberrant histocompatibility antigen expression in the pathogenesis of the TGF-beta I null mouse phenotype. Proc Natl Acad Sci USA 90:9944
32. Gharavi AE, Chu J, Elkon KB (1988) Autoantibodies to intracellular proteins in human systemic lupus erythematousus are not due to random polyclonal B cell activation. Arthritis Rheum 1:1337
33. Golbus J, Salata M, Greenwood J, Hudson J, Richardson BC (1988) Increased immunoglobulin response to gamma-interferon by lymphocytes from patients with systemic lupus erythematosus. Clin Immunol Immunopathol 46:129
34. Gordon C, Emery P (1993) Cytokines and the acute phase response in SLE. Lupus 2:345
35. Gordon C, Wofsy D (1990) Effects of recombinant murine tumor necrosis factor-α on immune function. J Immunol 144:1753
36. Gordon C, Ranges GE, Greenspan JS, Wofsy D (1989) Chronic therapy with recombinant tumor necrosis factor-α in autoimmune NZB/NZW F1 mice. Clin Immunol Immunopathol 52:42
37. Gordon C, Richards N, Howie AJ, et al. (1991) Urinary IL-6: a marker for mesangial proliferative glomerulonephritis. Clin Exp Immunol 86:145
38. Gottlieb AB, Lahita RG, Chiorazzi N, Kunkel HG (1979) Immune function in systemic lupus erythematosus. Impairment of in vitro T-cell proliferation and in vivo antibody response to exogenous antigen. J Clin Invest 63:885
39. Graninger WB, Hassfeld W, Pesau BB, Machold KP, Zielinski CC, Smolen JS (1991) Induction of systemic lupus erythematousus by interferon-gamma in a patient with rheumatoid arthritis. J Rheumatol 18:1621
40. Gray JD, Hirokawa M, Horwitz DA (1994) The role of transforming growth factor beta in the generation of suppression: an interaction between $CD8^+$ T cells and NK cells. (in press)
41. Gutierrez-Ramos JC, Andreu JL, Revilla Y, Vineula E, Martinez C (1990) Recovery from autoimmunity of MRL/lpr mice after infection with an interleukin-2/vaccinia recombinant virus. Nature 346:271
42. Gutierrez-Ramos JC, Andreu JL, Marcos MA, Vegazo IR, Martinez C (1991) Treatment with IL-2/vaccinia recombinant virus leads to serologic, histologic and phenotypic normalization of autoimmunity MRL/lpr-lpr mice, Autoimmunity 10:15
43. Hayakawa K, Hardy RR, Honda M, Herzenberg LA, Steinberg AD, Herzenberg LA (1984) Ly-1 B cells: functionally distinct lymphocytes that secrete IgM autoantibodies. Proc Natl Acad Sci USA 81:2494
44. Hefeneider SH, Cornell KA, Brown LE, Bakke AC, McCoy SL, Bennett RM (1992) Nucleosomes and DNA bind to specific cell-surface molecules on murine cells and induce cytokine production. Clin Immunol Immunopathol 63:245
45. Hefeneider SH, Brown LE, McCoy SL, Bakke AC, Cornell KA, Bennett RM (1993) Immunization of BALB/c mice with a monoclonal anti-DNA antibody induces an anti-idiotypic antibody reactive with a cell-surface DNA binding protein. Autoimmunity 15:187
46. Hirohata S, Miyamoto T (1990) Elevated levels of interleukin-6 in cerebrospinal fluid from patients with systemic lupus erythematosus and central nervous system involvement. Arthritis Rheum 33:644
47. Hirokawa M, Gray JD, Takahashi T, Horwitz DA (1992) Human resting B lymphocytes serve as accessory cells for anti-CD2 induced T cell activation. J Immunol 149:1859
48. Hirose T (1989) Spontaneous production of interleukin-1 and B cell stimulating factors by B cells from patients with systemic lupus erythematousus. Ryumachi 29:277
49. Hoffman M, Weinberg JB (1987) Tumor necrosis factor-α induces increased hydrogen peroxide production and Fc receptor expression, but not increased Ia antigen expression by peritoneal macrophages. J Leukoc Biol 42:704
50. Horwitz DA (1992) Systemic lupus erythematousus: generalized autoimmunity resulting from disordered immune regulation In: McCarty DJ, (ed) Arthritis and allied conditions 12th edn. Lea & Febiger, Philadelphia, pp 1185–1200
51. Horwitz DA, Wang H (1994) Cytokine gene profile in circulating blood mononuclear cells from patients with systemic lupus erythematousus : increased interleukin-2 but not interleukin 4 mRNA. Lupus 3:423

52. Huang FP, Stott DI (1993) Restoration of an early, progressive defect in responsiveness to T cell activation in lupus mice by exogenous IL-2. Autoimmunity 15:19
53. Huang YP, Miescher PA, Zubler RH (1986) The interleukin 2 secretion defect in vitro in systemic lupus erythematousus is reversible in rested cultured T cells. J Immunol 137:3515
54. Huang YP, Perrin LH, Miescher PA, Zubler RH (1988) Correlation of T and B cell activities in vitro and serum IL-2 levels in systemic lupus erythematosus. J Immunol 141:827
55. Ishida H, Kumagai S, Umehara H, Sano H, Tagaya Y, Yodoi J, Imura H (1987) Impaired expression of high affinity interleukin 2 receptor on activated lymphocytes from patients with systemic lupus erythematousus. J Immunol 139:1070
56. Ishida H, Hastings R, Kearney J, Howard M (1992) Continuous anti-interleukin 10 antibody administration depletes mice of Ly-1 cells but not conventional B cells. J Exp Med 175:1213
57. Ishida H, Hastings R, Thompson-Snipes L, Howard M (1993) Modified immunological status of anti-IL-10 treated mice. Cell Immunol 148:371
58. Ishida H, Muchamuel T, Sakaguchi S, Andrade S, Menon S, Howard M (1994) Continuous administration of anti-interleukin-10 antibodies delays onset of autoimmunity in NZB/W F_1 mice. J Exp Med 179:305
59. Jacob CO (1992) Studies on the role of tumor necrosis factor in murine and human autoimmunity. J Autoimmune 5:133
60. Jacob CO, McDevitt HO (1988) Tumor necrosis factor-α in murine autoimmune "lupus" nephritis. Nature 331:356
61. Jacob CO, McDevitt HO (1991) Interferon gamma and tumor necrosis factor in autoimmune disease models: implications for immunoregulation and genetic susceptibility. In Talal N (ed): Molecular autoimmunity. Academic Press, New York, pp 107–126
62. Jacob CO, Van Der Meide PH, McDevitt HO (1987) In vivo treatment of (NZB × NZW)F1 lupus-like nephritis with monoclonal antibody to γ-interferon. J Exp Med 166:798
63. Jacob CO, Fronek Z, Lewis GD, Koo M, Hansen JA, McDevitt HO (1990) Heritable major histocompatibility complex class II-associated differences in production of tumor necrosis factor-α: relevance to genetic predisposition to systemic lupus erythematosus. Proc Natl Acad Sci USA 87:1233
64. Jacob CO, Lewis GD, McDevitt HO (1991) MHC class II associated variation in the production of tumor necrosis factor in mice and humans: relevance to the pathogenesis of autoimmune diseases. Immunol Res 10:156
65. Jacob CO, Hwang F, Lewis GD, Stall AM (1992) Tumor necrosis factor-α in murine systemic lupus erythematosus disease models: implications for genetic predisposition and immune regulation. Cytokine 3:551
66. Jandl RC, George JL, Silberstein DS, Eaton RB, Schur PH (1987) The effect of adherent cell-derived factors on immunoglobulin and anti-DNA synthesis in systemic lupus erythematosus. Clin Immunol Immunopathol 42:344
67. Jongeneel CV, Acha-Orbea H, Blankenstein T (1990) A polymorphic microsatellite in the tumor necrosis factor α promoter identifies an allele unique to the NZW mouse strain. J Exp Med 171:2141
68. Kanayama Y, Kim T, Inariba H, Necoro N, Okamura M, Takeda T, Inoe T (1989) Possible involvement of interferon alpha in the pathogenesis of fever in systemic lupus erythematosus. Ann Rheum Dis 48:86
69. Kekow J, Wachsman W, McCutchan JA, Cronin M, Carson DA, Lotz M (1990) Transforming growth factor beta and noncytopathic mechanisms of immunodeficiency in human immunodeficiency virus infection. Proc Natl Acad Sci USA 87:8321
70. Kim T, Kanayama Y, Okamura M, Takeda T, Inoue T (1987) Serum levels of interferons in patients with systemic lupus erythematousus. Clin Exp Immunol 70:562
71. Kitani A, Hara M, Hirose T, Harigai M, Suzuki K, Kawakami M, Kawaguchi Y, Hidaka T, Kawagoe M, Nakamura H (1992) Autostimulatory effects of IL-6 on excessive B cell differentiation in patients with systemic lupus erythematousus: analysis of IL-6 production and IL-6R expression. Clin Exp Immunol 88:75
72. Klashman DJ, Martin RA, Martinez-Maza O, Stevens RH (1991) In vitro regulation of B cell differentiation by interleukin-6 and soluble CD23 in systemic lupus erythematosus B cell subpopulations and antigen-induced normal B cells. Arthritis Rheum 34:276
73. Knight JG, Adams DD (1978) Three genes for lupus nephritis in NZB × NZW mice. J Exp Med 147:1653

74. Kotzin BL, Palmer ED (1987) The contribution of NZW genes to lupus-like disease in (NZB × NZW)F1 mice. J Exp Med 165:1237
75. Laut J, Senitzer D, Petrucci R, Sablay LB, Barland P, Glicklich D (1992) Soluble interleukin-2 receptor levels in lupus nephritis. Clin Nephrol 38:179
76. Leeuwenberg JFM, van Damme J, Meager T, Jeunhomme TMAA, Buurman WA (1988) Effects of tumor necrosis factor on the interferon-γ induced major histocompatibility complex class II antigen expression by human endothelial cells. Eur J Immunol 18:1469
77. Linker-Israeli M, Bakke AC, Kitridou RC, Gendler S, Gillis S, Horwitz DA (1983) Defective production of interleukin 1 and interleukin 2 in patients with systemic lupus erythematosus (SLE). J Immunol 130:265
78. Linker-Israeli M, Bakke AC, Quismorio FP Jr, Horwitz DA (1985) Correction of interleukin-2 production in patients with systemic lupus erythematousus by removal of spontaneously activated suppressor cells. J Clin Invest 75:762
79. Linker-Israeli M, Quismorio FP Jr, Horwitz DA (1990) $CD8^+$ lymphocytes from patients with systemic lupus erythematousus lymphocytes sustain rather than suppress spontaneous polyclonal IgG production and synergize with $CD4^+$ cells to support autoantibody synthesis. Arthritis Rheum 33:1216
80. Linker-Israeli M, Deans RJ, Wallace DJ, Prehn J, Ozeri-Chen T, Klinenberg JR (1991) Elevated levels of endogenous IL-6 in systemic lupus erythematousus. A putative role in pathogenesis. J Immunol 147:117
80a. Llorente L, Richaud-Patin Y, Wijdenes J, Alcocer-Varela J, Maillot MC, Durand-Gasselin I, Fourrier BM, Galanaud P, Emile D (1993) Spontaneous production of interleukin-10 by B lymphocytes and monocytes in systemic lupus erythematosus. Eur Cytokine Netw 4:421
81. Loughlin AJ, Woodroofe MN, Cuzner ML (1993) Modulation of interferon-gamma-induced major histocompatibility complex class II and Fc receptor expression on isolated microglia by transforming growth factor-beta 1, interleukin-4, noradrenaline and glucocorticoids. Immunology 79:125
82. Lust JA, Donovan KA, Kline MP, Greipp PR, Kyle RA, Maihle NJ (1992) Isolation of an mRNA encoding a soluble form of the human interleukin-6 receptor. Cytokine 4:96
83. Machold KP, Smolen JS (1990) Interferon-gamma induced exacerbation of systemic lupus erythematosus. J Rheumatol 17:831
84. Malave I, Searles RP, Montano J, Williams RC Jr (1989) Production of tumor necrosis factor/cachetin by peripheral blood mononuclear cells in patients with systemic lupus erythematosus. Int Arch Allergy Appl Immunol 89:355
85. Malygin AM, Meri S, Timonen T (1993) Regulation of natural killer cell activity by transforming growth factor-beta and prostaglandin E2. Scand J Immunol 37:71
86. Manoussakis MN, Papadopoulos GK, Drosos AA, Moutsopoulos HM (1989) Soluble interleukin 2 receptor molecules in the serum of patients with autoimmune diseases. Clin Immunol Immunopathol 50:321
87. Matei I, Ghyka G, Savi I, Tudor A (1990) Correlation of serum interferon with some clinical and humoral signs of systemic lupus erythematousus. Med Interne 28:289
88. Maury CPJ, Teppo AM (1989) Tumor necrosis factor in the serum of patients with systemic lupus erythematosus. Arthritis Rheum 32:146
89. Meijer C, Huysen V, Smeenk RTJ, Swaak AJG (1993) Profiles of cytokines (TNF-α and IL-6) and acute phase proteins (CRP and $\alpha 1$ AG) related to the disease course in patients with systemic lupus erythematosus. Lupus 2:359
90. Metsarinne KP, Nordstrom CDe, Konttinen YT, Tepp AM, Fyhrquist FY (1992) Plasma interleukin-6 and renin substrate in reactive arthritis, rheumatoid arthritis and systemic lupus erythematosus. Rheumatol Int 12:93
91. Miyagi J, Minato N, Sumiya M, Kasahara T, Kano S (1989) Two types of antibodies inhibiting interleukin-2 production by normal lymphocytesin patients with systemic lupus erythematosus. Arthritis Rheum 32:1356
92. Miyasaka N, Nakamura T, Russell IJ, Talal N (1984) Interleukin-2 deficiencies in rheumatoid arthritis and systemic lupus erythematosus. Clin Immunol Immunopathol 31:109
93. Morris SC, Cheek RL, Cohen PL, Eisenberg RA (1990) Autoantibodies in chronic graft versus host result from cognate T-B interactions. J Exp Med 171:503
94. Mosmann TR, Coffman RL (1989) TH1 and TH2 cells: different patterns of lymphokine secretion lead to different functional properties. Annu Rev Immunol 7:145

95. Mullberg J, Dittrich E, Graeve L, Gerhartz C, Yasukawa K, Taga T, Kishimoto T, Heinrich PC, Rose-John S (1993) Differential shedding of the two subunits of the interleukin-6 receptor. FEBS Lett 332:174
96. Mullberg J, Schooltink H, Stoyan T, Gunther M, Graeve L, Buse G, Mackiewicz A, Heinrich PC, Rose-John S (1993) The soluble interleukin-6 receptor is generated by shedding. Eur J Immunol 23:473
97. Muller U, Jongeneel CV, Nedospasov SA, Lindahl KF, Steinmetz M (1987) Tumor necrosis factor and lymphotoxin genes map close to H-2D in mouse major histocompatibility complex. Nature 325:265
98. Murakawa Y, Takada S, Yueda Y, Suzuki N, Hoshino T, Sakane T (1985) Characterization of T lymphocyte subpopulations responsible for deficient interleukin-2 activity in patients with systemic lupus erythematousus. J Immunol 134:187
99. Murphy ED, Roths JB (1979) A Y-chromosome associated factor in strain BXSB producing accelerated autoimmunity and lymphoproliferation. Arthritis Rheum 22:1188
100. Nagafuchi H, Suzuki N, Mizushima Y, Sakane T (1993) Constitutive expression of IL-6 receptors and their role in the excessive B cell function in patients with systemic lupus erythematosus. J Immunol 151:6525
101. Nagai H, Sztein MB, Steeg PS, Hooks JJ, Oppenheim JJ, Steinberg AD (1984) Diminished peripheral blood monocyte DR antigen expression in systemic lupus erythematosus. Clin Exp Rheumatol 2:131
102. Naiki M, Chiang BL, Cawley D, Ansari A, Rozzo SJ, Kotzin BL, Zlotnik A, Gershwin ME (1992) Generation and characterization of cloned T helper cell lines for anti-DNA responses in NZB. H-2bm12 mice. J Immunol 149:4109
103. Nelson BJ, Ralph P, Green SJ, Nacy CA (1991) Effect of transforming growth factor-beta on early and late activation events in human T cells. J Immunol 146:1849
104. Nelson DL, Rubin LA, Kurmann CC, Fritz ME, Boutin B (1986) An analysis of the cellular requirements for the production of soluble interleukin-2 receptors in vitro. J Clin Immunol 6:114
105. Novick D, Engelmann H, Wallach D, Rubinstein M (1989) Soluble cytokine receptors are present in normal human urine. J Exp Med 170:1409
106. O'Garra A, Murphy K (1993) T-cell subsets in autoimmunity. Curr Opin Immunol 5:880
107. Owen KL, Shibata T, Izui S, Walker SE (1989) Recombinant interleukin-2 therapy of systemic lupus erythematousus in the New Zealand black/New Zealand white mouse. J Biol Resp Modif 8:366
108. Patton JS, Shepard MH, Wilking H, Lewis GD (1986) Interferons and tumor necrosis factor have similar catabolic effects on 3T3 L1 cells. Proc Natl Acad Sci USA 83:8313
109. Pelton BK, Speckmaier M, Hylton W, Farrant J, Denman AM (1991) Cytokine-independent progression of immunoglobulin production in vitro by B lymphocytes from patients with systemic lupus erythematousus. Clin Exp Immunol 83:274
110. Pelton BK, Hylton W, Denman AM (1992) Activation of IL-6 production by UV irradiation of blood mononuclear cells from patients with systemic lupus erythematosus. Clin Exp Immunol 89:251
111. Pfizenmaier K, Scheurich P, Schluter C, Kronke M (1987) Tumor necrosis factor enhances HLA-A, B, C and HLA DR gene expression in human tumor cells. J Immunol 138:975
112. Preble OT, Black RJ, Friedman RM, Klippel J, Vilcek J (1982) Systemic lupus erythematosus: presence in human serum of unusual acid labile leukocyte interferon. Science 216:429
113. Ragousis J, Bloemer K, Weiss EH, Ziegler A (1988) Localization of the genes for tumor necrosis factor and lymphotoxin between the HLA class I and Class III regions by field inversion gel electrophoresis. Immunogenetics 27:66
114. Raveche ES, Steinberg AD, Klassen KW, Tijo JH (1978) Genetic studies in NZB mice. J Exp Med 147:1487
115. Raz E, Watanabe A, Baird SM, Eisenberg RA, Parr TB, Lotz M, Kipps TJ, Carson DA (1993) Systemic immunological effects of cytokine genes injected into skeletal muscle. Proc Natl Acad Sci USA 90:4523
116. Remick DG, Nguyen DT, Eskandari MK, Strieter RM, Kunkel SL (1989) Cyclosporine-A inhibits TNF production without decreasing TNF messenger RNA levels. Biochem Biophys Res Commun 161:551
117. Rizzo LV, DeKruyff RH, Umetsu DT (1992) Generation of B cell memory and affinity maturation. Induction with Th1 and Th2 T cell clones. J Immunol 148:3733
118. Roennblom LE, Alm GV, Oberg K (1991) Autoimmune phenomena in patients with malignant carcinoid tumors during interferon-alpha treatment. Acta Oncol 30:537

119. Schlling PJ, Jurzrock R, Kantarjian H, Guttterman JU, Talpaz M (1991) Development of systemic lupus erythematousus after interferon therapy for chronic myelogenous leukemia. Cancer 68:1536
120. Seckinger P, Isaaz S, Dayer JM (1989) Purification and biologic characterization of a specific tumor necrosis factor alpha inhibitor. J Biol Chem 264:11966
121. Semenzato G, Bambara LM, Biasi D, Frigo A, Vinante F, Zuppini B, Trentin L, Feruglio C, Chilosi M, Pizzolo G (1988) Increased serum levels of soluble interleukin-2 receptor in patients with systemic lupus erythematousus and rheumatoid arthritis. J Clin Immunol 8:447
122. Sher A, Gazzinelli RT, Oswald IP, Clerici M, Kullberg M, Pearce EJ, Berzofsky JA, Mosmann TR, James SL, Morse HC (1992) Role of T-cell derived cytokines in the downregulation of immune responses in parasitic and retroviral infection. Immunol Rev 127:183
123. Shiozawa S, Kuroki Y, Kim M, Hirohata S, Ogino T (1992) Interferon-alpha in lupus psychosis. Arthritis Rheum 35:417
124. Shirakawa F, Yamashita U, Suzuki H (1985) Decrease in HLA-DR monocytes in patients with SLE. J Immunol 134:3560
125. Sierakowski S, Kucharz EJ, Lightfoot RW Jr, Goodwin JS (1987) Interleukin-1 production by monocytes from patients with systemic lupus erythematousus. Clin Rheum 6:403
126. Sims JE, Gayle MA, Slack JL, et al (1993) Interleukin 1 signaling occurs exclusively via the type I receptor. Proc Natl Acad Sci USA 90:6155
127. Spronk PE, ter Borg EJ, Limburg PC, Kallenberg CGM (1992) Plasma concentration of IL-6 in systemic lupus erythematousus. Clin Exp Immunol 90:106
128. Stall AM, Farinas MC, Tarlinton DM, Lalor PA, Herzenberg LA, Strober S, Herzenberg LA (1988) Ly-1 B cell clones similar to human chronic lymphocytic leukemias routinely develop in older mice and young autoimmune (New Zealand Blackrelated) animals. Proc Natl Acad Sci USA 85:7312
129. Steinberg AD, Kreig AM, Gourley MF, Klinman DM (1990) Theoretical and experimental approaches to generalized autoimmunity. Immunol Rev 118:129
130. Stohl W (1992) Impaired generation of polyclonal T cell-mediated cytolytic activity despite normal polyclonal T cell proliferation in systemic lupus erythematousus. Clin Immunol Immunopathol 63:163
131. Stolzenburg T, Binz H, Fontana A, Felder M, Wagenhaeuser FJ (1988) Impaired mitogen-induced interferon-gamma production in rheumatoid arthritis and related diseases. Scand J Immunol 27:73
132. Tada T, Ohzeki S, Utsumi K, Takiuchi H, Muramatsu M, Li XF, Shimizu J, Fujiwara H, Hamaoka T (1991) Transforming growth factor-beta-induced inhibition of T cell function. Susceptibility difference in T cells of various phenotypes and functions and its relevance to immunosuppression in the tumor-bearing state. J Immunol 146:1077
133. Tanaka T, Saiki O, Negoro S, Igarashi T, Kuritani T, Hara H, Suemura M, Kishimoto S (1989) Decreased expression of intererleukin-2 binding molecules (p7O/75) in T cells from patients with systemic lupus erythematousus. Arthritis Rheum 32:552
134. Tanaka Y, Saito K, Shirakawa F, Ota T, Suzuki H, Eto H, Yamashita U (1988) Production of B cell-stimulating factors by B cells in patients with systemic lupus erythematosus J Immunol 141:3043
135. Tanaka Y, Saito K, Suzuki H, Eto H, Yamashita U (1989) Inhibitory effect of anti-class II antibody on the spontaneous activation of B cells in patients with systemic lupus erythematosus. Analysis with IL-1 production and IL-1 receptor expression. J Immunol 143:1584
136. ter Borg EJ, Horst G, Limburg PC, Kallenberg CGM (1990) Changes in plasma levels of interleukin 2 receptor in relation to disease exacerbations and levels of anti-dsDNA and complement in systemic lupus erythematousus. Clin Exp Immunol 82:21
137. Theofilopoulos AN, Dixon FJ (1985) Murine models of systemic lupus erythematosus. Adv Immunol 37:269
138. Tsokos GC, Rook AH, Djeu JY, Balow JE (1982) Natural killer cells and interferon responses in patients with systemic lupus erythematousus. Clin Exp Immunol 5:239
139. Tsokos GC, Boumpas DT, Smith PL, Djeu JY, Balow JE, Rook AH (1986) Deficient gamma-interferon production in patients with systemic lupus erythematosus. Arthritis Rheum 29:1210
140. Via CS, Tsokos GC, Bermas B, Clerici M, Shearer GM (1993) T cell-antigen-presenting cell interactions in human systemic lupus erythematousus. Evidence for heterogeneous expression of multiple defects. J Immunol 151:3914
141. Von Wussow P, Jakschies D, Hartung K, Deicher H (1988) Presence of interferon and anti-interferon in patients with systemic lupus erythematosus. Rheumatol Int 8:225
142. Warrington RJ, Rutherford WJ (1990) Normal mitogen-induced suppression of the interleukin-6 response and its deficiency in systemic lupus erythematosus. J Clin Immunol 10:52

3. Watanabe Y, Jacob CO (1991) Regulation of MHC class II antigen expression: opposing effects of TNF-α on IFN-γ induced HLA-DR and Ia expression depends on the maturation and differentiation state of the cell. J Immunol 146:899
4. Wolf RE, Brelsford WG (1988) Soluble interleukin-2 receptors in systemic lupus erythematosus. Arthritis Rheum 31:729
5. Wong GHW, Goeddel DV (1986) Tumor necrosis factor-α and -β inhibit virus replication and synergize with interferons. Nature 323:819
6. Yasukawa K, Saito T, Fukunaga T, et al (1990) Purification and characterization of soluble human IL-6 receptor expressed in CHO cells. J Biochem 108:673
7. Yssel H, De Waal-Malefyt R, Roncarolo MG, Abrams JS, Lahesmaa R, Spits H, de Vries JE (1992) IL-10 is produced by subsets of human $CD4^+$ T cell clones and peripheral blood T cells. J Immunol 149:2378

Antibodies to CD45 and other cell membrane antigens in systemic lupus erythematosus

John B. Winfield[1], Philip Fernsten[1], Jan Czyzyk[1], Ena Wang[2], John Marchalonis[2]

[1]Division of Rheumatology and Immunology, University of North Carolina, Chapel Hill, 932 FLOB 231H CB#7280, Chapel Hill, NC 27599, USA
[2]University of Arizona, Tucson, Arizona 85724, USA

Introduction

At some point in their illness, most patients with systemic lupus erythematosus (SLE) develop cold-reactive IgM anti-lymphocyte autoantibodies, which appear to represent a type of natural autoantibody that exhibits a disease-related increase in titer. Increased levels of such autoantibodies are found during flares of SLE disease activity in association with lymphopenia [7, 61], suggesting a causal relationship with T cell depletion and various functional abnormalities of T cells, B cells, and monocytes. Addition of SLE serum or immunoglobulin with anti-lymphocyte autoantibody activity to in vitro cultures of normal peripheral blood mononuclear cells alters their function in ways closely paralleling that of freshly isolated lymphocytes and monocytes from patients with SLE. Mechanisms by which such functional effects could occur in vivo include: (a) elimination of cells by complement-mediated lysis, antibody-dependent, cell-mediated cytotoxicity [15], and/or opsonization; (b) alteration of lymphocyte migration patterns; (c) modulation of surface determinants [63]; (d) agonist, partial agonist, or antagonist effects on cell surface receptors [38, 39, 65]; and (e) interaction with soluble products of activated cells [18]. Thus, autoantibodies to lymphocyte and monocyte surface determinants may constitute one of the pathogenetically significant extrinsic elements that alters cellular immune function in this disorder.

This brief review discusses some of the general characteristics of anti-lymphocyte autoantibodies in SLE. Special emphasis is given to ongoing investigation in the authors' laboratories regarding CD45 as a potentially important target and to largely unpublished data concerning SLE IgG reactivity with T cell receptor peptides.

Correspondence to: J.B. Winfield

General characteristics of anti-lymphocyte autoantibodies

IgM autoantibodies, the major type detected in conventional two-stage complement-dependent cytotoxicity assays performed at colder temperatures, are broadly reactive with autologous lymphocytes and lymphocytes from unrelated donors [25, 54, 62] and are produced almost universally in disorders of persistent immune system stimulation. Originally described in patients with viral infections as "naturally occurring cold lymphocytotoxins" [53], cold-reactive IgM anti-lymphocyte autoantibodies are clearly distinct from "warm-reactive" IgG alloantibodies to HLA antigens that develop as a consequence of pregnancy or multiple transfusions. The thermal binding properties of IgM autoantibodies have been exploited for their isolation and purification by elution from cells at warm temperatures. Conversely, carry-over of cold-reactive IgM autoantibody bound to cells during lymphocyte isolation procedures performed at temperatures less than 37 C can be a source of artifact in studies of disease-related abnormalities in lymphocyte populations and function. IgG anti-lymphocyte autoantibodies in SLE have been less well characterized, primarily because they do not lyse lymphocytes in the presence of complement [62] and because immunofluorescence assays for their detection require special approaches to avoid artifactual Fc_{γ} or complement receptor binding, e.g. use of $F(ab')_2$ anti-immunoglobulin reagents and/or isolation of 7S monomeric IgG from serum or plasma using acid pH buffers to dissociate immune complexes.

Cell type specificity of anti-lymphocyte autoantibodies

Autoantibodies to T cells and T cell subsets

Early studies emphasized a relative specificity of lymphocytotoxic autoantibodies in SLE for T cells, especially thymocytes [17]. The existence of autoantibodies to discrete T cell subsets was suggested initially by the demonstration that T cells in a discrete layer of discontinuous Ficoll gradient-fractionated peripheral lymphocytes were reduced in patients with anti-lymphocyte autoantibodies in their serum directed to this fraction [11]. Autoantibodies to this lymphocyte fraction inhibited concanavalin A (Con A)-induced T cell suppression of the allogeneic mixed leukocyte reaction [58]. This observation, together with discoveries that (a) IgG anti-T cell autoantibodies in SLE serum inhibited the allogeneic MLR [59], (b) autoantibodies to $T\gamma$ cells (Fc_{γ} receptor positive) prevented the generation of Con A-stimulated non-specific T cell suppressor activity [44, 45], and (c) a T cell subset staining brightly with IgM from patient serum was markedly depleted in active SLE [47], were among the first to suggest a potential contribution of anti-lymphocyte autoantibodies to immune system dysfunction in this disorder.

Subsequent investigation using monoclonal antibodies to T cell receptors during the 1980s suggested that anti-T cell autoantibodies in SLE were more reactive with $CD8^+$ cells than with $CD4^+$ cells, a finding consistent with the idea that autoantibody-mediated $CD8^+$ cell depletion was responsible for reduced T cell suppressor function [26, 46]. When highly purified peripheral $CD4^+$ and $CD8^+$ T cells and $CD4^+$ and $CD8^+$ T cell clones are used as targets in complement-dependent cytotoxicity assays, however, overall cytotoxicity by SLE sera for these two subsets is similar, indicating that reactivity of T cells to classic cold-reactive anti-lymphocyte autoantibodies is determined primarily by the presence of antigen(s) that are shared by $CD4^+$ and $CD8^+$ subsets [66]. Superimposed on this major antigen/antibody system common to both subsets is a slight, but consistent, preferential reactivity with $CD4^+$ T cells [66], especially $CD4^+$ T cells expressing high levels of CD45RA [27, 50]. IgM autoantibodies to $CD4^+$,$CD45RA^+$ T cells have been associated with relative depletion of this subset in the circulation of patients with active disease [24, 52] and with a reduced capacity for suppressor-inducer function [28, 51, 52]. Additional complexity is suggested by recent observations that the relative cytotoxicity of SLE sera for $CD4^+$ and $CD8^+$ T cells varies with assay temperature [33], autoantibody titer, and SLE disease activity status [68].

Autoantibodies to activated T cells

Autoantibody binding to activated lymphocytes occurs preferentially at physiological temperatures and has been associated with suppression of mitogen and soluble antigen-induced T cell activation and proliferation [18, 60, 65]. SLE sera also contain IgG autoantibodies with the capacity to develop reverse hemolytic plaques in mitogen-activated T lymphocyte preparations, indicating reactivity with products released by activated T cells [18]. The elimination of the ability of SLE sera to develop plaques after absorption with viable T cell blasts, but not with resting cells, suggests that such autoantibodies are directed toward activation antigens shed from the surface membrane, but their exact nature has not been defined. Obvious candidates for future research in this area include the various soluble receptors for cytokines and adhesion molecules that are increased in the circulation of patients with SLE and other disorders.

Autoantibodies to B cells

SLE sera frequently contain cold-reactive IgM cytotoxic autoantibodies to B cells from various sources [23, 32, 54], which are at least partially distinct from autoantibodies to T cells. This type of IgM anti-B cell autoantibody develops in many immunological diseases other than SLE, and in normal individuals [32, 48]. IgG autoantibodies to B cells also have been reported [1, 49, 60], although at least some of this IgG B cell binding may represent IgG/Fc_γ receptor interactions rather than true antibody.

Autoantibodies to other cells

Relatively less emphasis has been directed toward autoantibodies to monocytes [2], NK cells [43], and to neutrophils, which occur in both neutropenic and non-neutropenic patients with SLE and a broad range of other diseases [19]. Autoantibodies to determinants shared by brain tissue or neuronal cell lines and lymphocytes have also been described, but their significance with respect to the pathogenesis of CNS manifestations in SLE is unclear [6].

Membrane targets

CD45

CD45 is a transmembrane protein expressed at high levels (> 10^6 molecules/cell) on hemopoietic cells and, interestingly, endothelial cells [10, 56, 57]. The extracellular portion of CD45 consists of three subdomains: a variable, highly O-glycosylated region and two cysteine rich subdomains. Its highly conserved intracytoplasmic segment consists of two internally homologous tyrosine phosphatase domains. CD45 is encoded by a single gene, which generates five different isoforms by alternative splicing of exons 4, 5 and 6 (also called exons A, B, and C). These isoforms have molecular masses of 180 kDa (4−, 5−, 6−), 190 kDa (4−, 5+, 6−), 205 kDa (4−, 5+, 6+), 205 kDa (4+, 5+, 6−), and 220 kDa (4+, 5+, 6+). The variable splicing of exons 4–6 alters the number of potential *N*- and *O*-glycosylation sites, and qualitative differences in the glycosylation patterns of the higher molecular weight isoforms have been demonstrated. The polymorphism of the *O*-glycosylated domain may allow specific associations with other cell surface receptors to regulate transmembrane signalling. Thus, the arrangement of the molecule suggests that the cytoplasmic enzymatic activity is under the control of extracellular ligand-binding structures with discrete ligands for the different CD45 isoforms, although their exact nature remains in question. Monoclonal antibodies (mAb) against restricted epitopes (CD45R) were initially considered to subdivide T cells into functionally distinct 'naive' and 'memory' subsets that express either the higher molecular weight p220 and p205 (CD45RA) isoforms or the p180 CD45R0) isoform [4], but more recent data suggest that CD45 phenotype shifts reflect activation status and different requirements for activation (reviewed in [3, 5].

That CD45 might be a target of IgM anti-lymphocyte antibodies was suggested initially by studies using the mAb anti-2H4 (anti-CD45RA), which showed (a) that patients with active SLE had significantly decreased percentages of circulating T cells bearing the $CD4^+$,$2H4^+$ phenotype [28], and (b) that anti-lymphocyte antibodies from these patients reacted preferentially with the $CD4^+$,$2H4^+$ subset [52]. In blotting experiments utilizing T cell glycoproteins isolated by lectin chromatography techniques, 25% of IgM anti-lymphocyte antibody-positive sera from 100 unselected patients with SLE contained anti-CD45 autoantibodies, primarily of the CD45RA isoform [24] and Winfield et al., unpublished results). The overall prevalence of anti-CD45 autoantibodies in this panel was ~ 15%. Preliminary analysis suggests an association of anti-CD45 autoantibodies with active SLE. At least some of the autoreactive epitopes appeared to be distinct from the CD45RA epitope(s) (expressed on p220 and p205 isoforms) and the CD45RO epitope(s) (expressed on the p180 isoform), recognized by mAb anti-2H4 and UCHL-1, respectively. Thus, of nine SLE sera studied in detail, four reacted with p220 and p205, but the others reacted with p205 alone (one serum), p220 alone (two sera), p205, p190, and p180 (one serum), and p220, p205, and p190 (one serum). This dominant specificity of SLE autoantibodies for the p220 and p205 isoforms suggested that they may recognize the CD45RA epitope encoded, at least in part, by exon 4.

As a first step in elucidating the fine specificity in autoantibodies in this system, recombinant *E. coli* fusion proteins encoded by CD45 exons 3–7 (p220 and p180 isoforms) were examined by Western blotting for reactivity with SLE IgM anti-CD45 autoantibodies (Fernsten et al., unpublished results). Although appropriately reactive with certain mouse mAb to CD45, CD45 polypeptides were recognized by none of 14 anti-CD45-positive SLE sera. These data suggested that anti-CD45 autoantibodies in SLE are directed against conformational and/or carbohydrate epitopes, rather than linear polypeptide epitopes. This issue was examined further using CD45 purified from T cells by lectin affinity chromatography with and without chemical or enzymatic deglycosylation as substrates. Treatment of CD45 with 25 mM sodium-*m*-periodate sufficient to abrogate binding to various lectins but without effect on reactivity with CD45RA-type mouse mAb directed against a linear polypeptide epitope, completely abolished the reactivity with SLE anti-CD45 autoantibodies. The reactivity of one serum was removed completely by treatment of CD45 with 50 mM borate and was restored by washing in 50 mM acetic acid pH 4.5. Conversely, *N*-glycosidase F, which increased the mobility of CD45 in Western blotting by cleavage of accessible *N*-linked sugars, did not reduce staining of CD45 by the SLE autoantibodies. Taken together, these results suggest that IgM anti-CD45 autoantibodies in SLE recognize carbohydrate determinants in the highly *O*-glycosylated polymorphic domains of CD45 primarily.

The isoform specificities of SLE autoantibodies suggests that they could mimic certain ligands and stimulate or inhibit phosphatase activity, a hypothesis consistent with earlier data showing that SLE anti-lymphocyte autoantibodies inhibit early phase activation events in the T cell proliferative response to tetanus toxoid [65]. Alternatively, such autoantibodies could sterically hinder ligand binding or influence the association of CD45 with other lymphocyte surface molecules.

CD45 is absolutely required for soluble antigen-induced T cell proliferation [34] and clearly plays a central role in the regulation of proximal signal transduction in lymphocytes and other cell types generally. In T cells, recent biochemical observations support a model in which CD45 exerts permissive effects on two members of Src family of tyrosine kinases, *lck* and *fyn*, and ZAP 70, a tyrosine kinase that associates with the T cell receptor (TCR) ζ chain (reviewed [14]. With respect to *lck*, for example, the action of CD45 in T cell signalling via the TCR appears to involve (a) engagement of the TCR with antigen bound to MHC molecules, which facilitates interaction of CD4/*lck* with CD45 and (b) CD45-mediated dephosphorylation of a tyrosine residue at the carboxy terminus of *lck*, which enables the *lck* to adopt a conformation suitable for association with its substrates. *lck* then rapidly phosphorylates tyrosine residues on several intracellular substrates in the ensuing cascade of T cell activation. CD45 also appears to act in analogous fashion in cellular activation involving many other receptors on lymphocytes and other cell types.

Depending on the nature of the activation signals, the experimental conditions of the assays, and the state of lymphocyte activation, different anti-CD45 mAb profoundly influence cell function. In some cases, such actions of anti-CD45 mAb have been related to their specificity for glycoproteins, which constitute a very heterogeneous molecular complex with epitopes that are selectively expressed by different cell types and at different stages of maturation. This raises the question that the apparent heterogeneity of SLE anti-lymphocyte autoantibodies for different cell types and their diverse functional effects both might reflect specificities for different forms of CD45. In other cases, the immunoglobulin class of the mAb may be important. For example, two anti-CD45 mAb that were found to have profound inhibitory effects on LFA-1-induced NK activation and cytolysis were both of the IgM isotype [36]; none of a large panel of IgG anti-CD45 mAb exhibited this capacity. This suggests that IgM anti-CD45 autoantibodies might be particularly active in perturbing CD45 regulatory effects in the immune system.

T cell receptor

IgM anti-lymphocyte autoantibodies in certain SLE sera react with T cells bearing either $\alpha\beta$ or $\gamma\delta$ TCR, but not with T cells that do not express TCR [HSB-2 and JRT3.T3.5, a CD3-TCR-Jurkat mutant that expresses most other surface determinants of peripheral T cells (Winfield et al., unpublished data)]. These data raise the possibility that SLE autoantibodies could be directed against the TCR. Indeed, given the frequency of rheumatoid factors and other anti-Ig autoantibodies in human disease, it would be surprising if such autoantibodies did not exist.

Recent data from the laboratory of John Marchalonis bear on this issue. First, healthy individuals and individuals suffering from autoimmune diseases have IgG autoantibodies against particular segments of their own TCR β chains [20]. Thus, in ELISA analyses of a series of overlapping 16-mer synthetic peptides derived from the sequence of the TCR β chain, different peptides exhibited interesting patterns of reactivity with human IgM and IgG from various population groups. Although SLE Ig binding was not increased relative to normal Ig binding, peptides corresponding to the first complementarity determining region (CDR1) and the third framework of the variable region (FR3) were much more reactive than other peptides, e.g., N terminus. In related studies [21, 22], IgM binding to CDR1 and FR3 was generally higher than IgG binding, an observation that was particularly striking in patients with rheumatoid arthritis. Age-related change in the degree of reactivity of normal IgG and IgM with CDR1 was noted, with IgM anti-CDR1 being highest in young adults and decreasing with increasing age. Synthetic peptides corresponding to CDR2 and the switch region of TCR $V\beta$ and $V\alpha$ chains have been studied in similar fashion (Marchalonis et al., unpublished data). IgG binding to $V\alpha$ CDR2 was consistently higher in SLE sera than in normal or pregnancy sera, whereas IgG reactivity with $V\beta$ and λ light chain CDR2 peptides was absent in all three of these groups. Of 30 SLE sera 2 also exhibited very high levels of IgG antibody to $V\alpha$, but not $V\beta$, switch region peptides.

Additional work will be required to determine the significance of these findings, especially with respect to the question of whether or not such antibodies in normal and autoimmune disease sera can recognize CDR3, which is most important for peptide binding (reviewed in [8]), and native TCR determinants on the cell surface. Nevertheless, different patterns of IgG or IgM reactivity with distinct peptides from exposed regions of the TCR are clearly demonstrable, raising the possibility, at least, that antibodies of this type may affect T cell function, either physiologically or pathogenetically. For example, recent data based on experiments with altered peptide ligands suggest that TCR signalling is not a simple "on-off" phenomenon, but rather is a continuum that encompasses: (a) full agonist triggering (complete signaling resulting in full T cell activation); (b) partial agonist triggering (partial T cell activation resulting in anergy induction, cytolysis without proliferation, or cytokine production without proliferation); and (c) inhibition of triggering that occurs when a stimulatory agonist (peptide, superantigen, or alloantigen) and an antagonist TCR ligand are simultaneously present [9]. This continuum of T cell triggering undoubtedly is part of the normal immune response and may, in autoimmune diseases such as SLE, contribute to well-recognized phenomena like T cell anergy in the setting of intense B cell production of autoantibodies. It will be particularly interesting to determine whether anti-TCR peptide autoantibodies can function as partial agonists or antagonists.

Other targets

Other anti-lymphocyte autoantibody specificities that have been reported in SLE include: the IL-2 receptor [13]; β_2 microglobulin [23, 31, 42, 67]; HLA class I heavy chains [23, 35]; a DR framework epitope [30]; IgM and IgD on B cells [37, 48]; determinants on plasma membrane molecules that cross-react with histones and DNA [12, 16, 39–41] and glycosphingolipids [29]. The latter appear to be targets of IgG autoantibodies and have been associated with lymphopenia. Cold agglutinins with I,i specificity also represent a type of IgM anti-lymphocyte autoantibody since I,i antigens are expressed on lymphocytes, but contribute relatively little to the lymphocytotoxic activity of SLE sera as detected in conventional assays performed at cold temperatures [55, 62]. Although vigorously pursued, neither viral antigens nor anti-viral antibodies have been convincingly implicated as part of the anti-lymphocyte autoantibody system.

Conclusions

The multivalency of cold-reactive IgM anti-lymphocyte autoantibodies, together with the local density of reactive antigens on the cell surface, may confer a capacity for a variety of immunoregulatory and non-specific physiological roles in the immune system and in SLE and other autoimmune diseases. Targets of interest in this regard include CD45, β_2 microglobulin, and surface immunoglobulin. IgG anti-lymphocyte autoantibodies, while more difficult to study, also exhibit interesting specificities. However, whether any of the mechanisms by which anti-lymphocyte autoantibodies could alter cellular function actually obtain in vivo remains speculative. Essentially all of the data in this regard derive from experiments in which anti-lymphocyte autoantibody-containing SLE serum or plasma, or purified Ig fractions thereof, is combined with peripheral blood mononuclear cells in short-term culture in vitro. Thus, it is possible that anti-lymphocyte autoantibodies in SLE, rather than contributing to pathogenesis, reflect a physiological attempt by the immune system to restore homeostasis in the face of aggressive autoimmune stimulation.

Acknowledgement. Some of the experimental work cited in this article was supported in part by National Institutes of Health grants AR30863, AR7416, AR30701 and CA42049, and #I103 from the Arizona Disease Control Research Commission.

References

1. Anderson CL, Stillman WS (1980) Raji assay for immune complexes. Evidence for detection of Raji-directed immunoglobulin G antibody in sera from patients with systemic lupus erythematosus. J Clin Invest 66:353
2. Arend WP, Emmerich TE, Sturge JC, Starkebaum GA (1977) Monocyte-reactive antibodies in patients with systemic lupus erythematosus. Arthritis Rheum 20:1049
3. Bell EB (1992) Function of CD4 T cell subsets in vivo: expression of CD45R isoforms. Semin Immunol 4:43
4. Beverley PC (1987) Human T cell subsets. Immunol Lett 14:26344.
5. Beverley PC (1992) Functional analysis of human T cell subsets defined by CD45 isoform expression. Semin Immunol 4:35
6. Bluestein HG, Zvaifler NJ (1976) Brain-reactive lymphocytotoxic antibodies in the serum of patients with systemic lupus erythematosus. J Clin Invest 57:509
7. Butler WT, Sharp JT, Rossen RD (1972) Relationship of the clinical course of systemic lupus erythematosus to the presence of circulating lymphocytotoxic antibodies. Arthritis Rheum 15:231
8. Chien Y-H, Davis MM (1993) How alpha beta T-cell receptors "see" peptide/MHC complexes. Immunol Today 14:597
9. Evavold BD, Sloan-Lancaster J, Allen PM (1993) Tickling the TCR: selective T-cell functions stimulated by altered peptide ligands. Immunol Today 14:602
10. Forsyth KD, Chua K-Y, Talbot V, Thomas WR (1993) Expression of the leukocyte common antigen CD45 by endothelium. J Immunol 150:3471
11. Glinski W, Gershwin ME, Steinberg AD (1976) Fractionation of cells on a discontinuous Ficoll gradient. Study of subpopulations of human T cells using anti-T cell antibodies from patients with systemic lupus erythematosus. J Clin Invest 57:604
12. Jacob L, Lety M-A, Louvard D, Bach J-F (1985) Binding of a monoclonal anti-DNA autoantibody to identical protein(s) present at the surface of several human cell types involved in lupus pathogenesis. J Clin Invest 75:315
13. Kagami M, Koike T, Takabayashi K, Tomioka H, Yoshida S (1987) Antibody to activated lymphocytes in patients with systemic lupus erythematosus. J Rheumatol 14:907
14. Koretzky GA (1993) Role of the CD45 tyrosine phosphatase in signal transduction in the immune system. FASEB J 7:420
15. Kumagai S, Steinberg AD, Green I (1981) Antibodies to T cells in patients with systemic lupus erythematosus can induce antibody-dependent cell-mediated cytotoxicity against human T cells. J Clin Invest 67:605
16. Lafer EM, Rauch J, Andrzejewski C Jr, Mudd D, Furie B, Schwartz RS, Stollar BD (1981) Polyspecific monoclonal lupus autoantibodies reactive with both polynucleotides and phospholipids. J Exp Med 153:897
17. Lies RB, Messner RP, Williams RC Jr (1973) Relative T-cell specificity of lymphocytotoxins from patients with systemic lupus erythematosus. Arthritis Rheum 16:369
18. Litvin DA, Cohen PL, Winfield JB (1983) Characterization of warm-reactive IgG anti-lymphocyte antibodies in systemic lupus erythematosus. Relative specificity for mitogen-activated T cells and their soluble products. J Immunol 130:181
19. Maher GM, Hartman KR (1993) Detection of antineutrophil autoantibodies by flow cytometry: use of unfixed neutrophils as antigenic targets. J Clin Lab Anal 7:334
20. Marchalonis JJ, Kaymaz H, Dedeoglu F, Schluter SF, Yocum DE, Edmundson AB (1992) Human autoantibodies reactive with synthetic autoantigens from T-cell receptor beta chain. Proc Natl Acad Sci USA 89:3325
21. Marchalonis JJ, Kaymaz H, Schluter SF, Yocum DE (1993) Human autoantibodies to a synthetic putative T cell receptor β -chain regulatory idiotype: expression in autoimmunity and aging. Exp Clin Immunogenet 10:1
22. Marchalonis JJ, Schluter SF, Wilson L, Yocum DE, Boyer JT, Kay MMB (1993) Natural human antibodies to synthetic peptide autoantigens: correlations with age and autoimmune disease. Gerontology 39:65
23. Messner RP, DeHoratius RJ, Ferrone S (1980) Lymphocytotoxic antibodies in systemic lupus erythematosus patients and their relatives. Reactivity with the HLA antigenic molecular complex. Arthritis Rheum 23:265

4. Mimura T, Fernsten P, Jarjour W, Winfield JB (1990) Autoantibodies specific for different isoforms of CD45 in systemic lupus erythematosus. J Exp Med 172:653
5. Mittal KK, Rossen RD, Sharp JT, Lidsky MD, Butler WT (1970) Lymphocyte cytotoxic antibodies in systemic lupus erythematosus. Nature 225:1255
6. Morimoto C, Reinherz EL, Abe T (1980) Characteristics of anti-T cell antibodies in systemic lupus erythematosus: evidence for selective reactivity with normal suppressor cells defined by monoclonal antibodies. Clin Immunol Immunopathol 16:474
7. Morimoto C, Letvin NL, Distaso JA, Aldrich WR, Schlossman SF (1985) The isolation and characterization of the human suppressor inducer T cell subset. J Immunol 134:1508
8. Morimoto C, Steinberg AD, Letvin NL, Hagan M, Takeuchi T, Daley J, Levine H, Schlossman SF (1987) A defect of immunoregulatory T cell subsets in systemic lupus erythematosus patients demonstrated with anti-2H4 antibody. J Clin Invest 79:762
9. Noguchi M, Iwamori M, Hirano T, Kobayashi S, Hashimoto H, Hirose S, Nagai Y (1992) Autoantibodies to T and B cell lines detected in serum samples from patients with systemic lupus erythematosus with lymphopenia and hypocomplementaemia. Ann Rheum Dis 51:713
0. Okudaira K, Searles RP, Ceuppens JL, Goodwin JS, Williams RC Jr (1982) Anti-Ia reactivity in sera from patients with systemic lupus erythematosus. J Clin Invest 69:17
1. Ooi BS, Ooi YM, Pesce AJ, Pollak V (1977) Antibodies to β_2 microglobulin in the sera of patients with systemic lupus erythematosus. Immunology 33:535
2. Ozturk GE, Terasaki PI (1979) Non-HLA lymphocyte cytotoxins in various diseases. Tissue Antigens 14:52
3. Peake PW, Greenstein JD, Timmermans V, Gavrilovic L, Charlesworth JA (1988) Lymphocytotoxic antibodies in systemic lupus erythematosus: studies of their temperature dependence, binding characteristics, and specificity in vitro. Ann Rheum Dis 47:725
4. Pingel JT, Thomas ML (1989) Evidence that the leukocyte-common antigen is required for antigen-induced T lymphocyte proliferation. Cell 58:1055
5. Pischel KD, Bluestein HG, Woods VL Jr (1984) Molecular characterization of lymphocyte cell surface proteins reactive with systemic lupus erythematosus (SLE) autoantibodies. Arthritis Rheum 27:83
6. Poggi A, Pardi R, Pella N, Morelli L, Sivori S, Vitale M, Revello V, Moretta A, Moretta L (1993) CD45-mediated regulation of LFA1 function in human natural killer cells. Anti-CD45 monoclonal antibodies inhibit the calcium mobilization induced via LFA1 molecules. Eur J Immunol 23:2454
7. Pope RM, Keightley R, McDuffy S (1982) Circulating autoantibodies to IgD in rheumatic diseases. J Immunol 128:1860
8. Ramirez F, Williams RC, Sibbitt WL, Searles RP (1986) Immunogloblin from systemic lupus erythematosus serum induces interferon release by normal mononuclear cells. Arthritis Rheum 29:326
9. Rekvig OP (1989) Intrinsic cell membrane antigen recognized by antichromatin autoantibodies; The membrane antigens do not derive from the nucleus. Scand J Immunol 29:7
0. Rekvig OP, Hannestad K (1977) Certain polyclonal anti-nuclear antibodies cross-react with the surface membrane of human lymphocytes and granulocytes. Scand J Immunol 6:1041
1. Rekvig OP, Hannestad K (1979) The specificity of human autoantibodies that react with both cell nuclei and plasma membranes: the nuclear antigen is present on core mononucleosomes. J Immunol 123:2673
2. Revillard JP, Vincent C, Rivera S (1979) Anti-β_2 microglobulin lymphocytotoxic autoantibodies in systemic lupus erythematosus. J Immunol 122:614
3. Rook AH, Tsokos GC, Quinnan GV Jr, Balow JE, Ramsey KM, Stocks N, Phelan MA, Djeu JY (1982) Cytotoxic antibodies to natural killer cells in systemic lupus erythematosus. Clin Immunol Immunopathol 24:179
4. Sakane T, Steinberg AD, Reeves JP, Green I (1979) Studies of immune functions of patients with systemic lupus erythematosus. J Clin Invest 63:954
5. Sakane T, Steinberg AD, Reeves JP, Green I (1979) Studies of immune functions of patients with systemic lupus erythematosus: T-cell subsets and antibodies to T-cell subsets. J Clin Invest 64:1260
6. Sakane T, Kotani H, Takada S, Murakawa Y, Ueda Y (1983) A defect in the suppressor circuits among OKT4+ cell populations in patients with systemic lupus erythematosus occurs independently of a defect in the OKT8+ suppressor T cell function. J Immunol 131:753
7. Steinberg AD, Klassen LW, Budman DR, Williams GW (1979) Immunofluorescence studies of anti-T cell antibodies and T cells in systemic lupus erythematosus. Selective loss of brightly staining cells in active disease. Arthritis Rheum 22:114

48. Takahashi H, Terasaki PI, Iwaki Y, Nakata S (1980) Identification of surface IgM as the target antigen of cold lymphocytotoxins. Tissue Antigens 16:176
49. Takeuchi T, Abe T, Kiyotaki M, Toguchi T, Koide J, Morimoto C, Homma M (1982) In vitro immune response of SLE lymphocytes. The mechanism involved in B-cell activation. Scand J Immunol 16:369
50. Takeuchi T, Rudd CE, Schlossman SF, Morimoto C (1987) Induction of suppression following autologous mixed lymphocyte reaction; role of a novel 2H4 antigen. Eur J Immunol 17:97
51. Takeuchi T, Tanaka S, Steinberg AD, Matsuyama T, Daley J, Schlossman SF, Morimoto C (1988) Defective Expression of the 2H4 Molecule after autologous mixed lymphocyte reaction activation in systemic lupus erythematosus patients. J Clin Invest 82:1288
52. Tanaka S, Matsuyama T, Steinberg AD, Schlossman SF, Morimoto C (1989) Antilymphocyte antibodies against $CD4^{+}2H4^{+}$ cell populations in patients with systemic lupus erythematosus. Arthritis Rheum 32:398
53. Terasaki PI, McClelland JD (1964) Microdroplet assay of human serum cytotoxins. Nature 204:998
54. Terasaki PI, Mottironi VD, Barnett EV (1970) Cytotoxins in disease. Autocytotoxins in lupus. N Engl J Med 283:724
55. Thomas DB (1973) Antibodies specific for human T lymphocytes in cold agglutinin and lymphocytotoxic sera. Eur J Immunol 3:824
56. Thomas ML (1989) The leukocyte common antigen family. Annu Rev Immunol 7:339
57. Tonks NK, Charbonneau H, Diltz CD, Fischer EH, Walsh KA (1988) Demonstration that the leukocyte common antigen CD45 is a protein tyrosine phosphatase. Biochemistry 27:8695
58. Twomey JJ, Laughter AH, Steinberg AD (1978) A serum inhibitor of immune regulation in patients with systemic lupus erythematosus (SLE). J Clin Invest 62:713
59. Williams RC Jr, Lies RB, Messner RP (1973) Inhibition of mixed leukocyte culture responses by serum and τ-globulin fractions from certain patients with connective tisue disorders. Arthritis Rheum 16:597
60. Williams RC Jr, Bankhurst AD, Montaño JD (1976) IgG anti-lymphocyte antibodies in SLE detected by ^{125}I protein A. Arthritis Rheum 19:1261
61. Winfield JB, Winchester RJ, Kunkel HG (1975) Association of cold-reactive anti-lymphocyte antibodies with lymphopenia in systemic lupus erythematosus. Arthritis Rheum 18:587
62. Winfield JB, Winchester RJ, Wernet P, Fu SM, Kunkel HG (1975) Nature of cold-reactive antibodies to lymphocyte surface determinants in systemic lupus erythematosus. Arthritis Rheum 18:1
63. Winfield JB, Shaw M, Minota S (1986) Modulation of IgM anti-lymphocyte antibody-reactive T cell surface antigens in systemic lupus erythematosus. J Immunol 136:3246
64. Winfield JB, Shaw M, Yamada A, Minota S (1987) Subset specificity of anti-lymphocyte antibodies in systemic lupus erythematosus. II. Preferential reactivity with T4+ cells is associated with relative depletion of autologous T4+ cells. Arthritis Rheum 30:162
65. Yamada A, Winfield JB (1984) Inhibition of soluble antigen-induced T cell proliferation by warm-reactive antibodies to activated T cells in systemic lupus erythematosus. J Clin Invest 74:1948
66. Yamada A, Cohen PL, Winfield JB (1985) Subset specificity of anti-lymphocyte antibodies in systemic lupus erythematosus. Preferential reactivity with cells bearing the T4 and autologous erythrocyte receptor phenotypes. Arthritis Rheum 28:262
67. Yamada A, Shaw M, Winfield JB (1985) Surface antigen specificity of cold-reactive IgM antilymphocyte antibodies in systemic lupus erythematosus. Arthritis Rheum 28:44
68. Yamada A, Minota S, Nojima Y, Yazaki Y (1993) Changes in subset specificity of anti-T cell autoantibodies in systemic lupus erythematosus. Autoimmunity 14:269

Antigenic specificities of "antiphospholipid" autoantibodies

Robert A. S. Roubey

Division of Rheumatology and Immunology, Thurston Arthritis Research Center, CB#7280, Room 932 FLOB, The University of North Carolina at Chapel Hill, Chapel Hill, NC 27599-7280, USA

Introduction

"Antiphospholipid" autoantibodies (aPL) are strongly associated with recurrent thrombosis, fetal loss, and thrombocytopenia [51]. This association has been termed the antiphospholipid antibody syndrome and may occur in patients with systemic lupus erythematosus (SLE) and related diseases, or as a primary syndrome in patients without other autoimmune diseases. Although direct evidence for the pathogenicity of aPL is lacking, a number of observations have led investigators to hypothesize that aPL may directly contribute to a thrombotic diathesis: (1) unlike antinuclear autoantibodies, aPL appear to target components of cells surface membranes that are accessible to circulating antibodies; (2) the putative antigens, anionic phospholipids, are critically involved in hemostatic and thrombotic reactions that occur on the surface of vascular endothelial cells, platelets, and other blood cells; (3) animal models of the aPL syndrome have been developed via passive transfer of human aPL [6, 9]; (4) a recent prospective study has demonstrated that the presence of aPL precedes the first episode of venous thrombosis by months to years in a population of apparently normal individuals [27]; and (5) the risk of developing clinical manifestations of the aPL syndrome correlates directly with the level of aPL [27, 30].

If aPL are directly pathogenic, elucidation of the antigenic specificity or specificities of these antibodies is essential to understanding the pathophysiology of the aPL syndrome. Until recently the conventional wisdom held that aPL were directed against anionic phospholipids. This paradigm, however, does not adequately explain important features of aPL, for example, the inconsistent overlap of groups of aPL defined by current clinical laboratory tests and the clinical heterogeneity of the aPL syndrome. Over the past several years studies using purified autoantibodies and serum- and plasma-free assay systems have demonstrated that aPL are, in fact, not directed against anionic phospholipids, but rather recognize certain phospholipid-binding plasma proteins or complexes of these proteins with negatively charged phospholipids. At present the best characterized antibodies are those directed against β_2-glycoprotein I (β2GPI) [1, 22, 40, 48, 50, 69, 82] and prothrombin [5, 21, 57]. These new data suggest that aPL are a subset of a larger, heterogeneous, linked group of autoantibodies to certain phospholipid-binding plasma proteins and associated proteins expressed on endothelial or platelet cell surfaces. For example, autoantibodies to protein C and protein S, although not detectable in standard "anticardiolipin" and lupus anticoagulant assays, may be associated with aPL and the aPL syndrome and have considerable pathophysiological relevance [57].

Background

Historically, "antiphospholipid" autoantibodies have been detected in three different types of clinical laboratory assays and categorized based upon the method of detection [51]. First, aPL may give false-positive reactions in nontreponemal serological tests for syphilis. The VDRL and RPR tests, commonly used for screening purposes, are flocculation assays utilizing an antigenic mixture of cardiolipin, phosphatidylcholine, and cholesterol. Second, in lupus anticoagulant assays, aPL may be detected based upon their ability to inhibit certain coagulation reactions that require an anionic phospholipid surface, for example, the conversion of prothrombin to thrombin. Third, antibodies are detected in enzyme-linked immunosorbent assays (ELISA) in which the putative antigen is cardiolipin or other anionic phospholipids dried onto plastic microtiter plates.

The overlapping reactivities of aPL detected in these assays give a confusing picture of antigenic specificities. Antibodies from patients with syphilis react in the VDRL and anticardiolipin ELISA, but uniformly lack lupus anticoagulant activity [36] and are not associated with the aPL syndrome. Many patients with the aPL syndrome and "anticardiolipin" antibodies have false-positive syphilis serology, although a significant proportion do not (this discrepancy is likely due to the significantly greater sensitivity of the anticardiolipin ELISA). Most patients with the aPL syndrome have both "anticardiolipin" antibodies and lupus anticoagulants, although some clearly have one specificity but not the other [51]. In some patients whose sera/plasma are reactive in both assays, "anticardiolipin" antibodies and lupus anticoagulants can be separated physicochemically [11, 17, 49], while in other patients a single antibody population appears to possess both activities [23, 29, 61]. Some investigators have emphasized the importance of the phospholipid-phase structure in the specificity of aPL [35]. For example, certain aPL, particularly lupus anticoagulants, have been reported to recognize the neutral phospholipid phosphatidylethanolamine in the hexagonal phase, but not the lamellar phase [64].

In retrospect, a number of older reports suggest that aPL may not be directed against phospholipids. Loeliger was among the first to describe the lupus anticoagulant "cofactor" phenomenon, i.e., that normal plasma contains a cofactor which potentiates lupus anticoagulant activity, and concluded that the cofactor was prothrombin [43]. Case reports of the coexistence of hypoprothrombinemia and the lupus anticoagulant from several groups suggested that lupus anticoagulants were directed against prothrombin [8, 32, 52]. In an elegant study published in 1965, Yin and Gaston [85] purified a lupus anticoagulant, identified it as a 6.6 S gammaglobulin (IgG), and, in coagulation assays using purified components, clearly demonstrated that the anticoagulant activity required a protein present in both normal and patient plasma. The cofactor in this patient, although not fully characterized, was not prothrombin.

Previous studies indicating the phospholipid specificity of aPL are difficult to interpret as almost all such experiments were performed in the presence of serum or plasma. Although a number of investigators utilized purified antibodies, anticoagulant activity was assessed in normal plasma and "anticardiolipin" ELISA were performed with bovine serum as the blocking agent and/or sample diluent. Further, purified antibody preparations were not specifically tested for contamination with proteins now thought to be of importance in these assays, e.g., β2GPI. The reported specificity of lupus anticoagulants for hexagonal-phase phospholipid structures [35] has not been demonstrated in the absence of serum or plasma.

Targets of "antiphospholipid" and associated autoantibodies (Table 1)

β_2-glycoprotein I

In 1990 two groups of investigators reported that IgG anticardiolipin antibodies affinity-purified from patient sera did not bind to solid-phase cardiolipin or cardiolipin liposomes in serum-free assay systems [22, 50]. Addition of normal serum restored antibody binding. The serum component required for the binding of "anticardiolipin" autoantibodies to cardiolipin was found to be β_2-glycoprotein I, a phospholipid-binding plasma protein.

Table 1. Antigenic specificities of "antiphospholipid" autoantibodies (aPL) and associated autoantibodies

Specificities of antibodies detected in standard "antiphospholipid" assays
"Anticardiolipin" ELISA
β_2-glycoprotein I
Cardiolipin (associated with syphilis and other infections)
Lupus anticoagulant assays
β_2-glycoprotein I
Prothrombin
Factor X
Specificities of other autoantibodies potentially associated with the aPL syndrome
Phospholipid-binding plasma proteins
Protein C
Protein S
140-kDa glycoprotein (antiphosphatidylethanolamine cofactor)
Phospholipase A_2?
Endothelial cell surface molecules
Thrombomodulin
Vascular heparan sulfate proteoglycan?

β2GPI, a 50-kD glycoprotein, is a non-complement member of the complement control protein family [66]. It has five of the consensus repeats, or so-called "sushi domains," characteristic of such proteins. The fifth domain may contain a phospholipid-binding region [33, 78]. The amino acid sequence of β2GPI was originally determined by Lozier [44] and a number of laboratories have reported the complete cDNA sequence [46, 77]. β2GPI has also been termed apolipoprotein H [42], as up to 40% may circulate bound to lipoproteins. However, β2GPI bears no structural similarity to other apolipoproteins. Genetic polymorphisms of β2GPI have been observed based upon isoelectric focusing patterns [39], but these have not yet been defined on a DNA basis. An unrelated polymorphism, a valine-leucine amino acid exchange at position 247, has been recently reported [79]. The plasma level of β2GPI is also under genetic control [12]. Approximately 94% of the population is homozygous for the normal allele, with a mean plasma concentration of $\sim$ 200 μg/ml, whereas approximately 6% are heterozygous with a mean concentration of $\sim$ 100 μg/ml. Homozygous deficiency of β2GPI is rare ($<$ 1 in 1000).

Although, its physiological role is not known, in vitro data suggest that β2GPI may play a role in coagulation. β2GPI binds to anionic phospholipids [84] and inhibits the contact phase of intrinsic blood coagulation [31, 75], ADP-dependent platelet aggregation [54], and the prothrombinase activity of platelets [53]. Recent preliminary data indicate that β2GPI may play a regulatory role in the protein C pathway by inhibiting the interaction between protein S and C4b-binding protein [83]. While these data imply an anticoagulant role for β2GPI, deficiency of this protein is not a clear risk factor for thrombosis. A recent study of familial thrombophilia demonstrated that heterozygous partial β2GPI deficiency (plasma levels of $\sim$ 60–140 μg/ml) is not associated with thrombosis [4]. Two brothers with homozygous β2GPI deficiency were identified; one had a history of venous thrombosis, while the other was asymptomatic at age 35. Patients with aPL appear to have normal or somewhat elevated levels of β2GPI [14, 24], and the β2GPI phenotype, as determined by isoelectric focussing, does not appear to differ with racially matched controls [67].

Several laboratories have confirmed the observation that β2GPI is required for the binding of "anticardiolipin" autoantibodies to cardiolipin [37, 45, 68]. Some investigators, however, have reported that β2GPI enhances the binding of these antibodies to cardiolipin, but that it is not an absolute requirement for such binding [63, 73]. Interestingly, the requirement for β2GPI clearly distinguishes the "anticardiolipin" antibodies that occur in the setting of autoimmune disease and the aPL syndrome from those that occur in the setting of syphilis and other infectious diseases [47, 68]. Syphilis-associated anticardiolipin antibodies bind to cardiolipin in the absence of β2GPI and this binding to cardiolipin is inhibited by human β2GPI, presumably because the antibodies and β2GPI bind to similar phospholipid structures. This difference in antigenic specificity may explain why the autoimmune type of "anticardiolipin" antibody is associated with the lupus anticoagulant and thrombosis, fetal loss, etc., while anticardiolipin antibodies associated with infection are not [36, 59].

Some controversy remains as to whether autoimmune "anticardiolipin" antibodies recognize β2GPI in its native conformation, a β2GPI-phospholipid complex, neo- or cryptic phospholipid antigens expressed as a result of the binding of β2GPI to phospholipid, or neo-or cryptic β2GPI antigens. A number of groups have now reported antibody binding to β2GPI in ELISA performed in the absence of phospholipid [1, 22, 34, 40, 48, 69, 82], although antibody binding to fluid-phase β2GPI has generally not been observed. Discrepancies among laboratories regarding antibody binding to β2GPI alone appear to be due to methodological differences, specifically the type of microtiter plate used in the ELISA. Patient antibodies bind β2GPI when it is coated on "high-binding" polystyrene plates, but not on plain polystyrene plates [48, 69]. "High-binding" plates are produced commercially by γ-irradiation (typically $\geq$ 3 mrad), which partially oxidizes the polystyrene surface, rendering the plate more anionic and significantly enhancing protein-binding capacity [55].

Two possible explanations for this observation and the absent or weak binding of antibodies to β2GPI in solution have been proposed. First, these antibodies may be specific for one or several conformational epitopes of β2GPI formed when the protein binds to an anionic surface, such as irradiated polystyrene or cardiolipin [48]. Circular dichroism data indicate that the conformation of β2GPI does change upon its interaction with anionic phospholipid vesicles [38]. An alternative explanation is that antibody binding may require a relatively high density of immobilized antigen, which cannot be achieved on untreated polystyrene. Data from our laboratory support this interpretation and suggest that IgG anti-β2GPI autoantibodies are of intrinsically low affinity, with detectable antibody binding in ELISA occurring only when the density of immobilized antigen is sufficient to allow engagement of both IgG antigen-binding sites [69]. The enhancement of the antigen-antibody interaction due to antibody bivalency may be quite marked, as overall avidity is directly related to the binding constant of one site raised to the power of the number of binding sites simultaneously engaged [13]. In vivo such antibodies may bind to β2GPI clustered on an anionic phospholipid surface, e.g., an activated platelet or endothelial cell, but would not bind to β2GPI in the circulation. In this way autoantibodies to β2GPI may be analogous to another autoantibody to a plasma protein, namely rheumatoid factor. IgM rheumatoid factors have low affinity for monomeric IgG in solution, but bind avidly to IgG that is aggregated or bound to particles, due to the enhancement provided by multivalency [16]. While our data indicate the importance of antibody affinity and antigen density, they do not exclude the possibility that antibodies may be specific for conformational epitopes as well. Hunt and Krilis [34] have recently demonstrated binding of aCL to native β2GPI, but not to a proteolytically "clipped" form of the molecule at equivalent antigen density. Although autoantibodies specific for conformational epitopes are common, an autoantibody response limited to one or a small number of conformational epitopes would be unusual [65].

Certain autoantibodies to β2GPI have lupus anticoagulant activity [23, 41, 56, 68]. β2GPI itself inhibits prothrombinase activity in vitro [53] and β2GPI-dependent lupus anticoagulants appear to enhance this anticoagulant effect of β2GPI. A number of monoclonal and polyclonal antibodies to β2GPI have similar lupus anticoagulant-like activity [2, 10, 68]. Autoantibody enhancement of the anticoagulant activity of β2GPI could be due the steric effect of antibodies bound to β2GPI on a phospholipid surface or to cross-linking of surface bound β2GPI. Theoretically, cross-linking could increase the strength of the β2GPI-phospholipid interaction, thereby effectively decreasing the amount of phospholipid available to participate in the prothrombinase complex. Recently, "antiphospholipid" autoantibodies were shown to enhance the binding of β2GPI to cardiolipin-coated microtiter plates [25]. The reason why some anti-β2GPI antibodies have lupus anticoagulant activity while others do not is unclear, but may be related to avidity and/or epitope specificity.

Prothrombin

Autoantibodies to prothrombin were first demonstrated by Bajaj et al. [3] in two patients with the lupus anticoagulant and acquired hypoprothrombinemia. These antibodies were of relatively high affinity, and hypoprothrombinemia was thought to be due to the clearance of prothrombin immune complexes. Circulating prothrombin-antibody complexes have also been observed in patients with lupus anticoagulants and normal prothrombin levels [15, 21]. Although autoantibodies to prothrombin were thought initially to be distinct from lupus anticoagulants [3], Fleck et al. [21] demonstrated that certain affinity-purified antiprothrombin autoantibodies had lupus anticoagulant activity. Based on the observation that these antibodies bind to immobilized prothrombin, but not to fluid-phase prothrombin in patient plasma, these authors concluded that, in some patients, autoantibodies to prothrombin were of relatively low affinity.

More recently, it has been demonstrated that some lupus anticoagulants are directed against phospholipid-bound prothrombin. Bevers et al. [5] incubated plasma samples from 16 patients with both "anticardiolipin" antibodies and lupus anticoagulants with cardiolipin-containing liposomes followed by centrifugation. In 11 of 16 patients, lupus anticoagulant activity remained in the supernatant while the anticardiolipin antibody activity pelleted with the liposomes, whereas in the remaining 5 patients, lupus anticoagulant activity co-sedimented with the anticardiolipin antibodies. In a prothrombinase assay using purified components, the 11 non-cardiolipin-binding lupus anticoagulants were shown to be specific for human prothrombin bound to phospholipid. Antibodies with both "anticardiolipin" and lupus anticoagulant were directed against β2GPI [23]. Oosting et al. [57] demonstrated that 4 of 22 lupus anticoagulants inhibited endothelial cell-mediated prothrombinase activity. The inhibitory activity could be absorbed by prothrombin-coated cardiolipin vesicles, but not by vesicles alone, or vesicles coated with β2GPI, factor Va, or factor Xa.

Taken together, the accumulated data strongly suggest that certain lupus anticoagulants are directed against immobilized or phospholipid-bound prothrombin. Analogous to the discussion of antibodies to β2GPI, such antibodies may recognize conformational epitopes formed when prothrombin binds to anionic phospholipid, and/or may be of intrinsically low affinity. The occurrence of hypoprothrombinemia in a small subset of patients with lupus anticoagulant suggests that the antiprothrombin antibodies in this group of patients are of high affinity and recognize native prothrombin. Whether some antibodies to prothrombin also recognize thrombin is unknown.

Protein C and protein S

Although inhibition of the protein C pathway has long been thought to contribute to the thrombotic diathesis associated with aPL, relatively little attention has been paid to the possibility that autoantibodies may be directed against the plasma components of this pathway, protein C and protein S. Recently Oosting et al. [57] investigated the effect of IgG fractions from 30 patients on the protein C-mediated inactivation of factor Va, in the presence and absence of protein S. Three IgG fractions inhibited Va inactivation independently of protein S, while an additional four IgG fractions inhibited only in the presence of protein S. This inhibitory activity could be adsorbed by protein C- or protein S-coated cardiolipin vesicles, respectively, but not by β2GPI-coated vesicles, or vesicles alone, suggesting that the inhibitory antibodies were directed against phospholipid-bound protein C or protein S. In another recent report, antibodies to protein C, detected in 12 of 108 SLE serum samples by an ELISA utilizing high-binding microtiter plates, were not associated with decreased protein C levels or functional protein C deficiency [71]. Parke et al. [60] did not detect autoantibodies to protein C or protein S by immunoblotting in 11 patients with the aPL syndrome, 7 of whom had low levels of free protein S.

Other potential antigens

Limited data suggests that several other phospholipid-binding proteins may be targets of autoantibodies in patients with aPL and the aPL syndrome. Anecdotally, a lupus anticoagulant specific for factor X has been identified in a patient with high titer anticardiolipin antibodies and a hemorrhagic diathesis (D. Triplett, personal communication). Autoantibodies with an apparent specificity for phosphatidylethanolamine have been reported in a few patients with the aPL syndrome [18, 76]. Sugi et al. [80] have shown that the binding of autoantibodies to phosphatidylethanolamine in ELISA requires a 140-kDa serum glycoprotein, which has not yet been further identified. Schorer et al. [74] have demonstrated that certain aPL inhibit phospholipase A_2 activity, potentially leading to decreased endothelial cell production of prostacyclin production and predisposing to thrombosis [74]. It has been suggested that these antibodies might be directed against a phospholipase A_2-phospholipid complex [81]. Although the fraction of phospholipase A_2 that mediates arachidonic acid release is thought to be predominantly intracellular, non-pancreatic secretory phospholipase A_2 may also contribute to the synthesis of arachidonic acid metabolites [7, 62]. At present there is no direct evidence of autoantibodies to any type of phospholipase A_2. Annexins are a family of calcium-dependent phospholipid-binding proteins thought to play important roles in membrane processes such as exocytosis. Sammaritano and coworkers [72] studied the potential interaction of aPL with annexin V (human placental anticoagulant protein I) but found no evidence of antibody reactivity to this protein.

Finally, certain molecules expressed on the luminal surface of vascular endothelial cells may be antigenic targets in patients with the aPL syndrome. Thrombomodulin, an endothelial cell receptor for thrombin, plays a critical in protein C activation. Autoantibodies to thrombomodulin have been identified in few patients [58, 70]. However, in a larger study, Gibson et al. [26] observed no significant differences in the incidence of antithrombomodulin antibodies detected by ELISA among 113 patients with lupus anticoagulants, 78 patients referred for lupus anticoagulant testing but found to be negative, and normal individuals. Vascular heparan sulfate proteoglycan is expressed on endothelial cells and plays an important role in vascular structure and function, including hemostasis. Importantly, vessel-wall heparan sulfate is required for the activation of antithrombin III. Fillit and coworkers have demonstrated autoantibodies to both heparan sulfate [19] and the protein core of vascular heparan sulfate proteoglycan [20] in the sera of certain patients with SLE. Given that sera were used in these assays and that β2GPI binds to heparin, it is possible that the apparent specificity of autoantibodies for heparan sulfate is, at least in part, due to antibodies to β2GPI.

Implications for clinical testing

The data summarized above strongly suggest that phospholipid-binding proteins and/or protein-phospholipid complexes are the targets of "antiphospholipid" autoantibodies. Currently used clinical laboratory tests detect some, but not all, of these autoantibodies (see Table 1). The standard "anticardiolipin" ELISA detects both autoantibodies to β2GPI and "true" anticardiolipin antibodies that are associated with syphilis and other infections. In this assay, β2GPI present in bovine serum used in the blocking buffer and in the patient's serum sample binds to the cardiolipin-coated microtiter plate and can subsequently be engaged by anti-β2GPI autoantibodies. Certain autoantibodies to β2GPI, as well as autoantibodies to prothrombin demonstrate lupus anticoagulant activity in assays such as the activated partial thromboplastin time and dilute Russell viper venom time. Antiprothrombin antibodies are probably not reactive in "anticardiolipin" ELISA due to several factors including the use of serum rather than plasma and the low concentration of Ca^{2+} in the assay. Neither type of aPL assay detects autoantibodies to protein C and protein S. Thus, the reactivity of autoantibodies with different antigenic specificities in the currently used "antiphospholipid" assays appears to explain much of the heterogeneity and inconsistent overlap of "anticardiolipin" antibodies and lupus anticoagulants. For example, it clarifies why, in some patients, "anticardiolipin" antibodies and lupus anticoagulants are the same antibodies (anti-β2GPI antibodies with anticoagulant activity), while in others they are clearly distinct (anti-β2GPI antibodies without anticoagulant activity and antiprothrombin antibodies).

These new data suggest ways in which clinical testing may be improved. The fact that the amount and quality of β2GPI are uncontrolled variables in standard "anticardiolipin" ELISA may partly explain the considerable inter- and intralaboratory variability of such tests. Anti-β2GPI ELISA performed in the absence of phospholipid do not detect infection-associated anticardiolipin antibodies and, therefore, would be expected to have greater specificity for the aPL syndrome than "anticardiolipin" ELISA in current use.

Hypothesis: a linked set of autoantibodies directed against proteins bound to, or expressed on, anionic phospholipid membranes

Immunologically, it is of interest that autoantibodies to different phospholipid-binding proteins occur together, in various combinations. As recently demonstrated by Oosting et al. [57], some patients may have autoantibodies to β2GPI, prothrombin, protein C, and protein S, while others may have antibodies against one, two, or three of these proteins in different combinations. Speculatively, this is similar to certain linked sets of antinuclear antibodies that occur in patients with SLE, e.g., antibodies to constituents of small nuclear ribonucleoprotein particles. Autoantibodies may be directed against different protein components of such particles, such as Sm and U1-RNP proteins, suggesting that the immune response is antigen driven [28]. By analogy, the co-occurrence of antibodies to different phospholipid-binding proteins suggests that the relevant antigenic particle in this instance may consist of a number of proteins bound to, or expressed on, an anionic phospholipid surface in close proximity to one another, perhaps a damaged vascular endothelial cell or an activated platelet.

Conclusions

Recent data indicate that "antiphospholipid" and associated autoantibodies recognize a number of phospholipid-bound plasma proteins and endothelial cell surface molecules involved with thrombosis and hemostasis, rather than anionic phospholipids alone. Although these recent findings provide potentially important insights into the pathophysiology of autoantibody-mediated thrombosis and fetal loss, it should be understood that these studies have involved relatively small numbers of patients with high levels of IgG autoantibodies. At this juncture it is not clear which, if any, of these autoantibodies are pathogenic. Promising future avenues of investigation include determining whether different antigenic specificities will explain the clinical heterogeneity of the aPL syndrome (why a particular patient might have arterial thrombosis versus venous thrombosis versus recurrent miscarriages) or whether certain specificities may not be related to any disease manifestation, explaining why many individuals with aPL are asymptomatic. The observation that certain autoantibodies to plasma proteins are of low affinity may provide insights into the mechanism of the loss of tolerance and the development of autoimmunity in patients with the aPL syndrome.

References

1. Arvieux J, Roussel B, Jacob MC, Colomb MG (1991) Measurement of anti-phospholipid antibodies by ELISA using β_2-glycoprotein I as an antigen. J Immunol Methods 143:223
2. Arvieux J, Pouzol P, Roussel B, Jacob MC, Colomb MG (1992) Lupus-like anticoagulant properties of murine monoclonal antibodies to β_2-glycoprotein I. Br J Haematol 81:568
3. Bajaj SP, Rapaport SI, Fierer DS, Herbst KD, Schwartz DB (1983) A mechanism for the hypoprothrombinemia of the acquired hypoprothrombinemia-lupus anticoagulant syndrome. Blood 61:684
4. Bancsi LFJMM, van der Linden IK, Bertina RM (1992) β_2-glycoprotein I deficiency and the risk of thrombosis. Thromb Haemost 67:649
5. Bevers EM, Galli M, Barbui T, Comfurius P, Zwaal RFA (1991) Lupus anticoagulant IgG's (LA) are not directed to phospholipids only, but to a complex of lipid-bound human prothrombin. Thromb Haemost 66: 629
6. Blank M, Cohen J, Toder V, Shoenfeld Y (1991) Induction of anti-phospholipid syndrome in naive mice with mouse lupus monoclonal and human polyclonal anti-cardiolipin antibodies. Proc Natl Acad Sci USA 88: 3069
7. Bomalaski JS, Lawton P, Browning JL (1991) Human extracellular recombinant phospholipase A_2 induces an inflammatory response in rabbit joints. J Immunol 146:3904
8. Bonnin JA, Cohen AK, Hicks ND (1956) Coagulation defects in a case of systemic lupus erythematosus with thrombocytopenia. Br J Haematol 2:168
9. Branch DW, Dudley DJ, Mitchell MD (1990) IgG fractions from patients with antiphospholipid antibodies cause fetal death in BALB/c mice:a model for autoimmune fetal loss. Am J Obstet Gynecol 163: 210
10. Brandt JT (1993) Antibodies to β_2-glycoprotein I inhibit phospholipid dependent coagulation reactions. Thromb Haemost 70:598
11. Chamley LW, Pattison NS, McKay EJ (1991) Separation of lupus anticoagulant from anticardiolipin antibodies by ion-exchange and gel filtration chromatography. Haemostasis 21:25
12. Cleve H (1968) Genetic studies on the deficiency of β_2-glycoprotein I of human serum. Humangenetik 5:294
13. Crothers DM, Metzger H (1972) The influence of polyvalency on the binding properties of antibodies. Immunochemistry 9:341
14. De Benedetti E, Reber G, Miescher PA, De Moerloose P (1992) No increase of β_2-glycoprotein I levels in patients with antiphospholipid antibodies. Thromb Haemost 68:624
15. Edson JR, Vogt JM, Hasegawa DK (1984) Abnormal prothrombin crossed-immunoelectrophoresis in patients with lupus inhibitors. Blood 64:807
16. Eisenberg R (1976) The specificity and polyvalency of binding of a monoclonal rheumatoid factor. Immunochemistry 13:355
17. Exner T, Sahman N, Trudinger B (1988) Separation of anticardiolipin antibodies from lupus anticoagulant on a phospholipid-coated polystyrene column. Biochem Biophys Res Commun 155:1001
18. Falcón CR, Hoffer AM, Carreras LO (1990) Evaluation of the clinical and laboratory associations of antiphosphatidylethanolamine antibodies. Thromb Res 59:383
19. Fillit H, Lahita R (1991) Antibodies to vascular heparan sulfate proteoglycan in patients with systemic lupus erythematosus. Autoimmunity 9:159
20. Fillit H, Shibata S, Sasaki T, Speira H, Kerr LD, Blake M (1993) Autoantibodies to the protein core of vascular basement membrane heparan sulfate proteoglycan in systemic lupus erythematosus. Autoimmunity 14:243

21. Fleck RA, Rapaport SI, Rao LV (1988) Anti-prothrombin antibodies and the lupus anticoagulant. Blood 72:512
22. Galli M, Comfurius P, Maassen C, Hemker HC, De Baets MH, van Breda-Vriesman PJC, Barbui T, Zwaal RFA, Bevers EM (1990) Anticardiolipin antibodies directed not to cardiolipin but to a plasma protein cofactor. Lancet 335:1544
23. Galli M, Comfurius P, Barbui T, Zwaal RFA, Bevers EM (1992) Anticoagulant activity of β_2-glycoprotien I is potentiated by a distinct subgroup of anticardiolipin antibodies. Thromb Haemost 68:297
24. Galli M, Cortelazzo S, Daldossi M, Barbui T (1992) Increased levels of beta-2-glycoprotein I (aca-cofactor) in patients with lupus anticoagulant. Thromb Haemost 67:386
25. Gharavi AE, Vindrola O (1993) Effect of antiphospholipid antibody on β_2-glycoprotein I- phospholipid interaction (abstract). Arthritis Rheum 36: S103
26. Gibson J, Nelson M, Brown R, Salem H, Kronenberg H (1992) Autoantibodies to thrombomodulin:development of an enzyme immunoassay and a survey of their frequency in patients with the lupus anticoagulant. Thromb Haemost 67:507
27. Ginsburg KS, Liang MH, Newcomer L, Goldhaber SZ, Schur PH, Hennekens CH, Stampfer MJ (1992) Anticardiolipin antibodies and the risk for ischemic stroke and venous thrombosis. Ann Intern Med 117:997
28. Hardin JA (1986) The lupus autoantigens and the pathogenesis of systemic lupus erythematosus. Arthritis Rheum 29:457
29. Harris EN, Gharavi AE, Tincani A, Chan JKH, Englert H, Mantelli P, Allegro F, Ballestrieri G, Hughes GRV (1985) Affinity purified anti-cardiolipin and anti-DNA antibodies. J Clin Lab Immunol 17:155
30. Harris EN, Chan JKH, Asherson RA, Aber VA, Gharavi AE, Hughes GRV (1986) Thrombosis, recurrent fetal loss, thrombocytopenia:predictive value of IgG anticardiolipin antibodies. Arch Intern Med 146: 2153
31. Henry ML, Everson B, Ratnoff OD (1988) Inhibition of the activation of Hageman factor (factor XII) by β_2-glycoprotein I. J Lab Clin Med 111: 519
32. Hougie C (1964) Naturally occurring species specific inhibitor of human prothrombin in lupus erythematosus. Proc Soc Exp Biol Med 116:359
33. Hunt JE, Simpson RJ, Krilis SA (1993) Identification of a region of β_2-glycoprotein I critical for lipid binding and anti-cardiolipin cofactor activity. Proc Natl Acad Sci USA 90:2141
34. Hunt J, Krilis S (1994) The fifth domain of β_2-glycoprotein I contains a phospholipid binding site (cys281-cys288), and a region recognised by anticardiolipin antibodies. J Immunol 152:653
35. Janoff AS, Rauch J (1986) The structural specificity of anti-phospholipid antibodies in autoimmune disease. Chem Phys Lipids 40:315
36. Johansson AE, Lassus A (1974) The occurrences of circulating anticoagulants in patients with syphilitic and biologically false-positive antilipoidal antibodies. Ann Clin Res 6:105
37. Jones JV, James H, Tan MH, Mansour M (1992) Antiphospholipid antibodies require β_2-glycoprotein I (apolipoprotein H) as cofactor. J Rheumatol 19:1397
38. Jones JV, Mansour M, James H, Anantharamaiah GM (1992) Antigenicity of β2GPI for anti-cardiolipin antibody depends on the presence of phospholipid (abstract). Arthritis Rheum 35:S117
39. Kamboh MI, Ferrell RE, Sepehrnia B (1988) Genetic studies of human apolipoproteins. IV. Structural heterogeneity of apolipoprotein H (beta-2-glycoprotein I). Am J Hum Genet 42:452
40. Keeling DM, Wilson AJG, Mackie IJ, Machin SJ, Isenberg DA (1992) Some 'antiphospholipid antibodies' bind to β_2-glycoprotein I in the absence of phospholipid. Br J Haematol 82:571
41. Keeling DM, Wilson AJG, Mackie IJ, Isenberg DA, Machin SJ (1993) Lupus anticoagulant activity of some antiphospholipid antibodies against phospholipid-bound β_2 glycoprotein I. J Clin Pathol 46:665
42. Lee NS, Brewer HB Jr, Osborne JC Jr (1983) Beta-2-glycoprotein I:molecular properties of an unusual apolipoprotein, apolipoprotein H. J Biol Chem 258:4765
43. Loeliger A (1959) Prothrombin as co-factor of the circulating anticoagulant in systemic lupus erythematosus? Thromb Diath Haemorrh 3:237
44. Lozier J, Takahashi N, Putnam FW (1984) Complete amino acid sequence of human plasma β_2-glycoprotein I. Proc Natl Acad Sci USA 81: 3640
45. Matsuura E, Igarashi Y, Fujimoto M, Ichikawa K, Koike T (1990) Anticardiolipin cofactor(s) and differential diagnosis of autoimmune disease. Lancet 336:177

46. Matsuura E, Igarashi M, Igarashi Y, Nagae H, Ichikawa K, Yasuda T, Koike T (1991) Molecular definition of human β_2-glycoprotein I (β_2-GPI) by cDNA cloning and inter-species differences of β_2-GPI in alteration of anticardiolipin binding. Int Immunol 3:1217
47. Matsuura E, Igarashi Y, Fujimoto M, Ichikawa K, Suzuki T, Sumida T, Yasuda T, Koike T (1992) Heterogeneity of anticardiolipin antibodies defined by the anticardiolipin cofactor. J Immunol 148:3885
48. Matsuura E, Igarashi Y, Yasuda T, Koike T, Triplett DA (1994) Anticardiolipin antibodies recognize β_2-glycoprotein I structure altered by interacting with an oxygen-modified solid-phase surface. J Exp Med 179:457
49. McNeil HP, Chesterman CN, Krilis SA (1989) Anticardiolipin antibodies and lupus anticoagulants comprise antibody subgroups with different phospholipid binding characteristics. Br J Haematol 73: 506
50. McNeil HP, Simpson RJ, Chesterman CN, Krilis SA (1990) Anti-phospholipid antibodies are directed against a complex antigen that includes a lipid-binding inhibitor of coagulation:β_2-glycoprotein I (apolipoprotein H). Proc Natl Acad Sci USA 87:4120
51. McNeil HP, Chesterman CN, Krilis SA (1991) Immunology and clinical importance of antiphospholipid antibodies. Adv Immunol 49:193
52. Medal LS, Lisker R (1959) Circulating anticoagulant in disseminated lupus erythematosus. Br J Haematol 5:284
53. Nimpf J, Bevers EM, Bomans PHH, Till U, Wurm H, Kostner GM, Zwaal RFA (1986) Prothrombinase activity of human platelets is inhibited by β_2-glycoprotein I. Biochim Biophys Acta 884:142
54. Nimpf J, Wurm H, Kostner GM (1987) β_2-glycoprotein-I (apo H) inhibits the release reaction of human platelets during ADP-induced aggregation. Atherosclerosis 63:109
55. Onyiriuka EC, Hersh IS, Herti W (1990) Surface modification of polystyrene by gamma-radiation. Appl Spectrosc 44:808
56. Oosting JD, Derksen RHWM, Entjes HTI, Bouma BN, De Groot PG (1992) Lupus anticoagulant activity is frequently dependent on the presence of β_2-glycoprotein I. Thromb Haemost 67:499
57. Oosting JD, Derksen RHWM, Bobbink IWG, Hackeng TM, Bouma BN, De Groot PG (1993) Antiphospholipid antibodies directed against a combination of phospholipids with prothrombin, protein C, or protein S:an explanation for their pathogenic mechanism? Blood 81:2618
58. Oosting JD, Preissner KT, Derksen RHWM, De Groot PG (1993) Autoantibodies directed against the epidermal growth factor-like domains of thrombomodulin inhibit protein C activation in vitro. Br J Haematol 85:761
59. Ordi J, Selva A, Monegal F, Porcel JM, Martinez-Costa X, Vilardell M (1993) Anticardiolipin antibodies and dependence of a serum cofactor. A mechanism of thrombosis. J Rheumatol 20:1321
60. Parke AL, Weinstein RE, Bona RD, Maier DB, Walker FJ (1992) The thrombotic diathesis associated with the presence of phospholipid antibodies may be due to low levels of free protein S. Am J Med 93:49
61. Pengo V, Thiagarajan P, Shapiro S, Heine MJ (1987) Immunologic specificity and mechanism of action of IgG lupus anticoagulants. Blood 70:69
62. Pfeilschifter J, Schalkwijk C, Briner VA, van den Bosch H (1993) Cytokine-stimulated secretion of group II phospholipase A_2 by rat mesangial cells:its contribution to arachidonic acid release and prostaglandin synthesis by cultured rat glomerular cells. J Clin Invest 92:2516
63. Pierangeli SS, Harris EN, Davis SA, DeLorenzo G (1992) β_2-glycoprotein 1 (β_2GP1) enhances cardiolipin binding activity but is not the antigen for antiphospholipid antibodies. Br J Haematol 82:565
64. Rauch J, Tannenbaum M, Tannenbaum H, Ramelson H, Cullis PR, Tilcock CPS, Hope MJ, Janoff AS (1986) Human hybridoma lupus anticoagulants distinguish between lamellar and hexagonal phase lipid systems. J Biol Chem 261:9672
65. Reeves WH, Blankson J, Chou C-H (1992) Molecular analysis of autoantibody production. Concepts Immunopathol 8:38
66 Reid KBM, Bentley DR, Campbell RD, Chung LP, Sim RB, Kristensen T, Tack BF (1986) Complement system proteins which interact with C3b or C4b:a superfamily of structurally related proteins. Immunol Today 7:230
67. Roubey RAS, Buyon JP, Winfield JB, Kamboh MI (1992) Phenotypic analysis of β_2-glycoprotein I in patients with antiphospholipid autoantibodies (abstract). Clin Exp Immunol 10:643
68. Roubey RAS, Pratt CW, Buyon JP, Winfield JB (1992) Lupus anticoagulant activity of autoimmune antiphospholipid antibodies is dependent upon β_2-glycoprotein I. J Clin Invest 90:1100

69. Roubey RAS, Eisenberg RA,Winfield JB (1994) "Anticardiolipin" autoantibodies recognize β_2-glycoprotein I in the absence of phospholipid. Importance of antigen density and bivalent binding (in press)
70. Ruiz-Argüelles GJ, Ruiz-Argüelles A, Deleze M, Alarcón-Segovia D (1989) Acquired protein C deficiency in a patient with primary antiphospholipid syndrome. Relationship to reactivity of anticardiolipin antibody with thrombomodulin. J Rheumatol 16:381
71. Ruiz-Argüelles A, Vazquez-Prado J, Deleze M, Perez-Romano B, Drenkard C, Alarcón-Segovia D, Ruiz-Argüelles GJ (1993) Presence of serum antibodies to coagulation protein C in patients with systemic lupus erythematosus is not associated with antigenic or functional protein C deficiencies. Am J Hematol 44:58
72. Sammaritano LR, Gharavi AE, Soberano C, Levy RA, Lockshin MD (1992) Phospholipid binding of antiphospholipid antibodies and placental anticoagulant protein. J Clin Immunol 12:27
73. Sammaritano LR, Lockshin MD, Gharavi AE (1992) Antiphospholipid antibodies differ in aPL cofactor requirement. Lupus 1:83
73. Schorer AE, Duane PG, Woods VL, Niewoehner DE (1992) Some antiphospholipid antibodies inhibit phospholipase A_2 activity. J Lab Clin Med 120:67
75. Schousboe I (1985) β_2-glycoprotein I:a plasma inhibitor of the contact activation of the intrinsic blood coagulation pathway. Blood 66:1086
76. Staub HL, Harris EN, Khamashta MA, Savidge G, Chahade WH, Hughes GR (1989) Antibody to phosphatidylethanolamine in a patient with lupus anticoagulant and thrombosis. Ann Rheum Dis 48:166
77. Steinkasserer A, Estaller C, Weiss EH, Sim RB, Day AJ (1991) Complete nucleotide and amino acid sequence of human beta-2-glycoprotein I. Biochem J 277:387
78. Steinkasserer A, Barlow PN, Willis AC, Kertesz Z, Campbell ID, Sim RB, Norman DG (1992) Activity, disulphide mapping and structural modelling of the fifth domain of human β_2-glycoprotein I. FEBS Lett 313:193
79. Steinkasserer A, Dorner C, Wurzner R, Sim RB (1993) Human beta 2-glycoprotein I:molecular analysis of DNA and amino acid polymorphism. Hum Genet 91: 401
80. Sugi T, Vanderpuye OA, McIntyre JA (1993) Partial purification of an anti-phosphatidylethanolamine antibody ELISA cofactor (abstract). Thromb Haemost 69:596
81. Vermylen J, Arnout J (1992) Is the antiphospholipid syndrome caused by antibodies directed against physiologically relevant phospholipid-protein complexes? J Lab Clin Med 120:10
82. Viard J-P, Amoura Z, Bach J-F (1992) Association of anti-β_2 glycoprotein I antibodies with lupus-type circulating anticoagulant and thrombosis in systemic lupus erythematosus. Am J Med 93:181
83. Walker FJ (1993) Does beta-2-glycoprotein I inhibit the interaction between protein S and C4b-binding protein? (abstract). Thromb Haemost 69:930
84. Wurm H (1984) β_2-glycoprotein I (apolipoprotein H) interactions with phospholipid vesicles. Int J Biochem 16:511
85. Yin ET, Gaston LW (1965) Purification and kinetic studies on a circulating anticoagulant in a suspected case of lupus erythematosus. Thromb Diath Haemorrh 14:89

Antiphospholipid antibodies and the antiphospholipid syndrome

E. Nigel Harris[1], **Silvia S. Pierangeli**[2]

[1] Department of Medicine, Division of Rheumatology, Ambulatory Care Building, 3rd floor, University of Louisville, Louisville, KY 40292, USA
[2] Antiphospholipid Standardization Laboratory, Louisville, Kentucky

Introduction

The term "antiphospholipid (aPL) antibodies" [47] will be used to describe antibodies detected by any one of the following tests: the anticardiolipin ELISA test [40], the lupus anticoagulant test [108], and standard tests for syphilis [47]. Currently, there are questions raised by some investigators as to whether these tests truly detect antibodies specific for phospholipids [75, 110], and this issue will be addressed in this review.

The term "antiphospholipid syndrome" (APS) was introduced and defined in 1987 [39] to achieve uniformity in identifying patients with clinical complications associated with positive lupus anticoagulant and/or positive anticardiolipin tests. The term APS has since been sub-divided into "primary" and "secondary" subgroups depending on whether patients present with clinical features of the disorder alone ("primary"), or whether other disease states such as systemic lupus erythematousus (SLE) are present ("secondary") [1, 5]. Distinction into "primary" and "secondary" subgroups may be useful for prospective clinical and laboratory studies, although there is little evidence to suggest that these are truly distinct entities [111]. Important questions regarding diagnosis, management, and the role of antiphospholipid antibodies in disease pathogenesis remain, as shall be discussed below.

Correspondence to: E.N. Harris

Antiphospholipid syndrome: clinical features, diagnosis, and management

Clinical features

APS may be defined as a disorder of recurrent venous and/or arterial thrombosis, pregnancy losses, and thrombocytopenia associated with positive anticardiolipin or lupus anticoagulant tests [39]. Since blood vessels of any size and at any site can be affected, patients can present in a variety of ways. Some authorities have suggested sub-grouping this disorder according to the site affected, e.g., myocardial infarction, adrenal insufficiency, stroke, renal vein thrombosis and so on, but there seems little to be gained by this approach since the causative agents, mechanisms, and thrombotic consequences appear to be the same regardless of site affected. However, the observation that patients with venous thrombosis tend to get recurrences at venous sites, arterial thrombosis get recurrences in the arterial circulation [92], and patients with pregnancy losses often do not get thrombosis [65] is important, since differences in presentation may reflect differences in subsets of aPL antibodies, or differences in host factors (e.g., in some instances, endothelial cells of arteries may be affected resulting in arterial thrombosis, whereas in others, protein C activation may be affected resulting in venous thrombosis).

An important question is whether clinical or laboratory features of APS are influenced by concomitant presence of SLE. A recent study by Vianna and colleagues suggests that the essential features of APS – diagnostic tests, management, and long term prognosis – are probably not affected by presence of SLE [111]. Indeed, Piette and colleagues have argued that complications such as thrombocytopenia and a false-positive test for syphilis would suffice as criteria either for SLE or APS [90]. In addition, their experience [90] and our own is that patients may present only with one or two complications of APS, but develop features of SLE later, or vice versa. Hence, for the practicing clinician, the distinction of patients into "pimary" and "secondary" groups may be unnecessary, since long-term management to prevent recurrent thrombosis, pregnancy losses, and thrombocytopenia will be the same.

A related question is whether "minor" features of APS such as livedo reticularis, leg ulcers, and cardiac valvular lesions [6] are a result of aPL antibodies or may be part of some broader connective tissue disease entity to which APS belongs. Gleason and colleagues [37] reported that the frequency of cardiac valvular lesions was the same in patients with primary antiphospholipid syndrome as in patients with anticardiolipin-negative SLE. This suggests that some factor other than aPL antibodies may be involved in the pathogenesis of cardiae valvular lesions. In a similar manner, livedo reticularis has been shown to occur as frequently in SLE as in primary antiphospholipid syndrome [111], although an earlier study showed an increased correlation with stroke and aPL antibodies [23].

Hence, APS may be a disorder which includes factors other than aPL antibodies, and these factors may be responsible for complications such as livedo reticularis and cardiac valvular vegetations. In addition, these factors may be present in other connective tissue diseases, suggesting that APS is a part of that group of disorders.

Diagnosis

Fulfillment of at least one major clinical and one laboratory feature listed in Table 1 should be a minimal requirement for diagnosing APS [39]. None of the clinical or laboratory features listed in Table 1 are specific to APS. Hence, there may be circumstances in which patients with one clinical feature, such as thrombosis, might have a low positive anticardiolipin or equivocal lupus anticoagulant test without necessarily having APS. Some of the following guidelines may be helpful in specifying the diagnosis – presence of more than one clinical and/or more than one laboratory feature (either at the time of evaluation or in the past); exclusion of other disorders which might cause venous or arterial thrombosis; a high positive IgG anticardiolipin test (> 80 GPL unit) [36, 49, 65]; a positive lupus anticoagulant test, particularly if the anticardiolipin test (any isotype) is also positive; and persistence of a positive test over several weeks.

Table 1.

*Clinical	+* Laboratory
Major features	
Venous thrombosis (DVT, PTE, etc)	IgG anticardiolipin (>20 GPL)
Arterial thrombosis (stroke, MI, gangrene)	IgM anticardiolipin (>20 GPL)
Pregnancy loss	IgA anticardiolipin (?)
Thrombocytopenia	
	Lupus anticoagulant
"Minor" features	
Heart valve abnormalities	
Coombs positive	
Livedo reticularis	
Migraine	
Leg ulcers	
Myelopathy	
Chorea	
?Pulmonary hypertension	
?Avascular necrosis	

* The more clinical and laboratory features, the more likely the diagnosis
+ Tests should be positive on more than one occasion 8 weeks apart

Treatment

Thrombosis. Until recently, there were few studies which served as guides to management of patients with APS. However, there is increasing evidence that a positive anticardiolipin antibody test, particularly at high levels [36, 49, 65], is a risk factor for thrombosis, and prophylactic anticoagulant therapy will prevent recurrence [22, 92].

Based on these studies [22, 92], it seems wise that patients with APS who have had venous or arterial thrombosis should be treated with Coumadin. International Ratio (INR) levels of 2.6–3.0 are recommended. In addition to Coumadin, we also prescribe 1/2 an adult aspirin daily for patients with arterial thrombosis.

The use of prednisone and immunosuppressive agents to prevent recurrent thrombosis does not appear justified except in patients with accelerated and widespread thrombosis despite adequate anticoagulant therapy. In the latter patients, plasmapheresis, high-dose prednisone, and pulse intravenous or oral cyclophosphamide have been utilized with varying success [42].

Pregnancy loss. Prevention of recurrent pregnancy losses in women with the APS has been a major reason for identifying these patients. Sufficient data has now been generated to offer tentative guidelines about management of these women during pregnancy. Beginning with studies of Lubbe and Liggins [67] and Branch et al. [12], high doses of prednisone and low-dose aspirin therapy seemed to reduce the risk of recurrent pregnancy losses. Although other investigators, utilizing modifications of this regimen, continue to report successful pregnancy outcome with this treatment, some found that it was not effective [65] or that steroids were associated with serious complications, such as infection [20], pre-eclampsia [20], gestational diabetes [20], and avascular necrosis (one case personally known to us).

Rosove et al. [93], Cowchock et al. [20] and Branch et al. [12] have all reported that treatment of women during pregnancy with subcutaneous heparin plus one baby aspirin daily results in improved pregnancy outcome. Efficacy with this treatment was equivalent to prednisone [12, 20]. Use of subcutaneous heparin is associated with fewer maternal complications than prednisone. There are also reports that the use of monthly pulses of intravenous gammaglobulin therapy during pregnancy may be effective in preventing pregnancy loss [82, 101, 107]. At the University of Louisville, 9 consecutive women have been treated with pulses of intravenous gammaglobulin (see regimen below), and all pregnancies have resulted in live births.

Based on the above data, the following recommendations can be made. Women with APS who are pregnant for the first time should receive no treatment or one low-dose aspirin daily. This recommendation is based on the report by Lockshin and colleagues that women with APS have a greater than 50% chance of a successful pregnancy outcome *without* treatment in their first pregnancy [65]. However, a history of previous pregnancy losses substantially increases the risk of losses in future pregnancies. Hence, affected women with histories of pregnancy losses require treatment in future pregnancies. We also recommend that women who are pregnant for the first time, but have a history of previous thrombosis and positive anticardiolipin or lupus anticoagulant tests, should be treated with therapeutic doses of heparin (for prophylaxis against thrombosis) during their first and any subsequent pregnancy. The latter recommendation is based on a report by Silver et al., who reported that thrombosis occurred in a number of women in their series during pregnancy [104].

In affected women with histories of pregnancy losses, heparin 5000–10000 units s.c. b.i.d. + one low-dose aspirin [12, 20, 93] initiated early in pregnancy is recommended to prevent pregnancy loss, even if these women have no history of thrombosis. If the woman suffers pregnancy loss despite treatment with heparin and aspirin, we recommend intravenous gammaglobulin therapy during the next attempted pregnancy – 0.4 g/kg per day for 5 days each month [101, 107]. If gammaglobulin fails, then prednisone 20–40 mg daily and one low-dose aspirin can be tried in the next pregnancy [12, 93].

Women with APS should be monitored carefully throughout pregnancy, regardless of what treatment is used. The risks of treatment and the possibility of an adverse outcome late in pregnancy should be carefully discussed with both woman and spouse, before the woman attempts to become pregnant.

Thrombocytopenia. This complication is treated as thrombocytopenia secondary to SLE or idiopathic thrombocytopenia purpura (ITP). High-dose steroids are used if platelet counts fall below 50000 and the patient has bleeding complications. If prednisone fails, immunosuppressive therapy, then splenectomy are utilized as necessary. Aspirin and oral anticoagulants are probably best avoided in patients with platelet counts below 100000.

Diagnostic tests

The anticardiolipin test

The anticardiolipin test is important in diagnosing APS [1, 5, 39, 111] and in exploring the specificity of aPL antibodies [40, 47, 75, 108, 110]. Considerable effort has been expended in standardizing the test [41, 50, 52]. Nevertheless, several problems remain, and it is our view that many of these issues can be settled if careful attention is paid to test protocols [52].

Details on performance of the anticardiolipin test are given in other reviews [44]. There are some technical points, however, which require a brief discussion. The first concerns the choice of ELISA plates. We have found a number of groups using "high-binding capacity" plates in which nonspecific antibody binding to the plates is significant – some samples bind empty wells in excess of wells coated with antigen. We suggest that when plates are selected, binding to empty wells be compared to binding to cardiolipin-coated wells, and plates with low nonspecific binding be selected (e.g. Titertek Linbro, or LKB by Labsystems). A second issue concerns coating plates with cardiolipin or other phospholipid antigens. It is important that the organic solvent in which the antigen is dissolved contains as little chloroform as possible (use of methanol:chloroform in a ratio of 4 or 5:1 is suitable for samples not soluble in methanol alone); chloroform dissolves plastic and can give false-positive readings if used in excess. A third point concerns use of adult (or fetal) bovine serum in PBS. The use of 10% adult bovine serum in PBS to block plates, as well as to dissolve serum samples and enzyme labeled antibodies is important since this buffer contains β_2 glycoprotein 1 (β_2 GP1) which enhances binding of aPL antibodies to cardiolipin [57, 74, 87, 95]. Fourth, it is important that all plates be run with isotype-specific calibrators to construct a calibration curve [40, 44]. Isotype-specific (IgG, IgM, or IgA) determination of anticardiolipin level enables geater uniformity and specificity in reporting test results. IgG anticardiolipin is reported in "GPL units", where 1 GPL unit is defined as the cardiolipin binding activity of 1 μg/ml of an affinitiy-purified IgG anticardiolipin antibody preparation [50]; IgM anticardiolipin is reported in "MPL units" where 1 MPL unit is defined as the cardiolipin binding activity of 1 μg/ml of an affinity-purified IgM anticardiolipin antibody preparation [50]; and IgA is reported in "APL units" where 1 APL unit is defined as the cardiolipin binding activity of 1 μg/ml of an affinity-purified IgA anticardiolipin antibody preparation.

Another commonly encountered problem is the use of "Tween" in PBS wash solutions, although more than one study has demonstrated that Tween (a soap) probably emulsifies phospholipids in ELISA plate wells. Tween should not be used in the anticardiolipin ELISA assay, since results are generally unreliable [33, 50].

Finally, utilization of at least one isotype-specific calibrator to stop the substrate color reaction is recommended; normally we utilize an IgG calibrator of about 90 GPL units, for the IgG anticardiolipin assay and an IgM of about 80–90 MPL units for the IgM assay [40, 44]. This method provides more reliable results than the use of a specific incubation period for the enzyme substrate.

Despite rigid adherence to the anticardiolipin ELISA protocol, there will inevitably be runs with poor results. To improve reproducibility of the assay, we currently include a positive control [usually medium positive, e.g., 20–40 GPL (for IgG), or 20–40 MPL (for IgM)], and if readings of the control fall outside certain defined limits (±10–15 GPL or ±10–15 MPL units for medium positive samples), the assay is discarded and the run repeated. Distribution and testing of a standard sample by a national body (e.g., College of American Pathologists in the USA) may also assist in improving test performance and in reducing interlaboratory variation.

A major problem with the anticardiolipin assay has been a lack of specificity for APS. Patients with syphilis [51, 76] and other infectious [15, 56], drug-induced [14, 62] and inflammatory [47] disorders, as well as normal individuals [47] may be positive – these results are usually IgM- or low IgG-isotype positive [49]. By studying various phospholipid antigens, our laboratory has found a phospholipid mixture which gives a more specific result than cardiolipin. Thus, sera from patients with syphilis and other miscellaneous disorders, which may give positive anticardiolipin test results, are now negative using the alternative phospholipid antigen. This modification will be incorporated into a new diagnostic kit; the kit has been calibrated so that results can be reported in the same units as the standard anticardiolipin test (distributed by Louisville APL Diagnostics, Louisville, Kentucky, USA).

The lupus anticoagulant test

The lupus anticoagulant test is also important in diagnosing APS [2, 108]. This and the anticardiolipin test should *both* be done in patients suspected of having the APS, since patients are sometimes positive for one but not the other test [21, 64]. If patients are receiving anticoagulant therapy, however, the lupus anticoagulant test is unreliable and only the anticardiolipin test can be used. The lupus anticoagulant test is a *functional* measure of aPL antibodies, since they are detected by their ability to inhibit phospholipid-dependent reactions in the clotting cascade – prothrombin-thrombin conversion [13, 38, 108] and factor X activation [13, 103, 108]. Patients with these antibodies have prolonged in vitro clotting tests and, as a rule, the degree of prolongation of the test is inversely proportional to the quantity of phospholipid in the test system [13, 38, 103]. Hence, confirmation of a positive lupus anticoagulant test is demonstrated by adding phospholipid to the test system and finding normalization of the clotting time [2, 108].

Standardization of the lupus anticoagulant test has proved elusive, but guidelines for test performance have been established, and these are reviewed elsewhere [64, 108]. The distribution of lupus anticoagulant test samples by the College of American Pathologists to laboratories in the USA is a useful first step to achieving greater uniformity in methodology.

Specifity of aPL antibodies

What are aPL antibodies – anticardiolipin? antiphospholipid? anti-β_2 glycoprotein 1?

Soon after introduction of the anticardiolipin test [45], investigators began determining the specificity of antibodies detected. Within the first few years, it seemed that these antibodies were specific for negatively charged phospholipids [47, 48, 84], but recently, some laboratories have reported that a plasma protein, β_2GP1, influences binding of anticardiolipin antibodies to cardiolipin [30, 57, 74, 87, 95]. To assess these recent findings, it is important to review all work on anticardiolipin specificity done to date. In a separate section, we shall discuss an equally important issue, lupus anticoagulant specificity, about which traditional views have also been challenged.

Initial work on anticardiolipin specificity showed these antibodies cross-reacted with negatively charged phospholipids (Fig. 1) [48, 84]. Thus, pre-incubation of anticardiolipin-positive sera with cardiolipin, phosphatidylserine (PS), phosphatidic acid (PA), or other negatively charged phospholipid liposomes caused a marked decrease in positivity of sera by ELISA [47, 48, 75, 84]. In a more recent study, Pierangeli et al. [88] showed that there was a decrease in cardiolipin binding activity when purified anticardiolipin immunoglobulins were pre-incubated with negatively charged phospholipids in 1% ovalbumin/PBS (w/v). The latter suggested that these antibodies bind phospholipids *independent* of β_2GP1 or other plasma proteins. In addition, purified anticardiolipin immunoglobulins in 1% ovalbumin/PBS (w/v) bound negatively charged phospholipids in ELISA plates [52, 87], but binding was enhanced by adding β_2GP1 to the buffer. In addition, immunoglobulins could be precipitated by cardiolipin liposomes from anticardiolipin-positive sera, and the antibodies eluted from the cardiolipin liposome-antibody complexes possessed both cardiolipin and negatively charged phospholipid binding activity [87]. Antibodies cross-reactive with negatively charged phospholipids can also be eluted off of cardiolipin or PS affinity column [74, 83]. Other data suggesting that anticardiolipin antibodies are phospholipid specific involve use of placental anticoagulant protein (PAP), a lipocortin which binds negatively charged phospholipids. PAP was shown to compete with anticardiolipin antibodies for binding to cardiolipin [96], suggesting that both molecules bind the same target antigen.

Zwitterionic phospholipids, such as phosphatidylcholine (PC), were not bound by anticardiolipin antibodies in any of the above experiments (Fig. 1) [48, 84, 88]. Based on the above data, it was reasoned that anticardiolipin antibodies did not only bind cardiolipin but cross-reacted with negatively charged phospholipids, perhaps by binding the phosphodiester moiety of the phospholipid [47] (Fig. 1). Thus, anticardiolipin antibodies should properly be called *antiphospholipid antibodies* [47]. Presumably, zwitterionic phospholipids are not bound because the positively charged head group (e.g., choline in PC) blocks antibody access to the phosphodiester group of the molecule [1, 47, 108].

aPL antibodies do not bind all molecules with phosphodiester groups. Thus, little or no binding to DNA is observed [48, 105], although DNA has a negatively charged phosphodiester-linked "backbone". One must conclude, therefore, that the glyceride portion of negatively charged phospholipids are also important in determining binding by aPL antibodies. The glyceride portion of the molecule, particularly the carbon chain of the fatty acid groups are important because they determine phospholipid confor-

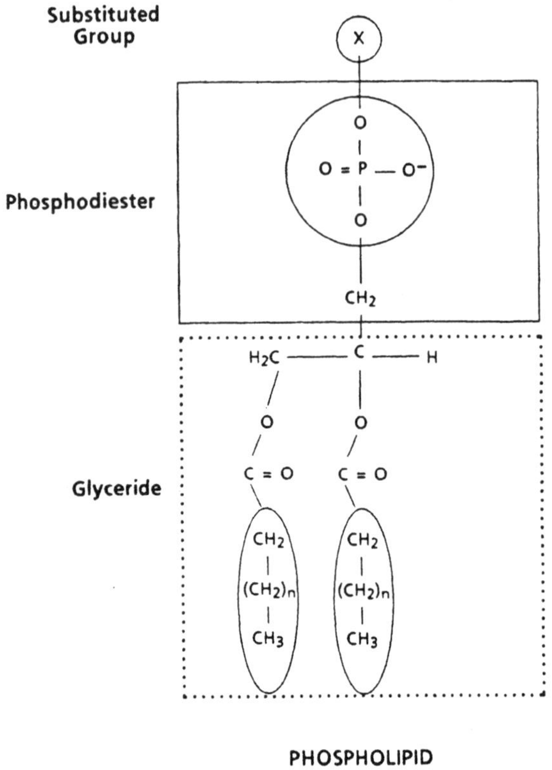

Fig. 1. The phospholipid structure. Phospholipids are made up of a phosphodiester group linked to a glyceride. The substituted group [X] may have a positive charge (e.g., choline) or no charge (e.g.,serine). It has been suggested that antibodies bind the phosphodiester group, but if [X] has a positive charge, antibody access to the phosphodiester group is blocked. Hence, phosphatidylserine is bound, but not phosphatidylcholine

mation in aqueous solution, and conformation may play an important role in antibody binding. It is noteworthy that phospholipids with fatty acid hydrocarbon chains of less than 16 carbon atoms are not bound by aPL antibodies [60]. This suggests either that phospholipids with short fatty acid chains do not form conformational structures recognized by aPL antibodies [40], or that the fatty acid chain is part of the epitope [60].

In 1990, Galli et al. [30] reported that they had affinity purified two anticardiolipin antibodies which bound the serum protein (β_2GP1). Almost simultaneously, McNeil et al. [74] reported that β_2GP1 was an essential cofactor for anticardiolipin binding to cardiolipin, although they saw no direct binding to β_2GP1. These observations were important since they might be relevant to the role of aPL antibody in thrombosis. β_2GP1 is a 50-kDa plasma protein which binds a variety of negatively charged molecules, including negatively charged phospholipids [99]. The protein was shown to inhibit prothrombin-thrombin conversion, presumably by binding the negatively charged phospholipid catalyst required for this reaction [38, 77, 103]. In addition, β_2GP1 was shown to inhibit contact activation of the clotting cascade, presumably by binding the negatively charged "activating surfaces" [100]. These data led to the hypothesis that β_2GP1 might serve as an anticoagulant in plasma. Thus, Galli et al.

[30] and McNeil et al. [74] proposed that aPL antibodies might favor thrombosis by interfering with the anticoagulant effects of β_2GP1 in vivo.

The reports of aPL binding to β_2GP1 has attracted considerable interest and controversy. Some authors have reported that aPL antibodies bind β_2GP1 [4, 71], or even that independent anti-β_2GP1 antibodies may exist that are associated with thrombosis [112]. Other authors have found no evidence of binding to β_2GP1 in ELISA assays [34, 57, 74, 87, 95]. More recently, there have been reports that the type of ELISA plate on which the β_2GP1 is presented may be important [71], although it should be noted that plates utilized to measure anti-β_2GP1 have varied considerably [4, 71, 112]. What is agreed by all authors is that in the ELISA test, β_2GP1 enhances binding of aPL antibodies to cardiolipin and other negatively charged phospholipids [52, 57, 74, 87, 95]. It was postulated that this might occur because of exposure of "neo-epitopes" on β_2GP1 [57], on cardiolipin [43], or on both molecules [74]. The latter view is supported by a recent study in which Borchman and colleagues used Fourier transform infra-red spectroscopy (FTIR) to study cardiolipin and β_2GP1 structure (Borchman et al., submitted). They demonstrated marked changes in spectra of both cardiolipin and β_2GP1 when the two molecules formed a complex. The effect of β_2GP1 on cardiolipin binding activity appears confined to ELISA plates. Pre-incubation of anticardiolipin-positive immunoglobulins with β_2GP1 did not inhibit anticardiolipin activity by ELISA [87, 88]; and pre-incubation of sera with cardiolipin liposomes plus β_2GP1 did not enhance the inhibition observed with cardiolipin liposomes alone [88].

One important observation with respect to the β_2GP1-cardiolipin interaction is that immunization of mice with human β_2GP1 alone induces both anti-β_2GP1 and anticardiolipin antibodies [35, 85]. These appear to be separate groups of antibodies. It has been postulated that β_2GP1 binds phospholipids in the mouse circulation making the phospholipids immunogenic [85]. This observation may be important to the generation of autoantibodies in general, in that immunization with an apparently unrelated molecule (β_2GP1) can induce autoantibodies to an unrelated antigen (e.g., cardiolipin and negatively charged phospholipids) [85].

No conclusions can be drawn with respect to the interaction of anticardiolipin antibodies with β_2GP1. Various authors believe that these antibodies bind β_2GP1 [4, 30, 71], a complex of β_2GP1-cardiolipin [57, 74, 95], or neo-epitopes on β_2GP1 [57] or on cardiolipin alone [43]. Determination of the true specificity of these antibodies may be important in understanding anticardiolipin pathogenesis in thrombosis.

Lupus anticoagulant: specificity

The specificity of antibodies responsible for lupus anticoagulant activity may also be important to pathogenesis of APS. A number of recent reports challenge traditional views that these are aPL antibodies [13, 38, 40, 47, 48, 75, 84, 108, 110]. Oosting et al. [78] reported that depletion of β_2GP1 from lupus anticoagulant-positive plasma, utilizing an affinity column, resulted in loss of lupus anticoagulant activity in the majority of samples examined. In a subsequent study, they suggested that immunoglobulins from patients with APS might bind coagulation protein-phospholipid complexes (e.g., prothrombin-phospholipid, protein C-phospholipid, etc.) [79]. The latter report led to speculation that one subgroup of antibodies specific for a prothrombin-phospholipid complex may prolong clotting in vitro and cause "lupus anticoagulant

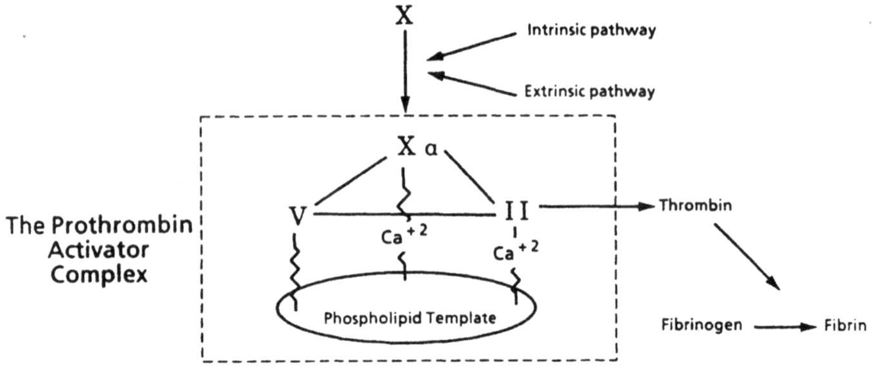

Fig. 2. The "prothrombinase complex" is required for conversion of prothrombin to thrombin in the clotting cascade. Thrombin goes on to convert fibrinogen to fibrin and a clot is formed. Antibodies with lupus anticoagulant activity inhibit formation of the prothrombinase complex and so delay thrombin generation and clot formation. Investigators now ask whether these antibodies are specific for prothrombin, prothrombin-phospholipid complex [8, 31, 79], phospholipids alone [13, 38, 45, 48, 83, 84, 88, 96, 103], or β_2 glycoprotein 1 (β_2GP1) [78,94]. Both β_2GP1 [38, 77] and antibodies with lupus anticoagulant activity [13, 38] have been shown to inhibit prothrombin-thrombin conversion

activity" (Fig. 2), whereas another subgroup specific for a protein C-phospholipid complex (Fig. 3) might be responsible for thrombosis in vivo [110]. In another study, Bevers et al. [8] reported that antibodies with lupus anticoagulant activity inhibited *human* but not *bovine* prothrombin-thrombin conversion [8]. They suggested that the lupus anticoagulant might be specific for epitopes on human prothrombin-phospholipid complex. Galli et al. [31] reported that absorption of lupus anticoagulant plasma with cardiolipin liposomes resulted in three categories of antibodies: one group with lupus anticoagulant activity not absorbed by cardiolipin, and another group, divisible into two subgroups, that can be absorbed by cardiolipin, one with lupus anticoagulant activity in the presence of β_2GP1 and another with no lupus anticoagulant activity. It might be argued that the "lupus anticoagulant only" group of Galli et al. [31] might bind a prothrombin-phospholipid complex and this would resemble the antibodies described by Bevers et al. [8] and by Oosting et al. [79]. Secondly, the anticardiolipin subgroup which requires β_2GP1 for lupus anticoagulant acivity, described by Galli et al. [31], resembles that described earlier by Oosting et al. [78]. Yet another formulation has been suggested by Roubey et al. [94], who described a monoclonal antibody specific for β_2GP1 alone which had lupus anticoagulant activity. This latter report suggested that antibodies with lupus anticoagulant activity might bind epitopes solely on β_2GP1. This would be a remarkable finding, since it suggests that both antibody (anti-β_2GP1) and antigen (β_2GP1) possess the same activity [38, 77, 94, 103], namely, inhibition of phospholipid-dependent coagulation reactions (Fig. 2).

During the past 3 years, our laboratory has carefully re-examined data on the specificity of antibodies with lupus anticoagulant activity. Thus far, our studies have been performed only with purified immunoglobulins or with plasma which have *both* lupus anticoagulant and anticardiolipin binding activitiy. As had been shown by other groups [34], we found that cardiolipin and PS liposomes absorb antibodies with cardiolipin binding *and* lupus anticoagulant activity [88], even in the absence of plasma as diluent (TRIS-buffered saline was used as diluent [88]). The same study showed that antibodies precipitated by cardiolipin liposomes have lupus anticoagulant activ-

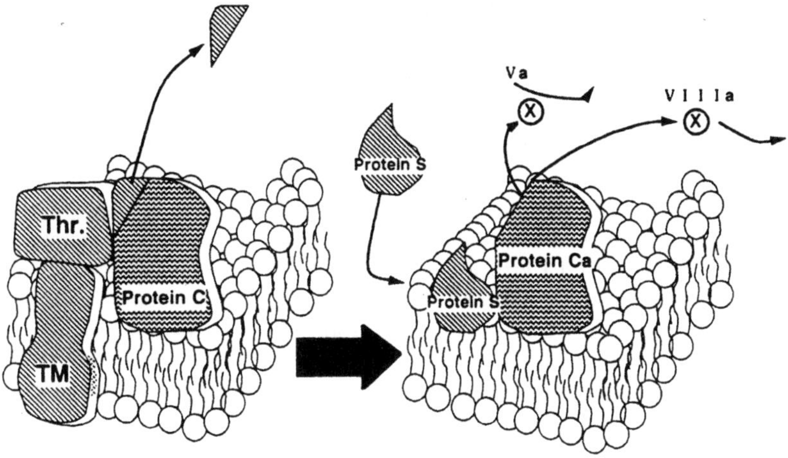

Fig. 3. The protein C activation system by which thrombin "turns off" its own generation. Thrombin binds thrombomodulin and this complex activates protein C. Activated protein C and its cofactor, protein S, inactivate factors Va and VIIIa. Inactivation of Va and VIIIa stops thrombin generation

ity [88]. These data suggested that anticardiolipin binding antibodies in the samples studied had lupus anticoagulant activity in the *absence* of β_2GP1.

A second study was done in which the inhibitory effects of these immunoglobulin preparations on the prothrombin-thrombin conversion reaction was investigated (Fig. 2). IgG purified from 11 consecutive patients with anticardiolipin and lupus anticoagulant activity were studied [38]. The reaction system contained only purified IgG immunoglobulins as well as purified prothrombin, Factors Va and Xa, and the prospholipid catalyst (PS/PC) (Fig. 2). The diluent used was 0.05% (w/v) human serum albumin in TRIS-buffered saline, ensuring the exclusion of other plasma proteins (including β_2GP1). All 11 IgG immunoglobulin preparations inhibited the prothrombin-thrombin conversion reaction, and the inhibitory effect decreased as phospholipid concentration in the sytem was increased [38]. In addition, affinity-purified anticardiolipin antibodies inhibited the prothrombinase reaction with an activity 25–50 times greater than that of whole IgG immunoglobulin preparations from the same patient samples [38]. These experiments suggested that the anticardiolipin antibody preparations studied had lupus anticoagulant activity. In a third study, the effect of PAP on the prothrombinase reaction system was studied (Dean et al., submitted). PAP is a lipocortin that binds negatively charged phospholipids [96]. PAP was shown to inhibit the prothrombinase reaction, probably by binding the phospholipid catalyst [96]. When both IgG anticardiolipin antibodies and PAP were added to the prothrombinase reaction system, there was additive inhibition of the prothrombinase reaction. PAP also inhibited cardiolipin binding activity (ELISA) of the IgG anticardiolipin preparations. These results imply that PAP and anticardiolipin antibodies bind common sites on phospholipids both in the prothrombinase reaction system and in the ELISA assay. This study confirms a previous report by Sammaritano et al. [96] in which PAP was shown to inhibit cardiolipin binding activity by ELISA, as well as cause additive prolongation of clotting times in lupus anticoagulant positive plasma.

In other studies, the effect of β_2GP1 and anticardiolipin antibodies on prothrombin-thrombin conversion or Factor Xa activation was investigated. β_2GP1 alone was found to inhibit prothrombin-thrombin conversion by most [38, 77, 103], but not all investigators [31], and it also inhibited Factor Xa generation [103]. When both anticardiolipin antibodies and β_2GP1 were added to the reaction system, there was additive inhibition of prothrombin-thrombin conversion in six of eight samples examined and competitive inhibition in the remaining two [38]. These results suggest that β_2GP1 and anticardiolipin bind similar (?phospholipid, ?phospholipid-prothrombin) sites [38]. Shi et al. [103] studied two preparations, one with lupus anticoagulant activity only, and another with β_2GP1-dependent cardiolipin binding activity only. They found that β_2GP1 inhibited factor Xa activation, and addition of the anticardiolipin antibody preparation partially interfered with the β_2GP1 effect. On the other hand, the lupus anticoagulant preparation competed with β_2GP1. These authors suggested that antibodies with lupus anticoagulant activity, and β_2GP1 bind similar (?phospholipid) sites, a conclusion similar to that of Goldsmith et al. [38]. However, Shi et al. [103] found that their anticardiolipin antibody preparation required β_2GP1 to inhibit factor Xa activation, whereas Goldsmith et al. [38] found inhibitory activity in the *absence* of β_2GP1 in all 11 samples studied.

One must regard the question of specificity of antibodies with lupus anticoagulant activity as unsettled. These antibodies may be specific for negatively charged phospholipids [48, 83, 84, 88], prothrombin-phospholipid complexes [8], or β_2GP1 [94].

Pathogenesis of the antiphospholipid syndrome

Thrombosis is a central clinical feature of APS. Both venous and arterial thrombosis can occur. However, patients with venous thrombotic events tend to get recurrences in the venous circulation, whereas those with arterial events tend to have recurrences in arteries, suggesting subtle differences in mechanisms of thrombosis [92]. These differences may be secondary to differences in causative factors (e.g., subtle autoantibody specificity differences), or differences in host factors, e.g., some patients may have a venous endothelium particularly susceptible to the causative factor(s), whereas in others the arterial circulation may be more subject to damage. Alternatively, there might be a variety of reactions in the hemostatic system that are influenced by aPL antibodies (see discussion below), and the outcome of these interactions may differ depending on the system affected. The occurrence of placental infarction and vascular thrombosis in women with recurrent pregnancy loss [80] suggests that this complication too may be part of a generalized thrombotic disorder. Since many women with APS have only recurrent pregnancy losses without systemic thrombosis [12, 65], it is possible that the hemostatic system in the placenta may be affected differently from the systemic vasculature.

Vascular thrombi are "bland" in APS and inflammatory cells in the vessel wall, characteristic of a vasculitis, are uncommon [61]. Hence, thrombosis is probably not secondary to an immune complex-mediated vasculitis, but due to some alteration of the hemostatic system (endothelium, platelets, coagulation reaction system) by aPL antibodies. Since thrombotic events are intermittent, while antibodies persist, it is likely that these antibodies alter the hemostatic system in such a way as to enhance thrombus formation, but some other "triggering event" is required to initiate the process.

There are several reasons to suggest that aPL antibodies play a role in thrombosis and pregnancy loss. Studies show that both anticardiolipin antibodies and the lupus anticoagulant are associated with thrombosis and pregnancy loss [47, 49, 66]. Some, but not all, studies show that the higher the antibody level, particularly that of the IgG isotype, the more likely is thrombosis and pregnancy loss, particularly when antibodies persist for prolonged periods of time [36, 49, 65]. Thirdly, there are now several mouse models in which pregnancy loss [7, 9, 11, 89] and thrombosis [89] have been induced by human aPL-positive immunoglobulins. In addition, these antibodies have a variety of effects on the hemostatic system in vitro, which would favor thrombosis if these same effects occurred in vivo. The ensuing discussion will summarize mouse models of APS and antibody effects on the hemostatic system in vitro.

Animal models

Pregnancy loss. Gharavi first observed that MRL/lpr mice with anticardiolipin antibodies had increased fetal wastage [32]. In 1990, Branch et al. [11] reported that pregnant BALB/c mice injected with purified immunoglobulins from five women with APS experienced 100% fetal death. In the following year, Blank et al. [9] reported that infusion of as little as 10 μg of IgG polyclonal or monoclonal antibody preparations into pregnant mice resulted in increased fetal resorption and thrombocytopenia. In follow-up experiments Bakimer et al. [7] reported that they were able to induce APS in mice by active immunization with a monoclonal anticardiolipin antibody (presumably by an idiotype-anti-idiotype mechanism), and these mice also had fetal resorptions. In other experiments by the same group, Fishman et al. [26] showed that splenocytes from these experimental mice produced decreased granulocyte-macrophage colony-stimulating factor and interleukin-3 (IL-3). Intraperitoneal injection of IL-3 prevented fetal loss and thrombocytopenia [27]. Since these cytokines support placental growth and development, reduction by aPL antibodies might result in fetal resorption. Thus, several studies suggest that aPL antibodies play a role in induction of pregnancy loss, perhaps by modulating cytokine production.

Thrombosis. Although work on a mouse model of pregnancy loss is well advanced, only recently has a mouse model of thrombosis been developed. Initially, Smith et al. [106] reported that two of eight MRL/lpr mice with anticardiolipin antibodies had cerebral infarction. However, MRL/lpr mice produce autoantibodies with a variety of specificities making it difficult to attribute thrombosis specifically to aPL antibodies. However, a mouse model of thrombosis has been developed at the University of Louisville which suggests a role for aPL antibodies in thrombus formation [89]. The mouse model of thrombosis involves induction of thrombus in the exposed femoral vein of an anesthetized mouse by a standardized, crush injury to the femoral vein. The forming thrombus can be visualized and recorded by fiber optic transillumination into a stereoscopic operating microscope equipped with a closed circuit video system [89]. Typically the induced thrombus grows rapidly between 1 and 5 min after injury followed by progressive reduction in size over the next 30 min. The rate of thrombus formation and disappearance, as well as thrombus area is measured by digitalizing the recorded video image and using computer-assisted gray-level analysis [89]. On days 1 and 2 prior to surgery, the CD1 mice were injected intraperitoneally with purified IgG or IgM immunoglobulins from patients with APS. High blood levels of anticardiolipin antibodies [50–80 GPL (for IgG) or 50–80 MPL units (for IgM)] were achieved. Control mice were injected with an equal quantity of purified IgG or IgM obtained from healthy humans. In experiments with IgG ($n = 3$) and IgM ($n = 3$) preparations, there was a significant increase in the *size* of thrombi, and the thrombi persisted *significantly longer* than in mice immunized with normal IgG or IgM [86, 89]. It was noteworthy that when postmortems were performed in the mice after surgery, no thrombi were noted in the systemic circulation [89]. This supports the hypothesis that aPL antibodies predispose to thrombosis, but another initiating event such as endothelial injury (achieved in these experiments by crush injury to the femoral vein) is required.

Mechanism of action

Over the past 15 years, there have been a variety of in vitro studies showing effects of aPL antibodies on the hemostatic system. Some of these effects might explain their ability to promote thrombosis or pregnancy loss in vivo. Effects on prostaglandin synthesis, endothelial cells, platelets, the coagulation system and on β_2GP1 have all been described. These will be briefly discussed.

Effect on prostaglandin synthesis. Carreras and Vermylen [17] reported that plasma from 8 of 14 lupus anticoagulant-positive patients inhibited prostacylin (PGI_2) production by rat aorta rings. Of the 8 patients with "inhibitory activity" 6 had a history of thrombosis. Since PGI_2 is a potent inhibitor of platelet aggregation, they speculated that aPL antibodies might induce thrombosis by decreasing PGI_2 synthesis by endothelial cells [17]. Other groups have examined this issue with different conclusions. For example, Hasselaar et al. [53] studied the effect of sera from 27 patients with aPL antibodies on PGI_2 production by cultured human umbilical vein endothelial cells (HUVEC); 4–19% of the sera inhibited PGI_2 production, whereas 4–28% stimulated PGI_2 production. In the same study, 4–30% sera increased thromboxane (TXA_2) production by platelets [53]. These investigators found no correlation between a history of thrombosis and effects on PGI_2 production by endothelial cells, or TXA_2 production by platelets. In contrast, Watson and Schorer [113] reported that in 26 patient plasma examined, decreased PGI_2 production occurred in the presence of lupus anticoagulant-positive plasma after stimulation of endothelial cells with 1 μg/ml thrombin. In a subsequent study, they performed experiments which suggested that these antibodies might inhibit the effect of phospholipase A_2 on membrane phospholipids, resulting in decreased PGI_2 production [98].

In a more recent study, Lellouche et al. [59] measured urinary excretion of metabolites of TXA_2 [11-dehydro thromboxane B_2 (TXB_2)] and prostacyclin (2,3-dinor-6-keto-prostaglandin F1α) in 25 patients with the lupus anticoagulant and 32 healthy controls. They reported a significant increase in the TXA_2 metabolite and a lesser increase in the PGI_2 metabolite. In this and a follow-up study [70], F$(ab')_2$ fragments from immunoglobulins of these patients enhanced both TXA_2 generation as well as ^{14}C-labeled serotonin release by platelets [70]. The effect of the F$(ab')_2$ fragments on platelets could be neutralized by phospholipids [70]. Thus, these workers proposed that antibodies specific for phospholipids may stimulate TXA_2 release from platelets. Such an effect would favor platelet aggregation and thrombosis.

Endothelial cells. Endothelial cells may also be targets for aPL antibodies and modification of endothelial cell function might conceivably induce thrombosis. Several groups have examined binding of anticardiolipin-positive sera to HUVEC in culture utilizing an ELISA technique [72, 109]. All studies have found that sera from some patients with the APS bind endothelial cells, but there was no correlation between anti-endothelial and anti-cardiolipin activity [72, 209], and endothelial binding activity was not inhibited by prior incubation of sera with cardiolipin liposomes. In one study, investigators reported that immunoglobulins from five of six patients immunoprecipitated a 70-kDa endothelial cell surface protein [72]. In addition, they reported that four of five preparations which bound the cell surface protein also caused an increased release of von Willebrand factor from endothelial cells. The same group reported that sera from women with the APS and pregnancy loss bound trophoblast cells in culture (20/29 women with anticardiolipin antibodies versus 1/20 healthy controls) [73]. The trophoblast binding antibody preparations immunoprecipitated a 62-kDa membrane protein. The latter antibodies reportedly inhibited arachnidonic acid and TXA_2 release by trophoblasts as well as binding of pro-urokinase to trophoblast urokinase receptors [73]. Hence, the studies by McCrae et al. [72, 73] suggest the existence of antibodies with specificities for endothelial cell and trophoblast proteins which alter endothelial and placental function to produce thrombosis and pregnancy loss, respectively.

In two other studies, antibodies from patients with APS appeared to increase "tissue factor activity" of endothelial cells. Hasselaar et al. [54] compared 15 aPL-positive SLE sera, 13 aPL-negative SLE sera, and 10 aPL-negative sera from patients without connective tissue disease (CTD). "Procoagulant activity" by cultured endothelial cells was increased in the presence of suboptimal doses of tumor necrosis factor in 14 of 15 aPL-positive SLE patients, 7/13 aPL-negative SLE, and 2/10 aPL-negative CTD patients [54]. In another study, Branch et al. [12] studied sera from 11 patients with the APS versus 8 normal controls and reported enhanced tissue factor expression by the APS sera; this activity resided in the IgG fraction of the sera.

Platelets. The association of aPL antibodies with thrombocytopenia led to speculation that these antibodies could bind platelet membranes resulting in increased uptake and destruction by the reticuloendothelial system [45]. Alternatively, binding to platelet membranes might result in platelet activation, increased aggregation, and thrombosis. Khamashta et al. [58] reported that cardiolipin binding activity could be inhibited by pre-incubation of sera with freeze-dried but not intact platelet. They suggested that these antibodies might bind phospholipids on the inner leaflet of the bimolecular platelet membrane such as PS and phosphatidylethanolamine (PE) [58]. Two studies reported that aPL antibodies which bind platelets may be specific for phospholipids, as well as for other antigens. Utilizing human hybridomas, Rauch et al. [91] reported that binding to platelets correlated with binding to PE, cardiolipin, and DNA. Hasselaar et al. [55] also reported that sera from patients with platelet and endothelial cell binding activity cross-reacted with a variety of negatively charged phospholipids as well as with DNA. In another study, Out et al. [81] reported that antibodies that eluted off of platelets from patients with APS cross-reacted with a variety of negatively charged phospholipids

In summary, sera from patients with APS may contain antibodies specific for a variety of platelet antigens. The antibodies may be specific for phospholipids [45], DNA [58, 91], or platelet membrane proteins [24]. By binding platelet membranes, there may be enhanced uptake by the reticuloendothelial system, resulting in thrombocytopenia.

Whether aPL antibodies can induce platelet activation is important since this might be one mechanism of thrombosis. As with other issues pertaining to these antibodies, quite separate conclusions have been reached by different investigators. Out et al. [81] reported that, although they were able to elute phospholipid-binding antibodies off platelets, these antibodies had *no* effect on platelet activation or aggregation. In contrast, Martinuzzo et al. [70] reported that $F(ab')_2$ fragments from IgG of patients with APS increased platelet aggregation and enhanced serotonin release in the presence of low doses of thrombin (0.01 U/ml). Piertangeli et al. (submitted) also demonstrated that three of six affinity-purified IgG anticardiolipin antibodies caused platelet activation, and that in the presence of subaggregating doses of thrombin, ADP, and collagen, all six affinity-purified antibodies enhanced platelet aggregation. Escolar et al. [24] reported that when anticardiolipin-positive plasma from SLE patients were perfused through annular chambers containing denuded arterial segments, deposition of platelets was statistically increased compared to plasma from anticardiolipin-negative SLE patients. This activity was reproduced by two affinity purified anticardiolipin antibody preparations where increasing concentrations of antibodies correlated with increasing platelet deposition [24].

In a series of elegant experiments, Lin and Wang [63] showed that affinity-purified anticardiolipin antibodies obtained from rabbits immunized with cardiolipin bound platelets, as assessed by flow cytofluorometric analysis and inhibition experiments. These antibodies were shown to cause irreversible shape changes of platelets as assessed by electron microscopy. The preparations also caused increased platelet aggregation as demonstrated by platelet aggregometry, as well as increased levels of TXA_2 formation, and increased cytosolic free calcium ion, 47-kDa protein phosphorylation, and serotonin secretion [63]. Subaggregatory concentrations of antibodies caused synergistic activation of platelets with low concentrations of thrombin, collagen, and epinephrine. Unlike studies utilizing human affinity-purified anticardiolipin antibodies, this study found that the rabbit affinity-purified anticardiolipin antibodies bound an 80-kDa plasma membrane protein [63]. Since the antibodies were affinity purified by cardiolipin liposomes, one must assume that these are cross-reacting antibodies.

In summary, some studies show that antibodies with phospholipid binding specificity cause platelet activation and aggregation in the presence of subaggregating doses of thrombin, collagen, ADP and epinephrine [24, 70]. Normally resting platelets may have too few negatively charged phospholipids in the outer leaflet of the membrane for anticardiolipin binding to take place. However, partial activation of platelets by agents such as thrombin may cause translocation of PS from the inner to the outer leaflet making this molecule available for aPL antibody binding. Increased platelet binding would result in platelet activation [63, 70]. Since aPL antibodies derived from various patient sera are heterogeneous, and techniques used to demonstrate platelet binding, activation, and aggregation are very different, it is likely that there will continue to be varying reports on the effects of antibodies on platelet function.

Coagulation. aPL antibodies can affect several sites in the coagulation cascade, in vitro, and if such effects occurred in vivo, thrombosis might be induced. When clotting is initiated, several reactions are set into play which counteract the clotting process. These include activation of antithrombin-III (AT III), fibrinolysis, protein C activation, and possibly, inhibitory effects of β_2GP1. By inhibiting any of these reactions, aPL antibodies may favor in vivo thrombosis.

Anti-thrombin III. Thus far, there is little evidence for an antibody effect on AT-III. Cosgriff and Martin [104] reported a single patient with lupus anticoagulant activity who had low AT-III functional activity [19]. However, studies by Boey et al. [10], and Tsakiris et al. [109] found no correlation between decreased AT-III level and presence of the lupus anticoagulant. In a recent study, Shaibata and colleagues reported that aPL antibodies from seven patients with APS cross-reacted with heparan sulfate and blocked heparin-accelerated formation of AT III-thrombin complexes [102]. Such action in vivo would promote thrombosis.

Fibrinolysis. Studies of antibody effects on the fibrinolytic pathway have yielded mixed results. In a report of 28 SLE patients, 12 of whom had the lupus anticoagulant, Angeles-Cano et al. [3] found increased von Willenbrand factor activity and decreased fibrinolytic activity after venous occlusion (by applying a tourniquet to the patient's arm). In contrast, Francis et al. [29] performing similar studies found no increase in tissue-type plasminogen activator (t-PA) nor in plasminogen activator inhibitor (t-PAI), and they concluded that there was no antibody effect on the fibrinolytic pathway. Tsakiris et al. [109] measured determinants of the fibrinolytic pathway in plasma of 20 lupus anticoagulant-positive patients and 24 normal controls. There was no statistical difference in plasminogen, α_2-antiplasmin, fibrinogen, D-dimer or t-PA activity, but t-PAI was increased. An increase in t-PAI would decrease plasminogen activation and so decrease fibrinolysis [109]. The effects of lupus anticoagulant (n = 10) and normal plasma (n = 9) on t-PA and t-PAI secretion by endothelial cells in culture was compared by Francis and Neely [28]. There was no difference in t-PA or t-PAI secretion observed [28]. Finally, Sanfelippo and Drayna [111] in a study of three lupus anticoagulant-positive plasma reported that contact activation of fibrinolysis by kaolin was impaired [97]. In summary, there are some studies which suggest lupus anticoagulant-positive plasma have no effect on fibrinolysis [28, 29], whereas others report that decreased fibrinolysis might occur because of inhibitory effects on plasminogen activator release [3], increased PAI levels [97] or inhibition of prekallikrein activity [97].

Protein C. The effect of aPL antibodies on protein C activation has been a subject of considerable interest, since protein C activation is catalyzed by phospholipids (Fig. 3). Initiation of the coagulation cascade causes thrombin generation, but in addition to converting fibrinogen to fibrin, thrombin turns off its own production by activation of the protein C system. Thrombin binds an endothelial membrane protein, thrombomodulin, and the thrombin-thrombomodulin complex activates protein C. Activated protein C and a cofactor, protein S, then act in consort to inactivate factors VIIIa and factor Va (Fig. 3). Inactivation of factors Va and VIIIa will turn off thrombin generation and interrupt the clotting process [25].

Several studies have shown that antibodies with lupus anticoagulant activity inhibit the protein C activation system. Comp et al. [18] first reported that immunoglobulin fractions from two of seven patients with the lupus anticoagulant inhibited thrombin-thrombomodulin mediated activation of protein C. In a subsequent study, Cariou et al. [16] found that both IgG fractions and $F(ab')_2$ fragments from eight lupus anticoagulant-positive patients inhibited protein C activation by cultured endothelial cells. The latter effect could be neutralized by pre-incubation of the antibodies with phospholipids. Marciniak and Romond [69] in a complex series of experiments demonstrated that lupus anticoagulant-positive plasma in 15 consecutive patients inhibited the inactivation of factor Va by activated protein C. Thus, the latter workers suggested that antibody inhibition occurs not at the level of protein C activation, but at a later step, after protein C is activated. Studies by Malia et al. [68] suggest that these antibodies inhibit the effect of the activated protein C-protein S complex on Va degradation. All of the above studies suggest that aPL antibodies may induce thrombosis by inhibition of the protein C activation system, but the site of action is uncertain. In contrast to the above reports, one recent study showed an inconsistent antibody effect on protein C activation [79].

The effects of aPL antibodies on the prothrombinase complex and protein C activation system may explain the "paradox" of antibodies causing in vitro prolongation of clotting yet being procoagulant in vivo. In vitro, these antibodies inhibit conversion of prothrombin to thrombin, so delaying clot formation, whereas in vivo, the predominant effect might be inhibition of protein C activation, which would favor thrombosis. As also discussed previously, effects on endothelial cells and platelets, or on the fibrinolytic system may all account for thrombosis in vivo.

β_2 glycoprotein 1. The role of β_2GP1 on anticardiolipin binding has been discussed in a previous section of this review. To summarize that discussion, β_2GP1 is a 50-kDa plasma protein which binds negatively charged phospholipids [99] and, in this manner, inhibits conversion of prothrombin to thrombin [77] and contact activation of the clotting cascade [103]. Some have suggested that this protein acts as a natural inhibitor of clotting [77, 103]. Various investigators have proposed that some aPL antibodies, by competing with β_2GP1 or even binding a β_2GP1-phospholipid complex [30, 57, 74], may neutralize the inhibitory effects of β_2GP1 and so favor thrombosis. However, β_2GP1 levels were not found to be decreased in patients with aPL antibodies, and patients with congenitally decreased or absent β_2GP1 do not appear to have excess thrombosis.

Summary

The study of aPL antibodies and the APS has appealed to large numbers of investigators over the last decade. This accounts, in part, for the great degree of apparently contradictory data being published. What seems certain is that these antibodies are associated with thrombosis and recurrent pregnancy loss, and animal data suggest a direct role in pathogenesis. In vitro studies demonstrate that these antibodies have a variety of functional effects on the hemostatic system, giving further credence to an antibody role in thrombosis. Further studies will doubtless give better insight into the mechanisms of antibody action and this will provide a more rational basis for treatment.

References

1. Alarcon-Segovia D, Sanchez-Guerrero J (1989) Primary antiphospholipid syndrome. J Rheumatol 16:482
2. Alving BM (1994) Lupus anticoagulants, anticardiolipin antibodies and the APS. In: Loscalzo J, Schafer AL (eds) Thrombosis and hemorrhage. Blackwell, Oxford, pp 749–765
3. Angeles-Cano E, Sultan Y, Clauvel JP (1979) Predisposing factors to thrombosis in systemic lupus erythematosus: possible relation to endothelial damage. J Lab Clin Med 94:312
4. Arvieux J. Pouzol P, Roussel B, Jacib MC, Colomb MG (1992) Measurement of anti-phospholipid antibodies by ELISA using β_2 glycoprotein 1 as an antigen. Br J Haematol 81:568

5. Asherson RA (1988) A "primary" antiphospholipid syndrome? J Rheumatol 15:1742
6. Asherson RA, Khamashta MA, Ordi-Ros J, Derksen RHWM, Machin SJ, Barquinero J, Out HH, Harris EN, Vilardell-Torress M, Hughes GRV (1989) The "primary" antiphospholipid syndrome: major clinical and serological features. Medicine 68:366
7. Bakimer R, Fishman P, Blank M, Srednc B, Djaidetti M, Shoenfeld Y (1992) Induction of primary antiphospholipid syndrome in mice by immunization with a human monoclonal anticardiolipin antibody (H-3). J Clin Invest 89:1558
8. Bevers EM, Galli M, Barbui T, Comfurius P, Zwaal RFA (1991) Lupus anticoagulant (LA) IgGs are not directed to phospholipids only but to a complex lipid-bound human prothrombin. Thromb Haemost 66:629
9. Blank M, Cohen J, Toder V, Shoenfeld Y (1991) Induction of antiphospholipid syndrome in naive mice with mouse lupus monoclonal and human polyclonal anticardiolipin antibodies. Proc Natl Acad Sci USA 88:3069
10. Boey ML, Loizou S, Colaco CB, Matkin JA, Hughes GRV (1984) Antithrombin III in systemic lupus erythematosus. Clin Exp Rheumatol 2:53
11. Branch DW, Dudley DJ, Mitchell MD (1990) Immunoglobulin G fractions from patients with antiphospholipid antibodies cause fetal death in BALB/c mice: a model for autoimmune fetal loss. Am J Obstet Gynecol 163:120
12. Branch WD, Silver RM, Blackwell JL, Reading JC, Scott JR (1992) Outcome of treated pregnancies in women with antiphospholipid syndrome: an update of the Utah experience. Obstet Gynecol 80:614
13. Brandt JT (1991) Assays for phospholipid-dependent formation of thrombin and factor Xa: a potential method for quantifying lupus anticoagulant activity. Thromb Haemost 66:453
14. Canoso RT, de Oliviera RM (1982) Chlorpromazine-induced lupus anticoagulant and associated immunologic abnormalities. Am J Hematol 13:121
15. Canoso RT, Zon LI, Groopman JE (1987) Anticardiolipin antibodies associated with HTLV-111 infection. Br J Haematol 65:495
16. Cariou R, Tobelin G, Belluci S, Soria J, Soria C, Maclouf J, Caen J (1985) Effect of the lupus anticoagulant on antithrombogenic properties of endothelial cells: inhibition of thrombomodulin-dependent protein C activation. Thromb Haemost 60:54
17. Cameras LO, Vermylen JG (1982) 'Lupus' anticoagulant and thrombosis: possible role of inhibition of prostacyclin formation. Thromb Haemost 48:28
18. Comp PC, DeBault LE, Esmon NL, Esmon CT (1983) Human thrombomodulin is inhibited by IgG from two patients with non-specific anticoagulants. Blood 62:299a
19. Cosgriff TM, Martin BA (1981) Low functional and high antigenic antithrombin III level in a patient with the lupus anticoagulant. Arthritis Rheum 24:94
20. Cowchock FS, Reece EA, Balaban D, Branch WD, Plouffe L (1992) Repeated fetal losses associated with antiphospholipid antibodies: a collaborative randomized trial comparing prednisone with low-dose heparin treatment. Am J Obstet Gynecol 166:1318
21. Derksen RH, Hasselaar P, Blokzijl L, Meyling FH, degroot PG (1988) Coagulation screen is more specific than the anticardiolipin antibody ELISA in detecting a thrombotic subset of lupus patients. Ann Rheum Dis 47:364
22. Derksen RHWM, deGroot PG, Kater L, Nieuwenhuis HK (1993) Patients with antiphospholipid antibodies and venous thrombosis should receive long-term anticoagulant treatment. Ann Rheum Dis 52:689
23. Englert HS, Loizou S, Derue GM, Walport MJ, Hughes GRV (1989) Clinical and immunological features of livedo reticularis in lupus: a case-control study. Am J Med 87:408
24. Escolar G, Font J, Reverter JC, Lopez-Soto A, Garrido M, Cervera R, Ingelmo M, Castillo R, Ordinas A (1992) Plasma from systemic lupus erythematosus patients with antiphospholipid antibodies promotes platelet aggregation: studies in a perfusion system. Arterioscler Thromb 12:196
25. Esmon CT (1989) The roles of protein C and thrombomodulin in the regulation of blood coagulation. J Biol Chem 264:4743
26. Fishman P, Bakimer R, Blank M, Shoenfeld Y (1992) The putative role of cytoldnes in the induction of primary APS in mice. Clin Exp Immunol 54:495
27. Fishman P, Fulach-Vaknine E, Zigelman R, Bakimer R, Sredni B, Djaletti M, Shoenfeld Y (1993) Prevention of fetal loss in experimental APS by in vitro administration of recombinant interleukin 3. J Clin Invest 91:1834

28. Francis RB, Neely S (1989) Effect of the lupus anticoagulant on endothelial fibrinolytic activity in vitro. Thromb Haemost 61:314
29. Francis RB, McGehee WG, Feinstein DI (1988) Endothelial-dependent fibrinolysis in subjects with the lupus anticoagulant and thrombosis. Thromb Haemost 59:412
30. Galli M, Comfurius P, Maasen C, Heinker HC, de Baets MH, Van-Breda Vriesman PJC, Barbui T, Zwaal RFA, Bevers EM (1990) Anticardiolipin antibodies (ACA) directed not to cardiolipin but to a plasma protein cofactor. Lancet 336:1544
31. Galli M, Comfurius P, Barbui T, Zwaal RFA, Bevers EM (1992) Anticoagulant activity of β_2-glycoprotein 1 is potentiated by a distinct subgroup of anticardiolipin antibodies. Thromb Haemost 68:297
32. Gharavi AE (1991) Anti-phospholipid syndrome in murine lupus. In: Harris EN, Exner T, Asherson RA, Hughes GRV (eds) Phospholipid binding antibodies. CRC Press, Boca Raton, pp 403–416
33. Gharavi A, Lockshin MD (1988) Enhancement of anti-phospholipid antibody activity by Tween 20. J Immunol Methods 114:277
34. Gharavi AE, Harris EN, Sammaritano LR, Pierangeli SS, Wen J (1993) Do patients with antiphospholipid syndrome have antibodies to β_2 glycoprotein 1? J Lab Clin Med 122:426
35. Gharavi AE, Sammaritano LR, Wen J, Elkon KB (1992) Induction of antiphospholipid autoantibodies by immunization with β_2 glycoprotein 1. J Clin Invest 90:1105
36. Ginsburg KS, Liang MH, Newcomer L, Goldhaber SZ, Schur PH, Hennekens CH, Stampler MJ (1992) Anticardiolipin antibodies and the risk for ischemic stroke and venous thrombosis. Ann Intern Med 117:997
37. Gleason CB, Stoddard NT, Wagner SG, Longaker RA, Pierangeli S, Harris EN (1993) A comparison of cardiac valvular involvement in the primary antiphospholipid syndrome versus anticardiolipin negative systemic lupus erythematosus. Am Heart J 125:1123
38. Goldsmith GH, Pierangeli SS, Branch DW, Gharavi AE, Harris EN (1995) Inhibition of prothrombin activation by antiphospholipid antibodies and β_2 glycoprotein 1. Br J Haematol 87:548
39. Harris EN (1987) Syndrome of the Black Swan. Br J Rheumatol 26:324
40. Harris EN (1990) Annotation. Antiphospholipid antibodies. Br J Haematol 74:1
41. Harris EN (1990) The second international anti-cardiolipin standardization workshop/the Kingston Antiphospholipid Antibody Study (KAPS) Group. Am J Clin Pathol 94:476
42. Harris EN, Bos K (1991) An acute disseminated coagulopathy-vasculopathy associated with the antiphospholipid syndrome. Arch Intem Med 151:231
43. Harris EN, Pierangeli S (1990) What is the "true" antigen for antiphospholipid antibodies (letter). Lancet 336:1550
44. Harris EN, Pierangeli SS (1991) The anticardiolipin ELISA. In: Bullock GR, Van Velzen D (eds) Techniques in diagnostic pathology, vol 2. Academic Press, New York, pp 21–39
45. Harris EN, Gharavi AE, Boey ML, Patel BM, Mackworth-Young CG, Loizou S, Hughes GRV (1983) Anti-cardiolipin antibodies: detection by radioimmunoassay and association with thrombosis. Lancet II:1211
46. Reference deleted
47. Harris EN, Gharavi AE, Hughes GRV (1985) Anti-phospholipid antibodies. Clin Rheum Dis 11:591
48. Harris EN, Gharavi AE, Tincani A, Chan JKH, Englert H (1985) Affinity purified anti-cardiolipin and anti-DNA antibodies. J Clin Lab Immunol 17:155
49. Harris EN, Chan JKH, Asherson RA, Aber VR, Gharavi AE, Hughes GRV (1986) Thrombosis, recurrent fetal loss and thrombocytopenia. Predictive value of the anti-cardiolipin antibody test. Arch Intern Med 146:215
50. Harris EN, Gharavi AE, Patel S, Hughes GRV (1987) Evaluation of the anticardiolipin antibody test: report of an international workshop held 4 April 1986. Clin Exp Immunol 68:215
51. Harris EN, Gharavi AE, Wasley GD, Hughes GRV (1988) Use of an enzyme-linked immunosorbent assay and of inhibition studies to distinguish between antibodies to cardiolipin from patients with syphilis or autoimmune disorders. J Infect Dis 157:23
52. Harris EN, Pierangeli S, Birch D (1994) Anticardiolipin wet workshop report: Vth Intemational Symposium on antiphospholipid antibodies. Am J Clin Pathol 101:616
53. Hasselaar P, Derksen RHWM, Blokzijl L, deGroot PG (1988) Thrombosis associated with antiphospholipid antibodies cannot be explained by effects on endothelial and platelet prostanoid synthesis. Thromb Haemost 59:80

54. Hasselaar P, Derksen RHWM, Oosting JD, Blokzijl L, deGroot PG (1989) Synergistic effect of low doses of tumor necrosis factor and sera from patients with systemic lupus erythematosus on the expression of procoagulant activity by cultured endothelial cells. Thromb Haemost 62:654
55. Hasselaar P, Derksen RHWM, Blokzijl L, deGroot PG (1990) Cross-activity of antibodies directed against cardiolipin, DNA, endothelial cells, and blood platelets. Thromb Haemost 63:169
56. Intrator L, Oksenhendler E, Desforges L, Brerling P (1988) Anticardiolipin antibodies in HIV infected patients with or without autoimmune thrombocytopenic purpura. Br J Haematol 67:269
57. Jones JV, James H, Tan NM, Mansour M (1992) Antiphospholipid antibodies require β_2 glycoprotein 1 (apolipoprotein H) as cofactor. J Rheumatol 48:484
58. Khamashta MA, Harris EN, Gharavi AE, Derue G, Hughes GRV (1988) Immune mechanism for thrombosis: antiphospholipid antibody binding to platelet membranes. Ann Rheum Dis 47:849
59. Lellouche F, Martinuzzo M, Said P, Maclouf J, Cameras LO (1 99 1) Imbalance of thromboxane/prostacyclin biosynthesis in patients with lupus anticoagulant. Blood 78:2894
60. Levy RA, Gharavi AE, Sammaritano LR, Habina L, Lockshin MD (1990) Fatty acid chain is a critical epitope for antiphospholipid antibody. J Clin Immunol 10:141
61. Lie JT (1994) Vasculitis in the antiphospholipid syndrome – culprit or consort. J Rheum 21:397
62. Lillicrap DP, Pinto M, Benford K, Ford PM, Ford S (1990) Heterogeneity of laboratory test results for antiphospholipid antibodies in patients treated with chlorpromazine and other phenothiazines. Am J Clin Pathol 93:771
63. Lin Y-L, Wang C-T (1992) Activation of human platelets by the rabbit anticardiolipin antibodies. Blood 80:3134
64. Lockshin MD, Qamar T, Druzin M, Goei S (1987) Antibody to cardiolipin, lupus anticoagulant, and fetal death. J Rheumatol 14:259
65. Lockshin MD, Druzin ML, Qamar T (1989) Prednisone does not prevent recurrent fetal death in women with antiphospholipid antibody. Am J Obstet Gynecol 160:439
66. Love PE, Santoro SA (1990) Antiphospholipid antibodies: anticardiolipin and the lupus anticoagulant in systemic lupus erythematosus (SLE) and in non-SLE disorders: prevalence and clinical significance. Ann Intern Med 12:682
67. Lubbe WF, Liggins GC (1988) Role of lupus anticoagulant and autoinununity in recurrent pregnancy loss. Semin Reprod Endocrinol 6:81
68. Malia RG, Kitchen S, Greaves M, Preston FE (1990) Inhibition of activated protein C and its cofactor protein S by antiphospholipid antibodies. Br J Haematol 76:101
69. Marciniak E, Romond EH (1989) Impaired catalytic function of activated protein C: a new in vitro manifestation of lupus anticoagulant. Blood 74:2426
70. Martinuzzo ME, Maclouf J, Cameras LO, Levy-Toledano S (1993) Antiphospholipid antibodies enhance thrombin-induced platelet activation and thromboxane formation. Thromb Haemost 70:667
71. Matsuura E, Igarashi Y, Yasuda T, Triplett DA, Koike T (1994) Anticardiolipin Antibodies recognize beta(2) glycoprotein 1 structure altered by interacting with an oxygen modified solid phase surface. J Exp Med 179:457
72. McCrae KR, DeMichele A, Samuels P, Roth D, Kuo A, Meng Q, Rauch J, Cines DB (1991) Detection of endothelial cell reactive immunoglobulin in patients with anti-phospholipid antibodies. Br J Haematol 79:595
73. McCrae KR, DeMichele AM, Pandhi P, Balsai MJ, Samuels P, Graham C, Lala PK, Cines DB (1993) Detection of antitrophoblast antibodies in the sera of patients with anticardiolipin antibodies and fetal loss. Blood 82:2730
74. McNeil HP, Simpson RJ, Chesterman CN, Krilis S (1990) Anti-phospholipid antibodies are directed against a complex antigen that includes a lipid-binding inhibitor of coagulation: β_2 glycoprotein 1 (apolipoprotein H). Proc Natl Acad Sci USA 87:4120
75. McNeil HP, Chesterman CN, Krills SA (1991) Immunology and clinical importance of antiphospholipid antibodies. Adv Immunol 49:193
76. Mouritsen S, Hoier-Madsen M, Wiik A, Orum 0, Standberg-Pedersen N (1989) The specificity of anti-cardiolipin antibodies from syphilis patients and from patients with systemic lupus erythematosus. Clin Exp Immunol 76:178
77. Nimpf J, Bevers EM, Bomans PHH, Till U (1986) Prothrombinase activity of human platelets is influenced by β_2 glycoprotein 1. Biochim Biophys Acta 884:142
78. Oosting JD, Derksen RHWM, Entjes TI, Bouma BN, deGroot PG (1992) Lupus anticoagulant activity is frequently dependent on the presence of β_2 glycoprotein 1. Thromb Haemost 67:499

79. Oosting JD, Derksen RHWM, Bobbink IWG, Hackeng TM, Bouma BN, deGroot PG (1993) Antiphospholipid antibodies directed against a combination of phospholipids with prothrombin, protein C, or protein S: an explanation for their pathogenic mechanism. Blood 81:2618
80. Out HJ, Kooijman CD, Bruinse HW, Derksen RHWM (1991) Histopathological findings in placental from patients with intra-uterine fetal death and anti-phospholipid antibodies. Eur J Obstet Gynecol Reprod Biol 41:179
81. Out HJ, deGroot PG, Van Vliet M, Degast GC, Nieumenhuis HK, Derksen RHWM (1991) Antibodies to platelets in patients with anti-phospholipid antibodies. Blood 77:2655
82. Parke A, Maier D, Wilson D, Andreoli J, Ballow M (1989) Intravenous gammaglobulin, antiphospholipid antibodies, and pregnancy. Ann Intern Med 110:495
83. Pengo V, Biasiolo A (1993) Purification of anticardiolipin and lupus anticoagulant activities by using cardiolipin immobilized on agarose beads. Thromb Res 72:423
84. Pengo V, Heine MJ, Thiagarajan P, Shapiro SS (1987) Immunological specificity and mechanism of action of IgG lupus anticoagulants. Blood 70:69
85. Pierangeli SS, Harris EN (1993) Induction of phospholipid binding antibodies in mice and rabbits by immunization with human β_2 glycoprotein 1 or anticardiolipin antibodies alone. Clin Exp Immunol 93:269
86. Pierangeli SS, Harris EN (1994) Antiphospholipid antibodies in an in vivo thrombosus model in mice. Lupus 3:247
87. Pierangeli SS, Harris EN, Davis SA, DeLorenzo G (1992) β_2 glycoprotein 1 enhances cardiolipin binding activity but is not the antigen for antiphospholipid antibodies. Br J Haematol 82:565
88. Pierangeli SS, Harris EN, Goldsmith G, Gharavi AE, Branch DW, Dean WL (1993) Are immunoglobulins with lupus anticoagulant activity specific for phospholipids? Br Haematol 85:124
89. Pierangeli SS, Barker JH, Stikovac D, Anderson G, Ackerman D, Barquinero T, Acland R, Harris EN (1994) Effect of human IgG antiphospholipid antibodies on an in vivo thrombosis model in mice. Thromb Haemost 71:670
90. Piette JC, Wechsler B, Frances C, Godeau P (1992) Systemic lupus erythematosus and the antiphospholipid syndrome: reflections about the relevance of ARA criteria. J Rheumatol 19:1835
91. Rauch J, Meng G, Tannenbaum H (1987) Lupus anticoagulant and antiplatelet properties of human hybridoma autoantibodies. J Immunol 139:2598
92. Rosove MH, Brewer PMC (1992) Antiphospholipid thrombosis: clinical course after the first thrombotic event in 70 patients. Ann Intern Med 117:303
93. Rosove MH, Tabsh K, Wasserstrum N, Howard P, Hahn BH, Kalunian KC (1990) Heparin therapy for pregnant women with lupus anticoagulant and anticardiolipin antibodies. Obstet Gynecol 75:630
94. Roubey RAS, Pratt CW, Buyon JP, Winfield JB (1992) Lupus anticoagulant activity of autoimmune antiphospholipid antibodies is dependent on β_2 glycoprotein 1. J Clin Invest 1100
95. Sammaritano LR, Lockshin MD, Gharavi AE (1992) Antiphospholipid antibodies differ in aPL cofactor requirement. Lupus 1:51
96. Sammaritano LR, Gharavi AE, Soberano C, Levy RA, Lockshin MD (1992) Phospholipid binding of antiphospholipid antibodies and placental anticoagulant protein. J Clin Immunol 12:27
97. Sanfelippo MJ, Drayna CJ (1982) Prekallikrein inhibition associated with the lupus anticoagulant: a mechanism of thrombosis. Am J Clin Pathol 77:275
98. Schorer AE, Duane PG, Woods VL, Niewoehnere DE (1992) Some antiphospholipid antibodies inhibit phospholipase A_2 activity. J Lab Clin Med 120:67
99. Schousboe I (1983) Characterization of the interaction between β_2-glycoprotein 1 and mitochondria, platelets, liposomes, and bile acids. Int J Biochem 15:1393
100. Schousboe 1 (1985) β_2-glycoprotein 1: a plasma inhibitor of the contact activation of the intrinsic blood coagulation pathway. Blood 66:1086
101. Scott JR, Branch WD, Kochenour NK, Ward K (1988) Intravenous immunoglobulin treatment of pregnant patients with recurrent pregnancy loss caused by antiphospholipid antibodies and Rh inmunization. Am J Obstet Gynecol 159:1055
102. Shaibata S, Harpel PC, Gharavi A, Rand J, Fillit H (1994) Autoantibodies to heparin from patients with antiphospholipid antibody syndrome inhibit formation of antithrombin III-thrombin complexes. Blood 83:2532
103. Shi W, Chang BH, Hogg PJ, Chesterman CN (1993) Anticardiolipin antibodies block the inhibition by β_2 glycoprotein 1 of the factor Xa generating activity of platelets. Thromb Haemost 70:342

04. Silver RM, Draper ML, Scott JR, Lyon JL, Reading J, Branch DW (1994) Clinical consequences of antiphospholipid antibodies – an historic cohort study. Obstet Gynecol 83:372
05. Smeenk PJT, Luccassen WAM, Swaak TJG (1987) Is anticardiolipin activity a cross-reaction of anti-DNA or a separate entity. Arthritis Rheum 30:607
06. Smith HR, Hansen CL, Rose R, Canoso RT (1990) Autoimmune MRL-1 pr/lpr mice are an animal model for the secondary antiphospholipid syndrome. J Rheumatol 17:911
07. Spinatto J, Clark A, Pierangeli SS, Harris EN (1994) Intravenous immunoglobulin therapy for the antiphospholipid syndrome in pregnancy. Am J Obstet Gynecol 1995 (in press)
08. Triplett DA (1989) Annotation. Laboratory identification of the lupus anticoagulant. Br J Haematol 73:139
09. Tsakiris DA, Marbet GA, Markris PE, Settas L, Duckert F (1989) Impaired fibrinolysis as an essential contribution to thrombosis in patients with lupus anticoagulant. Thromb Haemos 61:175
10. Vermylen J, Amaut J (1992) Is the antiphospholipid syndrome caused by antibodies directed against physiologically relevant phospholipid-protein complexes. J Lab Clin Med 120:10
11. Vianna JL, Khamashta MA, Ordi-Ros J, Font J, Cervera R, Lopezsoto A, Tolosa C, Franx J, Selva A, Ingelmo M, Vilardell M, Hughes GRV (1994) Comparison of the primary and secondary antiphospholipid syndrome – a European multicenter study of 114 patients. Am J Med 96:3
12. Viard JP, Amoura Z, Bach JF (1992) Association of anti-β_2 glycoprotein with lupus circulating anticoagulant and thrombosis in SLE. Am J Med 93:181
13. Watson KV, Schorer AE (1991) Lupus anticoagulant inhibition of in vitro prostacyclin release is associated with a thrombosis-prone subset of patients. Am J Med 90:47

Lupus pregnancies and neonatal lupus

Michael D. Lockshin

National Institute of Arthritis and Musculoskeletal and Skin Diseases, Building 31, Room 4C-32, National Institutes of Health, 9000 Rockville Pike, Bethesda, MD 20892, USA

Lupus pregnancies

In the past two decades the diagnosis of systemic lupus erythematosus (SLE) has become easier to make and more certain when made. Advances in treatment have permitted patients with SLE to live longer and healthier lives. New clinical research has also described the role that some autoantibodies associated with SLE have on fetal well-being. As a result, many women with SLE or SLE-like disease now attempt pregnancy, and obstetricians, perinatologists, and pediatricians now consider the diagnosis of SLE when pregnancy complications occur to apparently healthy women. There has been a growth in our knowledge and a change in our understanding of lupus pregnancies. These new data form the basis of this review.

Diagnosis: SLE and SLE variants

Most recent publications on pregnancy and rheumatic disease focus on SLE, but SLE variants affect pregnancy prognosis and pregnancy outcome in manners similar to that of classical SLE. Thus, it is appropriate to evaluate all symptomatic pregnant women. Patients with classical SLE usually fulfill four or more of the American Rheumatism Association classification criteria [75] and usually have or have had positive tests for anti-DNA and/or anti-Sm antibody. Criteria and clinical descriptions of SLE are widely available [52]. Patients with SLE variants fall into three clinical groups [43]. The first includes women with *sub-clinical* SLE [24]. These patients often have been evaluated for SLE because of joint pain, leukopenia, thrombocytopenia, or serositis but do not fulfill the serological or clinical criteria required to make a confirmed diagnosis; they may or may not be under treatment for their symptoms. A second group of women has *serological* disease only. By definition these women are well but, for reasons that may or may not be relevant, they have been found to have high titer antinuclear, antiphospholipid, or anti-Ro or anti-La antibodies. A third group has *a defined illness related to and often overlapping with SLE*, but not SLE itself.

Diagnoses in this latter group include Sjogren's syndrome, antiphospholipid antibody syndrome, discoid LE, and undifferentiated or mixed connective tissue disease.

Compared to the literature on pregnancy in patients with classical SLE, literature on pregnancy in patients with SLE variants is sparse and is more descriptive than analytical. In both SLE and SLE-variant pregnant patients, *fetal* prognosis reflects maternal antiphospholipid or anti-Ro/La antibodies and severity of maternal organ system damage more than it does the specific rheumatic disease diagnosis or the amount of maternal disease "activity". *Maternal* prognosis, on the other hand, reflects severity of maternal organ system damage (primarily renal) existing at the beginning of the pregnancy [44, 52]. From both the maternal and the fetal perspective monitoring the progress of the pregnancy depends on pregnancy-specific criteria for the fetus and organ-specific criteria for the mother rather than on whether the mother has confirmed SLE or has an SLE variant.

Assessment of disease activity: lupus flare during pregnancy

It is frequently stated that pregnancy induces lupus flare [61], but there is no single biological test or tool which unequivocally identifies SLE or SLE-like disease as "active" or "inactive". Rather, several clinical SLE activity scorecards have been devised and tested, with good internal consistency and moderate agreement among themselves [7, 41]. These scorecards primarily rely on commonly available laboratory observations, including urinary protein, serum creatinine, platelet count, and hemoglobin and on common rheumatic disease symptoms such as rash, alopecia, and arthritis. Valid in several clinical studies of non-pregnant patients, the scorecards have been applied in modified form in studies of lupus pregnancy [42, 46, 47, 61, 77]. The modifications are required because in an individual patient the treating physician must often make a judgement whether to attribute a given abnormality to lupus activity, to a non-lupus pregnancy complication, or to both. Since there are no consensus standards for making these judgements, such subjective decisions color the conclusions of all studies on lupus disease activity in pregnancy published to date.

Built-in study biases may also influence the conclusion that pregnancy does or does not induce flare. These include differences among studies in: study design; ethnic diversity of reported patients; reasons for referral to or accrual by the study team; measures (including quantitation and duration) of disease activity used; presence or absence of control populations and whether or not controls and study patients are matched; inclusion or exclusion of women first diagnosed to have SLE during pregnancy; proportion of patients seen because of prior fetal loss (antiphospholipid antibody) or because of lupus disease activity; and physician behavior in making recommendations to lupus patients against or for pregnancy. The effects of these biases have been discussed elsewhere [45, 46].

The built-in biases of recently published studies have led authors to contradictory conclusions as to whether or not pregnancy worsens the course of SLE. In our own experience, a multi-ethnic group of 80 SLE patients, who were for the most part well and who were frequently first seen prior to a new pregnancy but referred because of a past fetal loss, did not have more frequent clinical worsening of disease (that merited a treatment change of 10 or more mg prednisone/day) than did clinically, age- and race-matched control SLE patients [42, 47]. Petri et al. [61] examined a sicker population. Their 37 patients were approximately half African American; they had largely been referred, already pregnant, because they had SLE. These authors concluded that short-lasting (multiple flares recorded in each pregnancy) and mild (flare often was not treated) lupus flare occurs more frequently in the pregnant patients than it does in a non-matched clinic population or in the same patients when not pregnant [61]. Urowitz et al. [77] looking at a largely white population of 46 women referred because of SLE and stratified by disease activity at the start of pregnancy, concluded that clinically well women have less disease activity during pregnancy than do matched controls, whereas women beginning pregnancy with severe disease have continuing disease activity. Based on these contradictory conclusions as well as those of many other authors, it is not yet clear whether pregnancy alters the natural course of SLE. In the absence of consensus concerning the effect of pregnancy on SLE, a growing literature attributing changes in lupus clinical behavior to pregnancy-associated hormonal biology and immunobiology remains uninterpretable. However, data from two studies, albeit not on human lupus pregnancy, offer additional avenues of investigation. In human rheumatoid arthritis, a related disease in which disease activity is clearly measurable, which does remit in some patients during pregnancy, and which does flare after delivery, the probability of disease remission during pregnancy depends on the degree of HLA mismatch between mother and fetus rather than on pregnancy hormones or pregnancy-associated immunological change [57]. The greater the HLA mismatch the more likely it is that remission will occur. Similar studies have not been done in lupus pregnancy. In the NZB/NZW mouse model of lupus, pregnancy and suckling worsen the serological abnormalities but not the clinical outcome, while pseudopregnancy worsens the longevity of the mouse [55]. Hyperprolactinemia, present in the pseudopregnant mouse and in non-pregnant women with SLE, has been suggested as an inducer of lupus flare [38, 78] but its actual role in driving lupus activity is only speculative at this time.

Maternal prognosis: disease activity and organ system damage

Maternal prognosis during the pregnancy depends on which organ systems are affected in an individual patient, how severely they are affected, and whether or not toxemia or other pregnancy complication occurs.

Lupus renal disease and its accompanying hypertension predispose women to hypertensive complications of pregnancy. In our own studies, 7/19 (37%) women with pre-existing lupus nephritis during pregnancy experienced reversible hypertension, proteinuria, and/or decreased renal function, which we diagnosed as toxemia; 15/106 (14%) women without pre-existing lupus nephritis suffered the same complication. In this population the risk for toxemia was greater for women with pre-existing lupus nephritis, but because we saw a large number of women with normal renal function prior to pregnancy, the majority of lupus patients who developed toxemia had not had pre-existing lupus nephritis. However, in the study of Petri et al. [61], 16/37 (43%) patients developed renal worsening [61], of which no case was attributed to toxemia. Nephrologists, examining only patients with lupus nephritis, have attributed renal worsening during pregnancy more commonly to SLE activation than to toxemia [27, 58]. In some cases renal worsening during pregnancy is not reversible.

There is no simple way to distinguish SLE nephritis from toxemia during pregnancy. Since renal biopsy is rarely performed during pregnancy, the attribution of an individual patient's renal deterioration to SLE or to toxemia is most often based on the clinician's guess, itself often based on the simultaneous presence of extra-renal symptoms and signs and on the duration of pregnancy when renal deterioration first occurs. Serum complement levels, commonly low in active non-pregnant lupus nephritis and commonly elevated in non-lupus pregnancy, contribute heavily to this guess. However, the literature is unclear whether lowered C3, C4, and CH_{50} invariably indicate exacerbation in a pregnant lupus patient [14, 48, 49]. Patients with low values, pregnant or not, are often clinically well. We found normal levels of the complement activation products C4a and C1s-C1 inhibitor complex [49], despite lowered C3, C4, and CH_{50} values in pregnant lupus patients, and concluded that decreased synthesis of rate-limiting components rather than increased complement consumption had occurred. Others, studying ill patients, reached the opposite conclusion [14]. Buyon and Abramson attempted to resolve the controversy by looking at alternative pathway complement components [16], as have we [40]. Activation of the alternative pathway, measured by Bb and by alternative pathway hemolytic complement, occurs primarily in pregnant women who do have other clinical evidence of disease activity. Thus measurement of alternative pathway complement activation may be the best serological way to distinguish between lupus nephritis and toxemia of pregnancy. However, the numbers of patients reported to date is small, and measurement of alternative pathway complement activation is not readily available.

The effect of pregnancy on organ systems other than the kidney is less well studied. The pregnant SLE patient may suffer clinical deterioration if she has pre-existing cardiac, pulmonary, or vascular compromise, because her own vascular or pulmonary bed cannot accommodate the normal pregnancy increase in fluid volume and cardiac output or the normal decrease in lung volume. Reviews of normal pregnancy physiology are available [9], and a number of textbooks describe the effects of pregnancy on each organ system.

In the antiphospholipid antibody syndrome, catastrophic vascular occlusion is a rare complication [4]. There have been occasional reports of this type of event occurring in the peripartum period [5, 63] and other reports of peripartum strokes and other isolated vascular occlusions. Whether the risk of such an event is greater in the pregnant than in the non-pregnant patient is unknown.

Fetal prognosis

From the fetal standpoint, the short-term outcome reflects maternal autoantibodies and maternal renal function more than it does any other characteristic of SLE.

Prematurity is the commonest cause of fetal morbidity, occurring in approximately one-third of liveborn children of a large published series [60], depending on definition of prematurity and frequency of neonatal death. In most studies high maternal disease activity itself (measured by one of the SLE flare scales) is not associated with premature delivery, but its proxy, corticosteroid dose, is. Renal-hypertensive complications of SLE, toxemia, or both are also associated with prematurity. Antiphospholipid antibody appears to cause prematurity, fetal death, and/or severe intrauterine growth retardation (see below). In newborns and infants of mothers with SLE, prognosis for children who are either growth-retarded or premature appears to be similar to that of similarly compromised infants of mothers who do not have SLE. However, systematic studies of this question have not been published.

With the exception of neonatal lupus (described below), and subject to qualifications required by any individual woman's medication history, SLE does not confer risks for specifically identifiable congenital abnormalities.

Long-term (childhood to adolescence) prognosis for infants of mothers with SLE is just beginning to be reported. The risk of an infant itself developing SLE is thought to be the same as that of a parent or sibling of the mother, approximately 1% [6]. There have been in the past suggestions, not systematically studied, that male children of SLE mothers have abnormal intellectual development [37, 74]. To examine this further, Ross and colleagues identified 25 children, aged 7 1/2 to 15, of mothers with SLE. All had been monitored by the same team throughout the relevant pregnancies. These children were compared then to sex-, socioeconomic status-, and gestational age-matched controls of non-SLE mothers selected from the same perinatal unit [70]. The study specifically sought out children who had not been extremely premature. It was found that 48% of the studied children of SLE mothers and 20% of the control children met criteria for learning disability, even though 96% of the SLE children had at least normal intelligence (Wechsler Intelligence Scale for Children > 80) and 48% had superior intelligence (IQ > 120). The difference was statistically significant. Consistent with the prior anecdotes, the abnormalities were most frequent among male children and in the tested area of reading disability. Larger but similarly prospective studies from different clinical units will be necessary to confirm these findings.

Antiphospholipid antibody syndrome

Antiphospholipid antibody syndrome is defined by a characteristic antibody plus one or more of specific clinical events, such as recurrent fetal loss, occlusive vascular disease, livedo reticularis, and/or thrombocytopenia [72]. The antibody can be identified in three ways: by an enzyme-linked immunosorbent assay (ELISA) (generally referred to as anticardiolipin antibody), by a test for lupus anticoagulant, or by a test for syphilis. Implications of positive tests differ among the three assays. [In this review antiphospholipid refers to an antibody identified by any of the assays, anticardiolipin to that identified by the ELISA, lupus anticoagulant to antiphospholipid antibody identified by a coagulation assay, and BFP (biological false-positive) to antiphospholipid antibody identified by a test for syphilis.] Among assays, the ELISA is most sensitive and the lupus anticoagulant (identified by screening for an abnormal activated partial thromboplastin time, Russell viper venom time, or equivalent and confirming with a mixing test with normal plasma) most specific. In both the ELISA and the lupus anticoagulant tests there is wide laboratory variation among commercial laboratories [59, 76], but reasonable agreement among research laboratories. Unlike anticardiolipin antibody and the lupus anticoagulant, the BFP does not have an important predictive value.

A proportion of women with antiphospholipid antibody are at risk to suffer a pregnancy syndrome consisting of intrauterine growth retardation leading to emergency premature delivery or second or third trimester fetal death. First trimester spontaneous abortion may also be attributable to antiphospholipid antibody, but because spontaneous abortion is a very frequent event and has many alternative causes, such attribution is more problematic than it is for a second trimester loss [10].

Studies of apparently normal women who have had recurrent fetal losses show anticardiolipin antibody to be present in approximately 5%. Among apparently normal women with high-titer antibody, the risk for growth retardation or fetal death may be as high as one-third. Anticardiolipin antibody occurs at any titer in approximately 2% of normal pregnant women and at high titer in approximately 0.2% [26, 53]. In normal women without prior fetal loss low-titer antiphospholipid antibody does not predict fetal death [31].

Controversy regarding the importance of determining isotype or antigenic specificity of antiphospholipid antibody is great, but those studies that have systematically evaluated several isotypes and antigens simultaneously in pregnant women suggest that the greatest risk falls on those women with high-titer IgG antibody to cardiolipin [62]. In most studies risk is directly proportional to IgG antibody titer. High-titer IgM or IgA antibody alone likely also generates risk, but this is less well documented than is IgG. A number of investigators have attempted to assess antigenic specificity of antiphospholipid antibodies, focusing primarily on phosphatidylserine or phosphatidylethanolamine as alternative antigens [54, 71]. However, technical problems with the assay make quantitation of these antibodies more difficult than is quantitation of the assay for anticardiolipin, and systematic studies of antiphosphatidylserine or antiphosphatidylethanolamine in large numbers of pregnant patients are lacking. Recent data suggest that the antigenic target of antiphospholipid antibody is not in fact a phospholipid but rather the complex formed by a plasma cofactor, β_2-glycoprotein I (apolipoprotein H) and any negatively charged phospholipid [56]. Within that complex a specific peptide fragment of the cofactor is critical [28]. It is, therefore, likely that in the future the assay will be adjusted to account for the cofactor and that measurement of antiphosphatidylserine or antiphosphatidylethanolamine antibody will not be considered to provide additional information for the monitoring of lupus pregnancies.

Women may have anticardiolipin antibody, lupus anticoagulant, and BFP simultaneously present or present in the various possible combinations or singly. Based on current but not definitive data, a woman with all three antibodies does not have a worse risk than does a woman with only one or two of the antibodies, nor is there a difference in pregnancy risk for a woman with lupus anticoagulant alone compared to one with anticardiolipin antibody alone.

At all titers of anticardiolipin antibody, including normal levels, a woman's prior pregnancy history may be at least as good a predictor of fetal outcome as antiphospholipid antibody [51, 65]. SLE patients who have had prior fetal deaths for any reason have approximately double the fetal death risk of women who have not had prior fetal deaths. In women who have SLE, high-titer IgG antibody ($\geq$ 80 GPL units), and no prior fetal deaths the risk for fetal death may be as high as 40%; if there have been two or more prior fetal deaths the risk for an SLE patient with high-titer antibody may be as high as 80% [51]. Lower risks have been quoted in other series [12, 36]. Differences in fetal survival among published series frequently reflect selection criteria for entry (SLE or not, prior fetal death or not, cut-off level for anticardiolipin antibody) as well as the willingness of the obstetrical team to deliver threatened fetuses before 30 weeks.

Some women with SLE and with both anticardiolipin antibodies in high titer and lupus anticoagulant carry normal pregnancies; occasional women with neither antibody have had intrauterine growth retardation or fetal death similar to that described for patients with antiphospholipid antibody. Management of an individual patient must, therefore, consider her prior pregnancy history and current pregnancy health as well as her serological status.

Neonatal lupus

Neonatal lupus is a rare condition clearly linked to maternal autoantibody to the Ro/SSA, La/SSB or, extremely rarely, U1RNP antigens. Its major clinical manifestations are rash, cardiac conduction disturbances, hematological abnormalities (thrombocytopenia, anemia), and hepatitis [13]. Children may have any single manifestation or any combination. Rash without cardiac disease is most common, followed by complete congenital heart block with or without rash.

Serology and prediction

Essentially all children with neonatal lupus are born of mothers who have anti-Ro/SSA, anti-La/SSB and/or anti-U_1RNP autoantibodies, and these children if tested at birth also have their mothers' antibodies [13, 18, 21]. There is a loose correlation between maternal antibody titer and clinical illness in the child [64]. Although neonatal lupus occurring in infants of seronegative mothers has been claimed, when these sera have been retested by sensitive ELISA or immunoblot methods they have been found to be positive, indicating first that antibody is a required element of the illness and second that low-titer antibody may be associated with neonatal lupus.

There have been many attempts to predict from the mother's autoantibodies the probability that she will deliver a child with neonatal lupus. Neonatal lupus occurs in offspring of as many as one-fourth of mothers with anti-Ro/SSA antibody (identified by a relatively insensitive method) [50]. Risk may be greater in those mothers who bear the HLA type DR3. The risk of neonatal lupus recurring in a second child is also thought to be approximately one in four [39].

Patterns of maternal immunoreactivity do define risk for congenital complete heart block but do not define risk for cutaneous forms of neonatal lupus. In one study almost all children with congenital complete heart block were born of mothers with both anti-Ro/SSA and anti-La/SSB by ELISA. The Ro/SSA antigen has a 52- and a 60-kDa epitope and La/SSB a 48-kDa epitope. Mothers of infants with congenital heart block had antibodies to the 48-kdA La/SSB and to the 52-kDa Ro/SSA antigens, while mothers who lacked these two antibodies did not [18]. Absolute risk was not calculable from these data. Mothers who do not have antibodies to the 48- and 52-kDa antigens can be reassured regarding heart block; mothers who do have these autoantibodies should be closely monitored.

Although the illness is called neonatal lupus, a maternal diagnosis of SLE is less relevant to the occurrence of illness in a child than are the mother's autoantibodies. Neonatal lupus occurs in children of mothers with Sjogren's syndrome, discoid lupus, and no recognized rheumatic disorder. In Buyon's study of 58 children with congenital heart block whose mothers' rheumatic disease status was known, 20 (34%) mothers had SLE, 9 (16%) had Sjogren's syndrome, 13 (22%) had undifferentiated and 16 (28%) no recognizable rheumatic disease [18]. Thus, while the risk for neonatal lupus for the child of a mother who enters pregnancy with a diagnosis of SLE can be roughly calculated, since many mothers are well, the probability of identifying all affected children before birth is very low.

Clinical description and pathogenesis

Neonatal lupus, with the exception of its cardiac manifestations, is a transient illness. It most frequently appears at or shortly after birth and subsides as maternal autoantibody disappears from the infant's circulation. The rash is photosensitive. Widely scattered macules are more common than is the "butterfly" distribution of spontaneous (adult) SLE rashes. On biopsy the rash resembles adult SLE, and it usually does not scar. Neonatal lupus rash is thought to result from maternal antibody-antigen immune complexes depositing at the dermal-epidermal basement membrane [13, 39].

The presence of heart block is most frequently first diagnosed by recognizing fetal bradycardia at some time between 15 and 25 weeks gestation. An occasional fetus has been observed to progress from first to second to third degree heart block; claims have been made that first degree heart block occurs frequently in children of SLE patients [25]. Myocarditis (documentable by fetal echocardiography), pericardial effusion, congestive heart failure (hydrops fetalis), and death may occur in utero. Anatomic cardiac abnormalities, such as ventricular septal defect, are not associated with neonatal lupus.

The prognosis for a child with complete congenital heart block is variable, both in utero and after birth. Most fetuses found to have heart block maintain normal cardiac output and are delivered at term, well except for cardiac rate. (Monitoring and management of such pregnancies is discussed below.) Many of these children also grow normally, are not severely limited in activities, and do not require pacemakers. However, the prognosis remains guarded. In a recent survey, a minority of children eventually had pacemakers implanted, other cardiac symptoms, or sudden death [79]. There is one American report that a survivor of complete congenital heart block developed SLE in adult life [68], and a Japanese report that 5/60 children with neonatal lupus eventually developed SLE [34] but the probability of this happening in other populations is not otherwise known.

The pathogenesis of congenital complete heart block remains speculative. In autopsy material, cardiac inflammation is found in early gestation fetuses and scarring about the atrio-ventricular conduction system is found in late gestation fetuses [13]. Although maternal autoantibody to the Ro/SSA and La/SSB antigens is an invariate component of the syndrome, and although these antigens are expressed in fetal tissue, the failure of heart block to occur in all pregnancies of mothers with these antibodies, or even in subsequent pregnancies of the same mother, and the occurrence of twins discordant for heart block are findings inconsistent with what is known about fetal disease caused by transplacental passage of maternal antibody. On the other hand, evidence supporting the hypothesis that antibody directly injures cardiac tissue includes the ability of anti-Ro/SSA antibody to slow cardiac conduction in a tissue culture model [2] and the fact that mice induced to have autoantibodies produce pups with congenital heart block [33]. Direct toxic effect of maternal antibody on fetal cardiac tissue has not been shown in this model, however.

Pregnancy monitoring and treatment

For the lupus or lupus-like patient considering pregnancy an appropriate evaluation, in this reviewer's opinion, includes a detailed history of prior pregnancies and clinical experiences on oral contraceptives (which create a pseudopregnant state); a physical examination which notes blood pressure and evidence of fluid overload or cardiac abnormality; blood count including platelets, urinalysis, creatinine clearance; and tests for lupus anticoagulant, anticardiolipin, and anti-Ro/SSA and anti-La/SSB antibodies. Platelet count, urinalysis (24-h urine protein), creatinine clearance, blood pressure, and physical examination need to be monitored periodically throughout the pregnancy; if equivocal on first test, anticardiolipin and lupus anticoagulant may be repeated in the first and second trimester.

Fetal monitoring consists of ultrasonographic measurements of fetal growth rate and, as indicated, placental size and quality, amniotic fluid volume, and umbilical artery wave form velocity [1]. In those women who are Ro/SSA and La/SSB antibody positive, fetal echocardiography searching for evidence of myocarditis or heart block should be performed at approximately 15 weeks and again at 20 and 25 weeks [23]. Antepartum fetal heart rate testing (non-stress test) should be performed weekly after approximately week 25, particularly in women with antiphospholipid antibody and/or prior fetal deaths.

Treatment options are not extensive. In this author's opinion, there is no need to treat prophylactically against SLE flare [45]. Rather, it is sufficient to monitor SLE patients closely and respond to clinical abnormalities as one would for a non-pregnant patient, except that choice and routes of medication will be constrained by potential effects on the fetus. In general this means that oral prednisone is used but other drugs, including immunosuppressives, intravenous bolus medications, and antimalarials are not. (Azathioprine and cyclosporin may be safe [29, 66].) Reviews of medications in pregnancy are available elsewhere [11, 66, 67, 73]. If pregnancy complications such as toxemia, renal failure, severe anemia, or thrombocytopenia occur, they are treated in manners similar to the same complications in non-lupus pregnant women except to note and anticipate the possibility that SLE rather than pregnancy complication has caused the abnormality.

For women with antiphospholipid antibody and prior fetal losses, a regimen consisting of low-dose aspirin (80–85 mg/day) for the first 12 weeks, subcutaneous heparin 10,000–12,000 units twice daily for weeks 12–32, and aspirin after week 32 is the only one supported as effective in a published controlled trial and confirmed by a retrospective study from another institution [10, 20]. Less-well-supported claims have been made for the efficacy of aspirin alone, heparin for the entire pregnancy, intravenous immunoglobulin, and prednisone plus aspirin. In animal models of pregnancy loss, aspirin, heparin, and interleukin-3 have been effective [22, 30, 35]. High-dose prednisone alone is probably ineffective, and complications such as osteoporosis, osteonecrosis, diabetes, hypertension, and infection are common and serious [51]. Hence high-dose prednisone is not recommended as treatment for a threatened pregnancy, though it may be needed for SLE exacerbation. If fetal growth rate ceases, if the antepartum fetal heart rate test or its equivalent shows fetal compromise, and if the fetus is potentially viable, emergency delivery is the safest decision.

There is no proven effective therapy for neonatal lupus, and prophylaxis is not indicated. If fetal myocarditis is identified early, dexamethasone (to treat the fetus), plasmapheresis, and other treatments have been attempted, but documentation of efficacy is weak [15, 19, 69]. If a viable fetus develops congestive heart failure, emergency delivery is the treatment of choice.

Contraception, abortion, hormone replacement

Opinions vary widely regarding the safety of hormonal contraception, elective abortion, hormone-supported pregnancy, and post-menopausal estrogen replacement in patients with SLE. A number of uncontrolled studies have suggested that oral contraceptives induce SLE flare, but these studies are subject to the same biases that exist in reports regarding the role of pregnancy in inducing flare. Recent studies suggest that use of oral contraceptives in selected SLE patients does not cause harm [17, 32]. Because the early history of oral contraceptive use was replete with stories of induced migraine and of unanticipated thromboembolic disease including stroke, many physicians decline to prescribe oral contraceptives for women with antiphospholipid antibody.

Elective first trimester abortion has had no apparent effect on the course of the mother's illness beyond that anticipated from the pregnancy alone [47]. Second trimester abortion is rarely performed electively, and then primarily because of the mother's deteriorating health. Hence no specific data are available concerning late abortion. Prostaglandin induction of delivery following fetal death has been uneventful in lupus patients.

Several lupus patients known to the author or presented at round table discussions have undergone stimulated pregnancy with clomiphene or supported pregnancy with progesterone and estrogen without apparent ill effect, but no systematic study has yet been published regarding this group of patients.

With lupus patients now surviving long periods of time, and with many, especially those treated with cyclophosphamide, experiencing early menopause [8], whether it is safe to use estrogen replacement therapy to prevent osteoporosis is a frequently asked question. Arden recently retrospectively compared 30 post-menopausal lupus patients who used estrogen to 30 who did not and found no increase in disease activity among the users, no increase in thromboembolic events among those users who had antiphospholipid antibody, and significant improvement in migraine, depression, and libido among the estrogen users [3]. Thus, currently available data, although by no means definitive, suggest that prior proscriptions against hormonal therapy in female lupus patients are overly restrictive.

References

1. Adams D, Druzin ML, Edersheim T, Bond A, Kogut E (1992) Condition specific antepartum testing: systemic lupus erythematosus and associated serologicalabnormalities. Am J Reprod Immunol 28:159
2. Alexander E, Buyon JP, Provost TT, Guarnieri T (1992) Anti-Ro/SS-A antibodies in the pathophysiology of congenital heart block in neonatal lupus syndrome, an experimental model – in vitro electrophysiologic and immunocytochemical studies. Arthritis Rheum 35:176
3. Arden NK, Lloyd M, Spector T, Hughes GRV (1993) The safety of estrogen replacement therapy (ERT) in systemic lupus erythematosus (abstract). Arthritis Rheum 36:s64
4. Asherson RA (1992) The catastrophic antiphospholipid syndrome. J Rheumatol 19:508
5. Bendon RW, Wilson JW, Getahun B, van der Bel-Khan J (1987) A maternal death due to thrombotic disease associated with anticardiolipin antibodies. Arch Pathol Lab Med 111:370
6. Block SR, Winfield JB, Lockshin MD, D'Angelo WA, Christian CL (1975) Studies of twins with systemic lupus erythematosus. A review of the literature and presentation of 12 additional sets. Am J Med 59:533
7. Bombardier C, Gladman DD, Urowitz MB, Caron D, Chang CH (1992) Derivation of the SLEDAI – a disease activity index for lupus patients. Arthritis Rheum 35:630

8. Boumpas DT, Austin HA, Vaughan EM, Yarboro CH, Klippel JH, Balow JE (1993) Risk for sustained amenorrhea in patients with systemic lupus erythematosus receiving intermittent pulse cyclophosphamide therapy. Ann Intern Med 119:366
9. Branch DW (1992) Physiologic adaptations of pregnancy. Am J Reprod Immunol 28:120
10. Branch DW, Silver RM, Blackwell JL, Reading JC, Scott JR (1992) Outcome of treated pregnancies in women with antiphospholipid syndrome: an update of the Utah experience. Obstet Gynecol 80:614
11. Briggs GG, Freeman RK, Yaffer SJ (1986) Drugs in pregnancy and lactation – a reference guide to fetal and neonatal risk, 2nd edn. Williams & Wilkins, Baltimore
12. Buchanan NMM, Khamashta MA, Morton KE, Kerslake S, Baguley EA, Hughes GRV (1992) A study of 100 high-risk lupus pregnancies. Am J Reprod Immunol 28:192
13. Buyon JP (1992) Neonatal lupus syndromes. Am J Reprod Immunol 28:259
14. Buyon JP, Cronstein BN, Morris M, Tanner M, Weissman G (1986) Serum complement values (C3 and C4) to differentiate between systemic lupus activity and preeclampsia. Am J Med 81:194
15. Buyon JP, Swersky SH, Fox HE, Bierman FZ, Winchester RJ (1987) Intrauterine therapy for presumptive fetal myocarditis with acquired heart block due to systemic lupus erythematosus. Arthritis Rheum 30:44
16. Buyon JP, Tamerius J, Ordorica S, Young B, Abramson SB (1992) Activation of the alternative complement pathway accompanies disease flares in systemic lupus erythematosus during pregnancy. Arthritis Rheum 35:55
17. Buyon JP, Abramson S, Belmont HM (1993) Past and present usage of oral contraceptives and hormonal replacement in women with SLE (abstract). Arthritis Rheum 36:s229
18. Buyon JP, Winchester RJ, Slade SG, Arnett F, Copel J, Friedman D, Lockshin MD (1993) Maternal antibodies to the 48-kDa SSB/La and 52-kDa SSA/Ro antigens but not to the 60-kDa SSA/Ro antigen are associated with neonatal lupus syndromes. Arthritis Rheum 36:1263
19. Carreira PE, Gutierrez-Larraya F, Gomez-Reino JJ (1993) Successful intrauterine therapy with dexamethasone for fetal myocarditis and heart block in a woman with systemic lupus erythematosus. J Rheumatol 20:1204
20. Cowchock FS, Reece EA, Balaban D, Branch DW, Plouffe L (1992) Repeated fetal losses associated with antiphospholipid antibodies: a collaborative randomized trial comparing prednisone to low-dose heparin treatment. Am J Obstet Gynecol 166:1318
21. Dugan EM, Tunnessen WW, Honig PJ, Watson RM (1992) U1RNP Antibody positive neonatal lupus – a report of two cases with immunogenetic studies. Arch Dermatol 128:1490
22. Fishman P, Falach-Vaknine E, Zigelman R, Bakimer R, Sredni B, Djaldetti M, Shoenfeld Y (1993) Prevention of fetal loss in experimental antiphospholipid syndrome by in vivo administration of recombinant interleukin-3. J Clin Invest 91:1834
23. Friedman DM (1992) Fetal echocardiography in the assessment of lupus pregnancies. Am J Reprod Immunol 28:164
24. Ganczarczyk L, Urowitz MB, Gladman DD (1989) "Latent lupus". J Rheumatol 16:475
25. Goble MM, Dick M, McCune WJ, Ellsworth J, Sullivan DB, Stern AM (1993) Atrioventricular conduction in children of women with systemic lupus erythematous. Am J Cardiol 71:94
26. Harris EN, Spinnato JA (1991) Should anticardiolipin tests be performed in otherwise healthy pregnant women? Am J Obstet Gynecol 165:1272
27. Hayslett JP (1992) The effect of systemic lupus erythematosus on pregnancy and pregnancy outcome. Am J Reprod Immunol 28:199
28. Hunt JE, Simpson RJ, Krilis SA (1993) Identification of a region of beta2-glycoprotein-I critical for lipid binding and anti-cardiolipin cofactor activity. Proc Natl Acad Sci USA 90:2141
29. Hussein MM, Mooij JMV, Roujouleh H (1993) Cyclosporine in the treatment of lupus nephritis including 2 patients treated during pregnancy. Clin Nephrol 40:160
30. Inbar O, Blank M, Faden D, Tincani A, Lorber M, Shoenfeld Y (1993) Prevention of fetal loss in experimental antiphospholipid syndrome by low-molecular-weight heparin. Am J Obstet Gynecol 169:423
31. Infante-Rivard C, David M, Gauthier R, Rivard GE (1991) Lupus anticoagulants, anticardiolipin antibodies, and fetal loss. N Engl J Med 325:1063
32. Julkunen HA, Kaaja R, Friman C (1993) Contraceptive practice in women with systemic lupus erythematosus. Br J Rheumatol 32:227
33. Kalush F, Rimoin E, Mozes E (1992) Neonatal lupus erythematosus in offspring of mothers with systemic lupus erythematosus. Am J Reprod Immunol 28:264

34. Kaneko F, Tanji O, Hasegawa T, Ohto H, Yamazaki K (1992) Neonatal lupus erythematosus in Japan. J Am Acad Dermatol 26:397
35. Krause I, Blank M, Gilbrut B, Shoenfeld Y (1993) The effect of aspirin on recurrent fetal loss in experimental antiphospholipid syndrome. Am J Reprod Immunol 29:155
36. Kutteh WH, Lyda EC, Abraham SM, Wacholtz MC (1993) Association of anticardiolipin antibodies and pregnancy loss in women with systemic lupus erythematosus. Fertil Steril 60:449
37. Lahita RG (1988) Systemic lupus erythematosus: learning disability in the male offspring of female patients and relationship to laterality. Psychoneuroendocrinology 13:385
38. Lavalle C, Graef A, Baca V, Ramirez-Lacayo M, Blanco-Favela F, Ortiz O (1993) Prolactin and gonadal hormones: a key relationship that may have clinical, monitoring and therapeutic implications in systemic lupus erythematosus. Lupus 2:71
39. Lee LA (1993) Neonatal lupus erythematosus. J Invest Dermatol 100:9s
40. Levy RA, Qamar T, Lockshin M (1990) Alternative complement pathway in hypocomplementemic/normal C1s-C1 inhibitor complex patients with SLE. Clin Exp Rheumatol 8:11
41. Liang MH, Socher SA, Larson MG, Schur PH (1989) Reliability and validity of six systems for the clinical assessment of disease activity in systemic lupus erythematosus. Arthritis Rheum 32:1107
42. Lockshin MD (1989) Pregnancy does not cause systemic lupus erythematosus to worsen. Arthritis Rheum 32:665
43. Lockshin MD (1989) What is SLE? J Rheumatol 16:419
44. Lockshin MD (1992) Overview of lupus pregnancies. Am J Reprod Immunol 28:181
45. Lockshin MD (1992) Treatment of lupus pregnancy: can we reach consensus? Clin Exp Rheumatol 10:429
46. Lockshin MD (1993) Does lupus flare during pregnancy? Lupus 2:1
47. Lockshin MD, Reinitz E, Druzin ML, Murrman M, Estes D (1984) Lupus pregnancy: case-control prospective study demonstrating absence of lupus exacerbation during or after pregnancy. Am J Med 77:893
48. Lockshin MD, Harpel PC, Druzin ML, Becker CG, Klein RF, Watson RM, Elkon KB, Reinitz E (1985) Lupus pregnancy. II. Unusual pattern of hypocomplementemia and thrombocytopenia in the pregnant patient. Arthritis Rheum 28:58
49. Lockshin MD, Qamar T, Redecha P, Harpel PC (1986) Hypocomplementemia with low C1s-C1 inhibitor complex in systemic lupus erythematosus. Arthritis Rheum 29:1467
50. Lockshin MD, Bonfa E, Elkon K, Druzin ML (1988) Neonatal lupus risk to newborns of mothers with systemic lupus erythematosus. Arthritis Rheum 31:697
51. Lockshin MD, Druzin ML, Qamar T (1989) Prednisone does not prevent recurrent fetal death in women with anti-phospholipid antibody. Am J Obstet Gynecol 160:439
52. Lockshin MD, Druzin ML (1990) Rheumatic disease. In: Barron WM, Lindheimer MD, (eds) Medical disorders during pregnancy. Mosby Year Book, St. Louis, pp 366–399
53. Lockwood CJ, Romero R, Feinberg RF, Clyne LP, Coster B, Hobbins JC (1989) The prevalence and biologic significance of lupus anticoagulant and anticardiolipin antibodies in a general obstetric population. Am J Obstet Gynecol 161:369
54. Maneta-Peyret L, Biron C, Previsani C, Moreau P, Bezian JH, Cassagne C (1993) Demonstration that anti-phospholipid auto-antibodies react with both anionic and zwitterionic phospholipids. Imunol Lett 35:141
55. McMurray RW, Keisler D, Izui S, Walker SE (1993) Effects of parturition, suckling and pseudopregnancy on variables of disease activity in the B/W mouse model of systemic lupus erythematosus. J Rheumatol 20:1143
56. McNeil HP, Chesterman N, Krilis SA (1991) Immunology and clinical importance of antiphospholipid antibodies. Adv Immunol 49:93
57. Nelson JL, Hughes KA, Smith AG, Nisperos BB, Branchaud AM, Hansen JA (1993) Maternal-fetal disparity in HLA class II alloantigens and the pregnancy-induced amelioration of rheumatoid arthritis. N Engl J Med 329:466
58. Packham DK, Lam SS, Nicholls K, Fairley KF, Kincaid-Smith PS (1992) Lupus nephritis and pregnancy. Q J Med 83:315
59. Peaceman AM, Silver RK, MacGregor SN, Socol ML (1992) Interlaboratory variation in antiphospholipid antibody testing. Am J Obstet Gynecol 166:1780
60. Petri M, Allbritton J (1993) Fetal outcome of lupus pregnancy – a retrospective case-control study of the Hopkins lupus cohort. J Rheumatol 20:650

61. Petri M, Howard D, Repke J (1991) Frequency of lupus flare in pregnancy. The Hopkins lupus pregnancy experience. Arthritis Rheum 34:1538
62. Qamar T, Levy RA, Sammaritano L, Gharavi AE, Lockshin, MD (1990) Characteristics of high-titer aPL in women with and without fetal death. Arthritis Rheum 33:501
63. Rallings P, Exner T, Abraham R (1989) Coronary artery vasculitis and myocardial infarction associated with antiphospholipid antibodies in a pregnant woman. Aust NZ J Med 19:347
64. Ramsey-Goldman R, Hom D, Deng JS, Ziegler GC, Kahl LE, Steen VD, LaPorte RE, Medsger TA (1986) Anti-SS-A antibodies and fetal outcome in maternal systemic lupus erythematosus. Arthritis Rheum 29:1269
65. Ramsey-Goldman R, Kutzer JE, Kuller LH, Guzick D, Carpenter AB, Medsger TA (1992) Previous pregnancy outcome in women with systemic lupus erythematosus. Am J Reprod Immunol 28:195
66. Ramsey-Goldman R, Mientus JM, Kutzer JE, Mulvihill JJ, Medsger TA (1993) Pregnancy outcome in women with systemic lupus erythematosus treated with immunosuppressive drugs. J Rheumatol 20:1152
67. Rayburn WF (1992) Glucocorticoid therapy for rheumatic diseases: maternal, fetal and breast-feeding considerations. Am J Reprod Immunol 28:138
68. Reichlin M, Friday K, Harley JB (1988) Complete congenital heart block followed by anti-Ro/SSA in adult life. Studies of an informative family. Am J Med 84:339
69. Rider LG, Buyon JP, Rutledge J, Sherry DD (1993) Treatment of neonatal lupus – case report and review of the literature. J Rheumatol 20:1208
70. Ross G, Sammaritano LR, Nass R, Lockshin M (1993) Learning disabilities in offspring of women with systemic lupus erythematosus (abstract). Arthritis Rheum 36:s87
71. Rote NS, Dostal-Johnson D, Branch DW (1990) Antiphospholipid antibodies and recurrent pregnancy loss: correlation between the activated partial thromboplastin time and antibodies against phosphatidylserine and cardiolipin. Am J Obstet Gynecol 163:575
72. Sammaritano LR, Gharavi AE, Lockshin MD (1990) Antiphospholipid antibody syndrome: immunologic and clinical aspects. Semin Arthritis Rheum 20:81
73. Schoenfeld A, Bar Y, Merlob P, Ovadia Y (1992) NSAIDs: maternal and fetal considerations. Am J Reprod Immunol 28:141
74. Schur PH (1990) Fingerprint analysis of patients with systemic lupus erythematosus and their relatives. J Rheumatol 17:482
75. Tan EM, Cohen AS, Fries JF, Masi AT, McShane DJ, Rothfield NF, Schaller JG, Talal N, Winchester RJ (1982) The 1982 revised criteria for the classification of systemic lupus erythematosus. Arthritis Rheum 25:1271
76. Triplett DA (1992) Coagulation assays for the lupus anticoagulant: review and critique of current methodology. Stroke 23:I11
77. Urowitz MB, Gladman DD, Farewell VT, Stewart J, Mcdonald J (1993) Lupus and pregnancy studies. Arthritis Rheum 36:1392
78. Walker SE (1993) Prolactin: an immune-stimulating peptide that regulates other immune- modulating hormones. Lupus 2:67
79. Waltuck J, Copel J, Kleinman C, Buyon JP (1993) Approach to fetal identification and therapy of congenital heart block (abstract). Arthritis Rheum 36:s97

Systemic lupus erythematosus in children

Alan M. Rosenberg

Department of Pediatrics, Royal University Hospital, University of Saskatchewan, Saskatoon, Saskatchewan, Canada S7N 0X0

Introduction

A child with systemic lupus erythematosus (SLE) presents a constellation of diagnostic and management challenges seldom encountered in pediatric clinical medicine. Providing optimal care for the child afflicted with this multisystem disorder requires thorough medical knowledge, a comprehensive array of clinical skills and multidisciplinary collaboration. Also required is an appreciation that the normal physical and emotional growth and development of children and adolescents are very vulnerable to the unfavourable influences of a chronic multisystem disease such as lupus.

Recently, substantial advances in understanding and managing SLE have been made. Refinement of diagnostic criteria, identification of disease-specific serological markers and insight into immunopathogenesis have aided in achieving earlier diagnosis, more effective monitoring of disease activity and improved therapeutic strategies. Despite this progress, the etiology of SLE remains unknown, the pathogenesis not clearly understood and therapy is not completely effective.

With the emergence and maturation of rheumatology as a pediatric subspecialty the features of SLE occurring in childhood and adolescence are being characterized with increasing clarity and the special needs of the pediatric SLE patient are now more fully appreciated. This discussion provides an overview of pediatric SLE, highlighting clinical features of the disease that are of particular relevance and prominence in children and adolescents.

Historical perspective

The French physician Cazenave derived the term *lupus erythemateux* in 1851 from the two Latin words *lupus* meaning wolf and *erythematosus* meaning redness because the malar distribution of the rash was reminiscent of the markings of the wolf's face [38]. The term *lupus,* however, had been used by Rogeritus six centuries earlier to describe the facial rash that resembled a wolfs bite [59].

Kaposi, in 1872, recognized that lupus was not confined to the skin [31]. Osler distinguished purely cutaneous forms of lupus from disseminated lupus, recognized its fluctuating course, and suggested that vasculitis was a fundamentally important pathological feature [49]. By the early 1900s pathological studies had established that lupus could exist without associated cutaneous manifestations. Based on histopathological observations of altered collagen, Klinge [36], in 1933, proposed that SLE represented a disorder of connective tissue. By 1941, Klemperer and his colleagues suggested that pathological processes affecting collagenous tissue in SLE could account for the widespread organ and tissue involvement seen in patients with this disorder [35]. However, Klemperer himself later cautioned that "there is a danger that (collagen disease) may become a catch-all term for maladies with puzzling clinical and anatomical features" and that "these morphological disorders (of connective tissue) are only outward manifestations of morbid processes, the site and nature of which are still obscure" [34]. Despite these cautionary comments, the terms "connective tissue disease" and "collagen vascular disease" still prevail when referring to diseases such as SLE.

The distinguishing serological profiles found in patients with SLE first became evident in 1940 when SLE patients were found to have false-positive tests for syphilis. Discovery of the LE cell test in 1948 invoked the notion of autoimmunity as an integral component in the pathogenesis of SLE and fostered the search for other autoantibodies [26]. In the 1950s the use of indirect immunofluorescence to test the sera of lupus patients established that the presence of antinuclear antibodies (ANA) in essentially all patients with lupus was an important serological hallmark of the disease [20]. Subsequently, the presence of antibodies to native DNA and later antibodies to Smith (Sm) antigen were established as highly specific serological markers of SLE [60].

It is likely that lupus in children and adolescents has been identified for about as long as the disease has been recognized. Reports of SLE in children, appearing as early as 1892 [58], continued to appear sporadically during the early decades of this century [13, 14, 50, 55]. During the past four decades accelerated accumulation of contributions to the literature have provided an increasingly thorough understanding of childhood SLE [5, 10–12, 15, 19, 22–24, 33, 43, 46, 48, 62, 64].

Diagnostic and classification criteria for SLE

The SLE classification criteria developed by a subcommittee of the American College of Rheumatology are applied for the classification of children, although it must be acknowledged that this set of criteria has not been validated in the pediatric age group [61]. These criteria are useful for identifying groups of patients for study purposes and have aided in determining the relative importance of certain clinical and serological features of SLE. The criteria are not intended as diagnostic criteria, as not all patients with lupus, especially those with mild or atypical forms, will satisfy the criteria.

Epidemiology and demographics of childhood SLE

SLE comprises approximately 2% of the patient population of a pediatric rheumatic disease clinic [4] and accounts for 10% of those patients with newly diagnosed, discrete systemic rheumatic diseases [7].

Neither the incidence nor the prevalence of SLE in children is known as no definitive epidemiological studies have been done. Based on pediatric rheumatology clinic attendance, estimates of incidence and prevalence can be made, although such approximations would be expected to underestimate the true population demographics. The underestimation reflects, in part, those patients who are not referred to a rheumatology clinic at all or those adolescent patients who could as likely be seen in an adult rather than a pediatric clinic setting. An SLE incidence of approximately 0.6/100,000 children less than 19 years of age has been reported for the pediatric age group [27, 56].

Reported prevalences in unselected populations have ranged as high as 50/100,000 [18]. This wide variability is likely explainable, in part, by variations in referral patterns and in ethnic composition of the respective populations. Approximately 20% of patients with SLE have their onset during childhood or adolescence [32, 53]. Thus, at an unselected population prevalence of 50/100,000 the prevalence in the pediatric age group could be as high as 10/100,000.

SLE occurs worldwide but the occurrence varies geographically, presumably because of racial diversity. Individuals of Mongoloid and Negroid ancestry appear to be particularly predisposed to developing SLE.

In the pediatric age group the onset of SLE predominates in adolescence reflecting the peak age of onset of the disease, in general, in the second and third decades of life. Accurate estimates of age of disease onset in the pediatric age group are difficult to ascertain from the literature as there is inconsistency with which the older adolescents are seen in pediatric or in adult referral centres. The onset of SLE is rare in children of less than 5 years of age, uncommon in those of less than 10 years of age and then becomes increasingly prevalent during later childhood and adolescence [7].

SLE is predominantly a disease of females especially in the older age childhood onset. This predominance is particularly striking in later adolescence. Generally, females are affected four to five times more frequently than males but the sex ratio varies with age. The female to male ratio varies from 4:3 in the under 10 age group and 4:1 in the 10–14-year age group. The ratio is approximately 5:1 in the 15–19-year age group which is comparable to the gender ratio in the adult population [7]. Thus, while the disease affects females more frequently than males in all age groups the ratio is substantially less disparate in children than it is in older adolescents and adults.

Why females are more affected than males is unclear but hormonal influences have been implicated. Patients with SLE, including males, express more exuberant conversion by hydroxylation of estrone to 16-hydroxyesterone, a potent oestrogen [39, 40]. The associations of onset and exacerbation of SLE with menarche, pregnancy, parturition and oestrogenic oral contraceptive usage further support the view that oestrogenic hormones influence disease expression. Furthermore, the association of SLE with Klinefelter's syndrome suggests that an X chromosome gene product contributes to disease expression [57]. A subset of SLE that occurs in males is characterized by transmission from father to son and presumably represents a genetically distinctive entity [41]. Maternal anti-Ro(SS-A) antibodies have been shown to be associated with male sex in children with SLE, but the immunopathogenic significance of this observation has not been established [42].

The influence of gender, race and age on the prevalence of childhood SLE can be appreciated by comparing disease prevalences in selected populations. In black, Asian, Hispanic and North American Indian children the prevalence of SLE is significantly greater than in whites [7]. In males the prevalence of SLE increases by 60% from the first decade (1/100,000 children aged 1 to 9 years) to the second decade (1.6/100,000 children aged 10–19 years) [43].

In females variability of prevalences relating to race and puberty are striking. The prevalence of SLE in pubescent white females (4.4/100,000) is approximately 3.5 times greater than the prevalence in pre-pubescent white females [43]. In other races the increased prevalence with puberty is more dramatic. The prevalence in blacks increases from 1.3/100,000 to 19.9/100,000 after puberty. In Orientals the increase is from 6.1/100,000 to 31.1/100,000 and in Hispanics from 4.6/100,000 to 13/100,000 [43]. Thus, gender, race and age combine to influence the prevalence of SLE in children and adolescents.

Etiology and pathogenesis

SLE is a prototypic autoimmune disorder. Understanding its pathogenic intricacies will assuredly contribute fundamentally important insights into normal immune functions and aberrant immune functions pertinent to other diseases. That SLE remains an enigmatic disorder reflects the complexity of the disease and suggests the possibility that the disease is etiopathogenically more disparate than the similar clinical expressions would suggest.

The etiology of SLE is unknown. It is probable that multiple factors combine to cause the disease in a genetically predisposed host. Insight into the etiopathogenesis of SLE may be more effectively achieved by studying pediatric patients rather than adults. Factors in adults such as the ageing process, associated diseases and accumulated exposure to a heterogeneous collection of potentially unfavourable exogenous influences are all less likely to confound the analysis of SLE in children. Furthermore, studying genetic and environmental influences on disease can be facilitated by comparison of affected children with parents and siblings residing in the same household environment.

Genetic predisposition is evidently a fundamentally integral factor in the pathogenesis of SLE. The familial aggregation of SLE reflects the genetic influences that predispose to developing the disease. The striking concordance of SLE in identical twins is particularly supportive of a genetic basis; more than two-thirds of identical twins are concordant for the disease [3]. Twins who both develop SLE may be more likely to do so during childhood or adolescence than in adulthood. Twins are more likely to develop the onset of disease at a younger and more similar age than non-twin siblings concordant for SLE [30]. Families in which the proband has SLE are more likely to include subjects with SLE, other connective tissue and autoimmune diseases, malignancies and immunodeficiencies [7]. Certain immune response genes predominate in SLE patients. As examples, HLA-DR2 and -DR3 haplotypes are frequent in SLE and histocompatibility profiles that include HLA-DR2, -DQw1 and -DQB1 confer a risk for developing lupus nephritis [21, 52].

SLE is more likely to occur in children with associated genetically acquired aberations of normal host defence mechanisms. Thus, perturbations of the complement and humoral and cell-mediated immune systems prevail in SLE [28]. There is a clear association between inherited deficiencies of complement components and the development of SLE [2]; such deficiencies can be associated with severe SLE in children [54]. IgA deficiency, the most common primary immune deficiency, occurs in approximately 5% of children with SLE, a frequency that is more than 100 times greater than in the normal population [9].

Although a multitude of quantitative and qualitative aberrations of immune functions characterize SLE, it is not always clear if such abnormalities occur as a result of inheritance, are of primary pathogenic importance or arise as secondary epiphenomena.

Clinical manifestations

The remarkable variability with which the characteristics of SLE are manifest suggests that an assortment of etiopathogenic factors may be operative, and that clinically distinctive subsets of SLE may vary more greatly etiopathogenically than their collective name suggests. The extensive variability of disease manifestations in childhood SLE precludes making precisely accurate generalizations about typical constellations of features. Based on accumulated publications of childhood SLE, estimates of the frequencies with which certain manifestations occur in children and adolescents with SLE can be determined [1, 5, 10, 12, 16, 17, 19, 22, 29, 33, 37, 43, 62–64] (Figs. 1, 2).

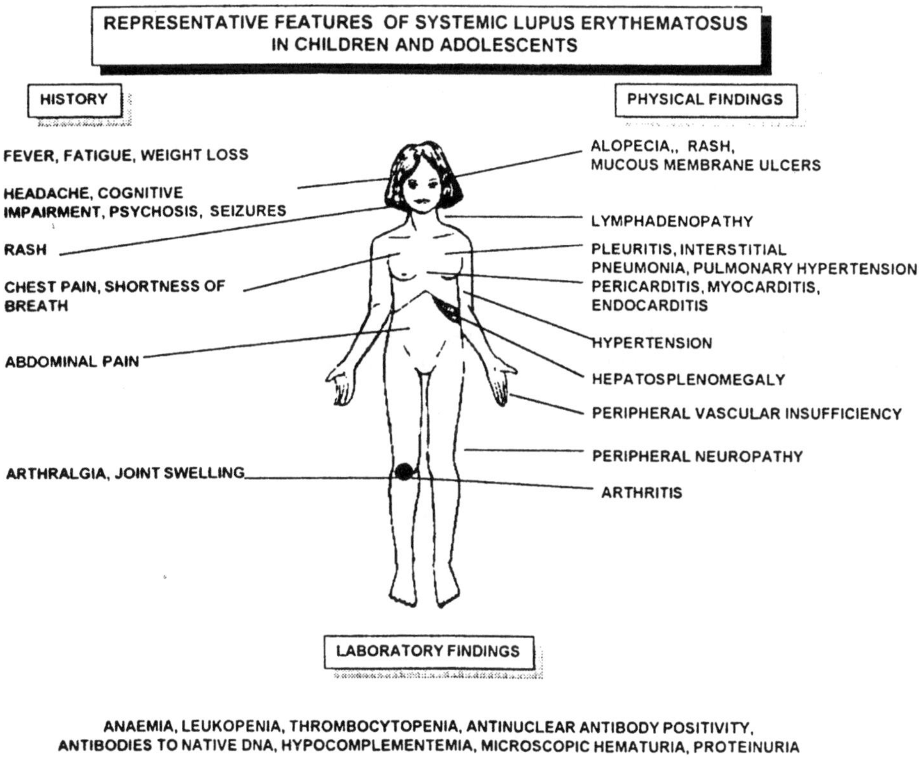

Fig. 1. An illustration of representative symptoms, signs and laboratory features seen in children and adolescents with systemic lupus erythematosus (SLE)

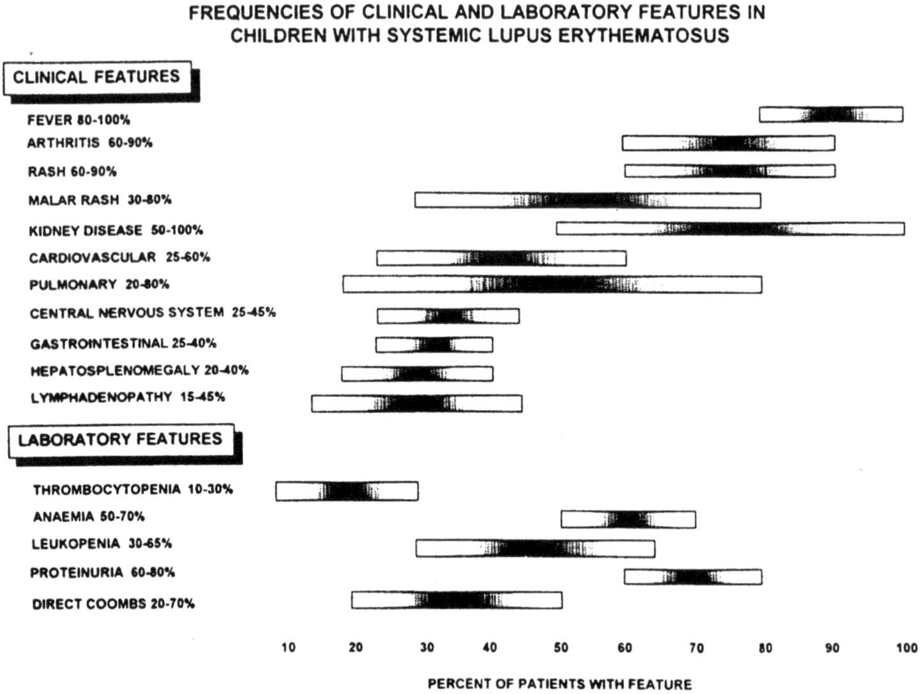

Fig. 2. The frequencies with which characteristics of SLE are manifest in children and adolescents. Values for the frequency ranges are derived from analysis of published series of pediatric SLE patient

The onset of SLE in children may vary from fulminant to insidious. Earlier analyses have indicated that less than half of children with SLE are diagnosed within the first 6 months after onset and, even though most patients have been diagnosed by 1 year, longer delays in diagnosis can occur. In general, the clinical and serological features with which the child initially presents tend to recur in the same way with future disease exacerbations. Multiple system involvement is the hallmark of SLE, although some patients may have more confined disease.

Constitutional features

Non-specific constitutional symptoms and signs such as fever, fatigue, anorexia and weight loss are frequent in children with SLE. Fever is the most common presenting feature occurring in almost all children. Although fever is usually only low, it can on rare occasions be very high. Approximately one-third of children will have mild weight loss of less than 10% of body weight. More substantial weight loss can occur but is unusual.

Mucocutaneous manifestations

The butterfly rash, so typical of SLE, is present in only approximately one-third to one-half of children with SLE. The distribution of the rash in the malar regions and over the bridge of the nose with sparing of the nasolabial folds reflects its photosensitive origins, although a definite history of photosensitivity is noted in less than half of patients. The rash may be macular, papular, or simply an erythematous blush. More dramatically florid eruptions may occur comprising nodular, vesicular or bullous lesions. Effective management of photosensitivity-induced rashes can generally be achieved by judicious sunlight avoidance, use of topical ultraviolet light-blocking agents and, if necessary, the use of hydroxychloroquine. Ordinarily, no residual scarring occurs.

Subcutaneous vasculitis may manifest as generalized maculopapular rashes or livedo reticularis. Telangiectasia, hypopigmentation, hyperpigmentation and erythema nodosum have been described. Petechial and purpuric lesions may occur even in the absence of coagulopathies and suggest an underlying cutaneous vasculitis. As a result of arteritis, ulcerations resulting from infarction due to small vessel disease occurs particularly on the palms and digits and usually in association with Raynaud's phenomenon. Approximately 20% of children will have oral mucous membrane lesions characterised by shallow ulcers, bullous lesions or areas of superficial erythema on the buccal mucosa, gingiva or palate.

Alopecia, a feature in approximately one-fifth of children with SLE, is characterized by generalized thinning of the scalp hair or patchy hair loss and is ordinarily reflective of active disease. Brittleness of the hair in the anterior hairline may also be noted. The use of cytotoxic agents, particularly cyclophosphamide, will induce hair loss that is not related directly to the activity of the underlying disease.

Nail ridging and periungual capillary dilatation and tortuosity can be seen.

Musculoskeletal manifestations

Arthritis, arthralgia, myositis and myalgia are frequent manifestations of childhood SLE occurring in approximately 50% of patients. The arthritis may be reminiscent of the articular manifestations seen in polyarticular juvenile rheumatoid arthritis with prominent involvement of small joints of the hands and feet. However, the joint deformities that can occur in SLE, such as swan neck deformities of the phalanges or ulnar deviation of the metacarpalphalangeal joints, are not fixed deformities as they are in juvenile rheumatoid arthritis. Rather, the deformities are reducible. Premature fusion of the epiphyses and growth disturbances of bones in the vicinity of the articular inflammation, characteristic of juvenile rheumatoid arthritis, tend not to be seen in children with SLE. Cartilage destruction and, therefore, bone erosions are not seen in SLE. The eponym Jacoud's arthritis has been used to designate a chronic, nonfixed, deforming arthritis seen in SLE.

Although rare, the acquisition of SLE as a second disease in a child with an antecedent history of definite, deforming, erosive seropositive polyarticular juvenile rheumatoid arthritis can occur [51]. This uncommon event, occurring usually in adolescent girls, suggests the possibility of a shared predisposition to the two diseases at least in a select population.

When they are acutely ill children with SLE may experience muscle pain. True myositis, as evidenced by weakness and elevation of muscle enzymes, may represent a subset of SLE patients having features of an overlapping connective tissue disease in which myositis is a component. Corticosteroid induced myopathy may account for muscle weakness in children receiving chronic steroid therapy.

Avascular necrosis of hips and knees may occur in up to 40% of children with longstanding SLE particularly those treated with corticosteroids. Axial spine pain can reflect vertebral osteoporosis and associated vertebral compression fractures secondary to steroid therapy.

Manifestations of underlying peripheral vascular disease

SLE is an immune complex-mediated vasculopathy that affects predominantly small caliber blood vessels such as arterioles and venules. Raynaud's phenomenon is seen in approximately one-quarter of children with SLE.

Venous and arterial thrombosis occur rarely in children with SLE and, when present, are usually in association with a hypercoaguable state secondary to the presence of antiphospholipid antibodies.

Lymphoid tissue

In children, hypertrophy of lymphoid tissue characteristically occurs when the child is afflicted with certain infectious, autoimmune or malignant disorders. The exuberant lymphoid response in children as compared to adults is a reflection of the lymphoid phase of the normal growth patterns of children; lymphoid tissue continues to grow throughout early childhood, peaking in late childhood and adolescence and then beginning to involute in later adolescence. Thus, prominence of lymphoid tissue may be more characteristic of the child with lupus than of adults with the disease. Lymphadenopathy is present at onset in approximately 40% of children with SLE. Up to three-quarters of patients may have lymphadenopathy at some time during the course of the disease. The first presentation of a child with fatigue, fever and lymphadenopathy raises concerns about an underlying malignancy. Infections, particularly with viruses including Epstein-Barr virus and human immunodeficiency virus, must also be excluded.

Splenomegaly, present in one-quarter of children with SLE, may reflect generalized lymphoid hyperplasia or may reflect hypersplenism secondary to lupus-induced autoimmune thrombocytopenia or leukopenia. Moderate splenomegaly is a feature of active disease. Splenic infarcts may occur and be associated with recurrent left hypochondrial pain. Rarely, functional asplenia occurs and can become associated with overwhelming pneumococcal sepsis. The presence of Howell-Jolly bodies in the peripheral blood smear and an abnormal spleen scan indicate functional asplenia.

Gastrointestinal manifestations

Approximately one-quarter to one-half of children will have gastrointestinal involvement. Abdominal pain can be due to serositis, mesenteric or mucosal vasculitis, pancreatitis, lymphadenitis, or peritonitis. Vasculitis may be associated with more ominous events such as bowel ischemia and perforation. Pancreatitis occurs in SLE most commonly as a complication of corticosteroid therapy. Anti-inflammatory and immunosuppressive therapy can mask the typical signs of impending serious intra-abdominal events.

Hepatomegaly occurs in approximately half of children with SLE but uncommonly is it associated with substantial liver dysfunction. Hyperbilirubinemia in children with SLE is more likely to be secondary to autoimmune hemolytic anemia than to intrinsic hepatopathy.

Lupoid hepatitis, usually a disease of older adolescent and young adult women, presents with features similar to SLE [25]. These patients can have ANA but lack antibodies to native DNA or Sm antigen. Occasionally, a positive family history of SLE may be found in patients with lupoid hepatitis, suggesting the possibility of an immunopathogenic basis common to both systemic lupus and lupoid hepatitis.

Kidney involvement

It is probable that virtually all children with SLE have renal involvement, although the degree of involvement and the overt clinical expression may vary substantially. Clinically apparent nephritis, manifested by hematuria, proteinuria and occasionally hypertension, is evident in three-quarters of children with SLE, usually manifesting clinically within the first 2 years after first presentation. It has been suggested that nephritis in children may be more frequent and severe than in adults. A classification of lupus nephritis based on glomerular histopathology has been devised by the World Health Organization [8].

Mesangial nephritis is a relatively mild form of kidney involvement. Routine light histopathology in this form of nephritis is generally normal, although a slight increase in the number of mesangial cells may be recognized. Direct immunofluorescence, however, reveals mesangial deposits of IgG and C3 and electron microscopy shows deposits in the mesangial and at the capillary basement membranes. Overt signs of renal disease are minimal and renal function is normal but may be associated with minimal, unsustained microscopic hematuria and proteinuria. Uncommonly, mesangial disease may be progressive although, theoretically, well-controlled systemic disease should prevent such occurrences.

Focal and segmental proliferative glomerulitis is characterized by increased cellularity in fewer than 50% of glomeruli, proliferation of the glomerular tufts and immunoglobulin and complement deposition along basement membranes. Mild proteinuria and microscopic hematuria may occur but biochemical evidence of renal insufficiency and progression to renal failure are uncommon.

Diffuse proliferative glomerulonephritis represents a more extensive (greater than 50% of the glomeruli involved) and intense nephritis. Deposition of immunoglobulin and complement on the peripheral capillary walls and the mesangium is characteristic. Extraglomerular, interstitial infiltrates may also be seen. Proteinuria, often sufficient to produce the nephrotic syndrome, and hematuria are present. Red cell casts, indicative of active glomerular inflammation, are often present. When the extent of glomerular damage is sufficient to allow larger molecules to be lost in the urine, such as IgG, circulating autoantibodies including anti-DNA antibodies may be lost in the urine, thus contributing to a deceptive lowering of anti-DNA antibody titers. Diffuse proliferative glomerulonephritis is present in more than half of children with lupus who are biopsied because of abnormal urinary sediment. Of all children with SLE, unselected by urinary sediment findings, 20% have diffuse proliferative glomerulonephritis.

Membranous lupus glomerulonephritis is characterized by deposition of immune complexes along the subepithelial surface of the glomerular basement membrane. Proteinuria and hematuria are present and the nephrotic syndrome is usual.

The WHO classification does not include extraglomerular changes that can include interstitial nephritis and necrotizing angiitis. Interstitial glomerulonephritis is typified by inflammatory interstitial infiltrates, tubular necrosis and interstitial fibrosis. Peritubular capillaritis is seen and the tubular basement membranes display deposits of IgG and complement. Renal tubular acidosis may be an associated finding. These features of interstitial glomerulonephritis are reminiscent of those seen in Sjögren's syndrome and those resulting from drug-induced (analgesic) nephropathy. Glomerular sclerosis, which is characterized by focal glomerulosclerosis associated with immune complex deposition, may be a stable process or may progress to more severe disease. Necrotizing angiitis is ordinarily associated with systemic arteritis that includes renal vasculature and may be associated with rapidly progressive renal failure. Based on cumulative experiences of kidney biopsies in children with lupus, approximately 40% will have diffuse proliferative glomerulonephritis, 25% will have focal glomerulonephritis, 25% will have normal to mild glomerulonephritis and less than 10% membranous disease.

In children, the value of renal biopsy is limited [45]. The biopsy can help distinguish between membranous nephritis and diffuse proliferative glomerulonephritis. In the former the prognosis is better and corticosteroid therapy is not especially efficacious. The decision to introduce cytotoxic therapy may be influenced by the biopsy. Deteriorating renal function with a still active inflammatory pathology would support the use of aggressive cytotoxic therapy, whereas end-stage histopathology would support a less aggressive approach and resignation that impending renal failure is inevitable and that aggressive therapy would be predictably ineffective. However, the assessment of renal histopathology relies on evaluation of a single, minute tissue sample at a single point in time. There can be no indication from the biopsy alone as to how pervasive the histopathological changes are throughout the kidney and whether the renal disease is in a state of arrest or is continuing to progress. The results of biopsy do not appear to accurately predict the prognosis more effectively than other clinical and laboratory signs.

Occasional children will develop chronic renal insufficiency progressing to renal failure. Hemodialysis and eventual renal transplantation are required. Recurrence of lupus in the transplanted kidney is unusual. In part, this may be due to the fact that the therapy required to prevent homograft rejection is sufficient to control any exacerbation of lupus activity. The development of end-stage renal disease as a consequence of lupus nephritis is usually insidious in onset. More abrupt onset of renal failure suggests the possibility of renal vascular thrombosis, especially in the child with hypercoaguability relating to the presence of anti-phospholipid antibodies or of the induction of renal failure by potentially nephrotoxic therapy.

The goal in treating children with lupus nephritis is to prevent progressive deterioration in renal function and, thus, prevent impedance of profound growth and development retardation that occurs with substantial renal insufficiency in children.

The optimal therapeutic strategy for treating children with lupus nephritis has not been established. The use of corticosteroid therapy alone or in combination with azathioprine and the use of cyclophosphamide are thought to have contributed to an improved prognosis for lupus nephritis [44].

Nervous system manifestations

Up to 50% of children with SLE may manifest one or more neurological manifestations. Usually, neurological signs of childhood SLE occur early in the course of the illness. Later neurological manifestations are more likely to represent events secondary to cerebrovascular accidents, uremia or infection.

Both central and peripheral neurological pathology occur. Ascertaining the nature of neuropsychiatric features occurring in the child with lupus can at times be challenging. The protean features may reflect underlying organic disease, superimposed infection or psychological reaction to the illness.

Cognitive impairment, believed to occur in 80% of adults with SLE, is probably much more prevalent in children and adolescents with SLE than has been appreciated previously [6]. Deterioration in school performance, mood changes, aberrant behavior and memory impairment may be indicators of nervous system involvement. In children it is often difficult to distinguish between primary disease as a cause for cognitive aberrations from effects of therapy and the psychological impact of a chronic disease. Controlled studies, utilizing pediatric appropriate psychometric measuring instruments, will be required for a more comprehensive evaluation of the frequency and specificity of cognitive impairment in childhood lupus.

Headaches occur in approximately 20% of children with SLE. Relatively severe and persistent headaches typify that associated with active disease. Although usually no definitive cause for the headache in children with SLE is found, it can reflect ominous disease complications including hypertensive encephalopathy, increased intracranial pressure due to pseudotumor cerebri, intracranial hemorrhage or complicating infection.

Approximately 10–20% of children with lupus have seizures either as a presenting manifestations or as a feature manifesting later. Seizures may be generalized or, less commonly, focal, temporal lobe, petit mal or Jacksonian. Seizures may occur as a result of cerebral vasculitis, cerebral vascular insufficiency, intracranial bleeding associated with coagulopathy, uremia, fluid and electrolyte imbalances, hypertension or central nervous system infection. When evaluating a child suspected of having SLE who has been treated with anticonvulsants for a pre-existing seizure disorder, one must consider that the emerging signs of lupus reflect anticonvulsant drug-induced lupus rather than idiopathic lupus. Serological discriminators such as the absence of anti-DNA and anti-Sm antibodies in the presence of a lupus-like illness in a patient treated with hydantoins, trimethadione or ethosuximide should suggest the drug-induced lupus syndrome.

Tremulousness, ataxia, and chorea are among the movement disorders associated with childhood SLE. One-fifth of children may often manifest dyskinesia well before the diagnosis of SLE is made. Chorea, present in only 10% or less of children with SLE, occurs more frequently in association with childhood lupus than in adults, and may antedate by years the manifestations of other features of lupus.

Approximately 10% of children with SLE have cranial or peripheral neuropathies as an isolated neurological sign. Cranial nerve involvement most often affects ocular nerves but facial and trigeminal cranial nerve involvement has been reported. The genesis of peripheral neuropathy may be either vascular insufficiency of nutrient supply to peripheral nerves or degenerative changes of the posterior roots of the spinal ganglia.

Paraesthesia, paraparesis, and paraplegia of the legs, urinary retention, and fecal incontinence should raise concerns about the possibility of transverse myelitis even in a child who does not yet manifest any other features of SLE.

Cardiac manifestations

Cardiac involvement occurs in approximately 10–30% of children with SLE most commonly involving pericarditis, myocarditis or valvulitis. Pericarditis is the most frequent single cardiac abnormality in childhood lupus. Constrictive pericarditis is uncommon. Myocarditis, occurring in approximately 25% of children with lupus, is ordinarily accompanied by signs of congestive heart failure. Valvular insufficiency, particularly involving the aortic valve, results from valve root dilatation or rupture. Endocarditis of the Libman-Sacks type is characterized by fibrinoid necrotic nodules on the aortic, pulmonary or tricuspid valves. Children so affected are predisposed to bacterial endocarditis and should receive appropriate antimicrobial prophylaxis.

Pulmonary manifestations

Pulmonary involvement has been found in more than three-quarters of children with lupus. Pleuritis is the single most common pulmonary manifestation of childhood SLE occurring in up to 30% of children with lupus. More ominous pulmonary manifestations include pneumonia, pneumothorax, pulmonary hypertension, chronic restrictive lung disease and acute pulmonary hemorrhage.

Bacterial pneumonia, due most frequently to *Escherichia coli, Klebsiella* or *Staphylococcus aureus*, might be the most common cause of death in children with SLE. Non-bacterial infectious agents such as *Pneumocystis carinii* can occur and reflect the immunocompromised state of the child with SLE. Aggressive antimicrobial therapy is required to manage children with SLE who manifest signs of associated pulmonary infection.

As control of renal and neurological manifestations of lupus has improved, pulmonary disease is attaining increased prominence as a cause of both morbidity and mortality in childhood lupus.

Laboratory features (Fig. 3A,B)

Laboratory studies in children with SLE are more likely to be helpful in diagnosing and managing the child than are laboratory studies undertaken in the context of other childhood rheumatic disease. In particular, the availability now of serological studies that are disease specific, that correlate with disease activity and that can provide accurate and sensitive measurements has contributed substantially to optimizing the management of the pediatric SLE patient.

Many children with SLE will present with laboratory studies indicative of anemia, leukopenia, thrombocytopenia, hypergammaglobulinemia and elevation of acute-

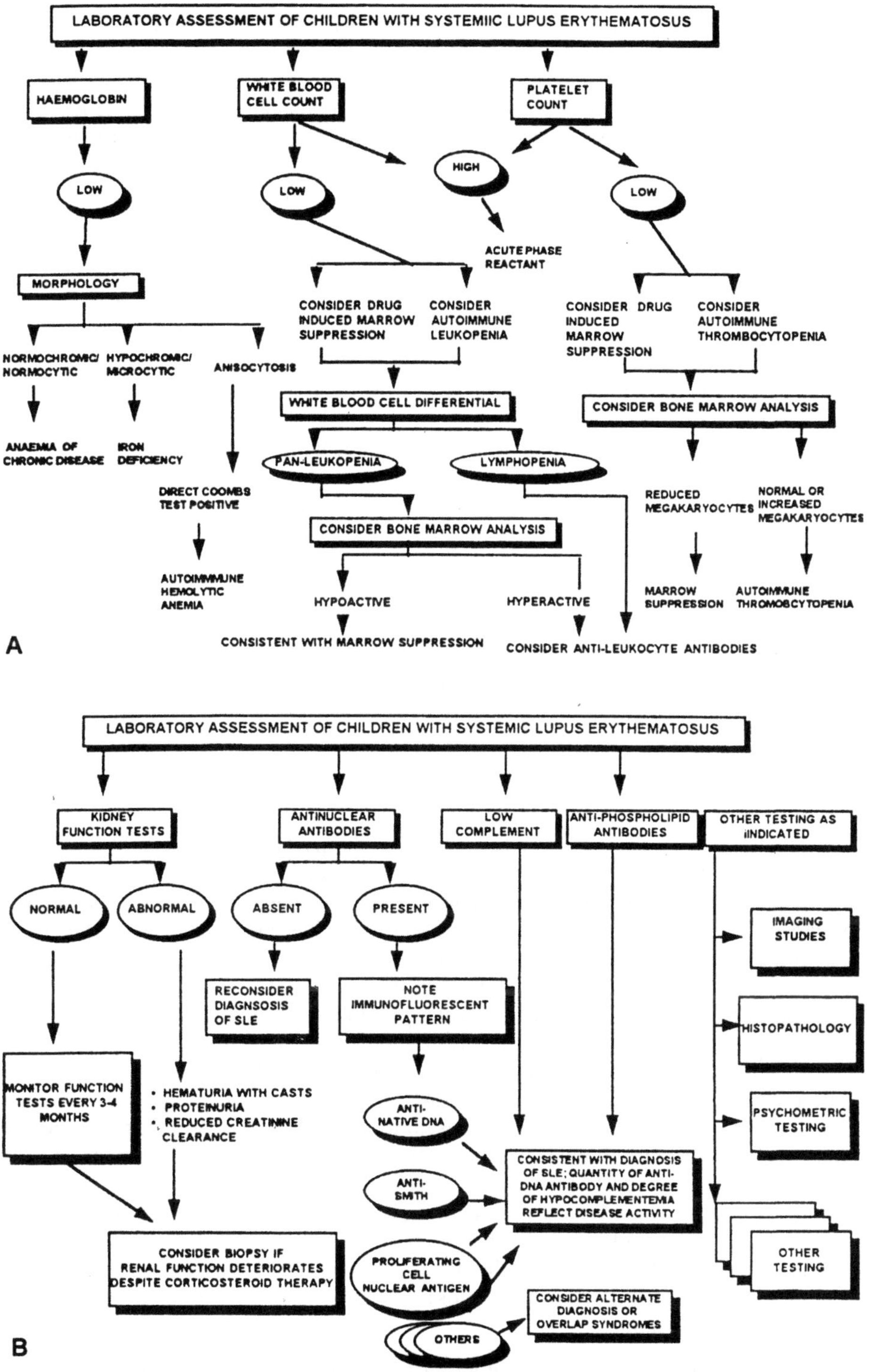

Fig. 3A,B. A general overview of the approach to the laboratory investigation of the child with SLE

phase reactants. Virtually all children with lupus will have positive tests for ANA; a negative ANA test requires careful reconsideration of the diagnosis of SLE. As detected by immunofluorescence the ANA pattern is ordinarily characterized by a dense, homogenous pattern displayed by interphase cells and localization of the immunofluorescence to the chromosomal regions of metaphase cells. This pattern usually reflects reactivity with native DNA. Antibodies to native DNA, the serological hallmark of SLE, are almost always present in children with SLE. Assuming the assay for the detection of anti-DNA antibodies is precise in detecting antibodies to only pure double-stranded DNA, with no contaminating single strands, the test is specific for SLE. When detected by quantitative assays, such as enzyme-linked immunosorbent assay or radioimmunoassay, the assay is helpful in monitoring the clinical course as the level of anti-DNA antibodies fluctuates with systemic disease activity. Hypocomplementemia, particularly a low C3, is also characteristic of active systemic SLE. C4 is also frequently low in association with a low C3 and, like reduced C3, may reflect active disease. However, a low C4 may also be noted in isolation both in the patient and in family members and, in these circumstances, indicates the likelihood of a C4 null allele.

Treatment

Among the most important improvements in pediatric SLE patient prognosis has been the emergence and dissemination of dedicated pediatric rheumatology programs. Such programs offer continuity of care and consistent monitoring from a pediatric perspective by experienced multidisciplinary teams of health care providers.

Children and adolescents, who are especially dependant on family and reliant on peer group interactions, cannot be cared for effectively if family needs and psychosocial ramifications of the illness are ignored. The effective management of SLE in the pediatric age group requires attentiveness to the psychosocial needs of the physically and emotionally maturing child and awareness of the impact of the illness on the family. By educating, supporting and guiding the patient and family, health care providers ease the burden of illness, facilitate effective coping skills and minimize non-compliance. Adhering to sensible lifestyle habits, so important for all children and adolescents, is especially vital for the those with SLE. Issues relating to diet and nutrition should be addressed particularly in those children in whom steroid therapy can contribute to deviant eating habits. The stimulatory effect on appetite that corticosteroids have can result in the child eating foods of poor nutritional quality. Alternatively, the child and particularly the adolescent may severely restrict caloric intake in a misguided attempt to compensate for steroid-induced weight gain. Special diets may be necessary to manage those patients with, for example, hypertension, hypoproteinemia and hyperlipidemia associated with chronic renal insufficiency. Maintaining an appropriate exercise program, regular school attendance and participation in extracurricular activities contributes to both the physical and emotional well-being of the pediatric SLE patient. For the adolescent the added issues of realistic career planning and counselling regarding smoking, alcohol and illicit drug use and sexual activity cannot be ignored.

Patients must be monitored closely to detect the earliest symptoms and signs of an impending exacerbation or complication. Close surveillance by health care providers is especially important in the pediatric patient as the children themselves may not easily appreciate the significance of fluctuating symptoms and signs.

Drug therapies must be individualized for each child depending on disease manifestations and severity. Those with mild musculoskeletal complaints such as arthralgia, arthritis, or myalgia may benefit from non-steroidal anti-inflammatory medications. Judicious use, however, of even this first line class of medication is required. Indiscriminate use of certain non-steroidal anti-inflammatory medications can result, for example, in salicylate-induced hepatotoxicity or ibuprofen-induced aseptic meningitis. Alternate non-steroidal agents, therefore, should be employed.

Troublesome photosensitivity is managed by sensible sun avoidance and the use of sunscreens. Anti-malarial agents, such as hydroxychloroquine sulfate, can be useful therapy for the cutaneous manifestations of SLE as well as being potentially helpful as a steroid-sparing agent. Because of the remote possibility of hydroxychloroquine-induced retinal toxicity, it is essential that pre-treatment and semi-annual ophthalmological examinations be performed to monitor for contraindications to or complications of therapy with anti-malarial agents.

Despite the predictable and potential adverse effects of corticosteroid therapy, steroids remain a mainstay of therapy for the child with lupus. Both oral and intravenous routes of administration are employed. Optimally, the goal is to to use the lowest dose possible to achieve disease control without inducing toxicity and adverse psychological effects. Intravenous pulse methylprednisolone is indicated when prompt control of acute exacerbations of central nervous system, hematological and renal manifestations is required. Low-dose prednisone (< 0.5 mg/kg per day) is often sufficient to achieve control of relatively mild disease. Higher doses (1–2 mg/kg per day) may be required to achieve prompt control of ominous disease manifestations such as central nervous system disease, acute hemolytic anemia or acute exacerbations of lupus nephritis. With the establishment of clinical remission and normalization of the anti-DNA antibodies and complement levels, tapering of the steroid dose can commence. Gradual and cautious dose reduction strives to achieve the lowest possible dose to maintain a balance between efficacy and minimization of toxic effects.

The inconsistency with which corticosteroid therapy has been effective in treating certain forms of lupus nephritis, the uncertainty about long-term prognosis using only steroid therapy and the predictable toxicity of steroids in children prompted a search for a more reliably effective therapy. Consequently, more potent immunosuppressive agents, particularly azathioprine and cyclophosphamide, have been introduced to treat children with SLE [44]. Legitimate concerns exist, however, with respect to potential long-term toxicities including a heightened risk of infection, bone marrow suppression, infertility and neoplasia. Even so, because of the adverse effects of poor disease control on survival rates and on quality of life, and growth and development, these agents continue to be used to achieve more effective disease control.

Prognosis

The long-term prognosis for children with SLE has progressively improved such that 10-year-survival rates now exceed 80%. Earlier diagnosis and diagnosis of milder disease may contribute somewhat to this improved statistic but, unequivocally, true prognostic improvements have occurred.

Among the most important factors contributing favorably to prognosis is the psychosocial environment in which the child exists. The effectiveness with which the child and family cope with the chronicity and fluctuating course of the disease, the consistency of compliance with health care monitoring and pharmacotherapy, and the receptiveness to education about the disease are integral elements in optimal management. As the life expectancy and quality of life of children with SLE has improved so dramatically, the necessity to address psychosocial adaptation to such a chronic and serious disease increases in importance.

SLE tends to display a remitting and relapsing course. Exacerbations tend to comprise manifestations which characterized disease onset. Exceptions to this generalization, however, are central nervous system manifestations which may first develop later in the course. In addition, deteriorating renal function or disease complications may influence the nature and severity of future disease exacerbations.

While long-term survival is clearly a discrete and desirable measurable endpoint, attentiveness to maintaining a tolerable quality of life is imperative. The immediate and long-term adverse consequences of disease therapy must always be balanced against the adverse consequences of inadequately controlled disease activity. When evaluating the prognosis of childhood lupus, more than half of children will continue to have chronic active disease despite therapy. Renal failure occurs in approximately 15%, severe central nervous system disease in 10%, chronic thrombocytopenia in 7% and death in 17% [47]. Infection and the complications of renal failure are the most likely to cause death but there is an increasing awareness of the potential seriousness of central nervous system, cardiac and pulmonary complications as a cause of both morbidity and mortality.

Conclusions

The special needs of children and adolescents afflicted with SLE are being recognized with increasing clarity. The development of pediatric rheumatology programs that are dedicated to caring for children and adolescents with SLE has been a vitally important development in heightening awareness of the special needs, characteristics and management strategies for the pediatric patient. While there has been substantial improvement in survival and quality of life as a result of earlier diagnosis and more effective and judicious therapy, it must be acknowledged that we are still fundamentally far away from understanding and optimally manageing SLE in children. Through collaborative research efforts improved understanding of SLE in children and adolescents can be achieved. The patients served will be the ultimate beneficiaries of such cooperative initiatives.

References

1. Abeles M, Urman JD, Weinstein A, Lowenstein M, Rothfield NF (1980) Systemic lupus erythematosus in the younger patient: survival studies. J Rheumatol 7:515
2. Agnello V (1987) Complement deficiency and systemic lupus erythematosus. In: Lahita RG (ed) Systemic lupus erythematosus. Wiley, New York, pp 565–589
3. Block SR, Winfield JB, Lockshin MD, D'Angelo WA, Christian CL (1975) Studies of twins with systemic lupus erythematosus. A review of the literature and presentation of 12 additional sets. Am J Med 59:533

4. Bowyer S, Pruett L, Roettcher P (1993) National pediatric rheumatology disease registry: first year data – diagnosis. Arthritis Rheum 36:S172
5. Caeiro F, Michielson FMC, Bernstein R, Hughes GR, Ansell BM (1981) Systemic lupus erythematosus in children. Ann Rheum Dis 40:325
6. Carbotte RM, Denburg SD, Denburg JA (1986) Prevalence of cognitive impairment in systemic lupus erythematosus. J Nerv Ment Dis 174:357
7. Cassidy JT, Petty RE (1990) Textbook of pediatric rheumatology, 2nd edn. Churchill Livingston, New York, pp 263–267
8. Cassidy JT, Petty RE (1990) Textbook of pediatric rheumatology, 2nd edn. Churchill Livingston, New York, pp 280–290
9. Cassidy JT, Burt A, Petty R, Sullivan D (1969) Selective IgA defiency in connective tissue diseases, N Engl J Med 280:275
10. Cassidy JT, Sullivan DB, Petty RE, Ragsdale C (1977) Lupus nephritis and encephalopathy. Arthritis Rheum 20 [Suppl]:315
11. Coleman WP, Coleman WP, Berbes VI, Jolly HW, Nosbitt LT (1977) Collagen disease in children. A review of 71 cases. JAMA 14:237
12. Cook CD, Wedgwood RJP, Craig JM, Hartmann JR, Janeway CA (1960) Systemic lupus erythematosus. Description of 37 cases in children and a discussion of endocrine therapy in 32 of the cases. Pediatrics 26:570
13. Deicher HR, Holman HR, Kunkel HG (1959) The precipitin reaction between DNA and a serum factor in SLE. J Exp Med 109:97
14. Denzer BS, Blumenthal S (1937) Acute lupus erythematosus disseminatus. Am J Dis Child 53:525
15. Downing JG, Messina SJ (1942) Acute disseminated lupus erythematosus associated with finger lesions resembling lupus pernio. N Engl J Med 227:408
16. El-Garf A, Salah S (1990) Juvenile systemic lupus erythematosus among Egyptian children. J Rheumatol 17:1168
17. Emery H (1986) Clinical aspects of systemic lupus erythematosus in childhood. Ped Clin N Am 33:1177
18. Fessel WJ (1988) Epidemiology of systemic lupus erythematosus. Rheum Dis Clin North Am 15
19. Fish AJ, Blau EB, Westberg NG, Burke BA, Vernier RL, Michael AF (1977) Systemic lupus erythematosus within the first two decades of life. Am J Med 62:99
20. Friou GJ (1957) Clinical application of lupus serum: nucleoprotein reaction using fluorescent antibody technique. J Clin Invest 36:890
21. Fronek Z, Timmerman LA, Alper CA, Hahn BH, Kalunian K, Peterlin BM, McDevift HO (1990) Major histocompatibility complex genese and susceptibility to systemic lupus erythematosus. Arthritis Rheum 33:1542
22. Glidden RS, Mantzouranis EC, Borel Y (1983) Systemic lupus erythematosus in childhood: clinical manifestations and improved survical in fifty-five patients. Clin Immunol Immunopathol 29:196
23. Gold AP, Yahr MD (1960) Childhood lupus erythematosus. Trans Am Neurol Assoc 85:96
24. Gribetz D, Henley WL (1959) Systemic lupus erythematosus in childhood. Mount Sinai J Med 26:289
25. Hall S, Czaja AJ, Kaufman DK, Markowitz H, Gisburg WW (1986) How lupoid is lupoid hepatitis? J Rheumatol 13:95
26. Hargraves MM, Richmond H, Morton R (1948) Presentation of two bone marrow elements: The tart cell and the LE cell. Mayo Clinic Proc 23:25
27. Hochberg MC (1985) The incidenc e of systemic lupus erythematosus in Baltimore, Maryland 1970–1977. Arthritis Rheum 28:80
28. Horwitz DA (1993) Systemic lupus erythematosus: generalized autoimmunity arising from disordered immune regulation. In: Mcarty DJ, Koopman WJ (eds) Arthritis and allied conditions. Lea & Febiger, Philadelphia, pp 1185–1199
29. Jacobs JC (1963) Systemic lupus erythematosus in childhood: report of thrity-five cases with discussion of seven apparently induced by anticonvulsant medication, and of prognosis and treatment. Pediatrics 32:257
30. Kaplan D (1984) The onset of disease in twins and siblings with sytemic lupus erythematosus. J Rheumatol 11:648
31. Kaposi MK (1872) Neue Beitrage zur Kenntnis des Lupus erythematosus. Arch Dermatol Syphitol 4:36

32. Kaufman DB, Laxer RM, Silverman ED, Stein L (1987) Systemic lupus erythematosus in childhood and adolescence – the problem, epidemiology, incidence, susceptibility, genetics and prognosis. Curr Prob Pediatr 16:555
33. King KK, Kornreich HK, Bernstein BH, Singsen BH, Hanson V (1977) The clinical spectrum of systemic lupus erythematosus in childhood. Arthritis Rheum 20 [Suppl]:287
34. Klemperer P (1950) Concept of collagen diseases. Am J Pathol 26:505
35. Klemperer P, Pollack AD, Baehr G (1941) Pathology of disseminated lupus erythematosus. Arch Pathol 32:569
36. Klinge F (1933) Der Rheumatismus. Ergeb Allg Pathol Pathol Anat 27:1
37. Lacks S, White P (1990) Morbidity associated with childhood systemic lupus erythematosus. J Rheumatol 17:941
38. Lahita RG (1987) Introduction. In: Lahita RG (ed) Systemic lupus erythematosus. Wiley, New York, pp 1–3
39. Lahita RG, Bradlow HL, Kunkel GH, Fishman J (1979) Alterations of estrogen metabolism in SLE. Arthritis Rheum 22:1195
40. Lahita RG, Bradlow HL, Fishman J. Kunkel HG (1982) Estrogen metabolism in systemic lupus erythematosus patients and family members. Arthritis Rheum 25:843
41. Lahita RG, Chiorazzi N, Gibofsky A, Winchester RJ, Kunkel HG (1983) Familial systemic lupus in males. Arthritis Rheum 26:39
42. Lehman TJA, Reichlin M, Santner TJ, Silverman E, Petty RE, Spencer CH, Harley JB (1989) Maternal antibodies to Ro (SS-A) are associated with both early onset of disease and male sex among children with systemic lupus erythematosus. Arthritis Rheum 32:1414
43. Lehman TJA, McCurdy DK, Bernstein BH, King KK, Hanson V (1989) Systemic lupus erythematosus in the first decade of life. Pediatrics 83:235
44. Lehman TJA, Sherry DD, Wagner-Weiner L, McCurdy DK, Emery HM, Magilavy DB, Kovalesky A (1989) Intermittent intravenous cyclophosphamide therapy for lupus nephritis. J Pediatr 114:1055
45. Malleson PN (1989) The role of renal biospy in childhood onset systemic lupus erythematosus: a viewpoint. Clin Exp Rheumatol 7:563
46. Meislin AG, Rothfiled N (1968) Systemic lupus erythematosus in childhood. Analysis of 42 cases with comparative data on 200 adult cases followed concurrently. Pediatrics 42:37
47. McCurdy DK, Lehman TJA, Bernstein B, Hanson V, King KK, Nadodra R, Landing BH (1992) Lupus nephritis: prognostic factors in children. Pediatrics 89:240
48. Norris DG, Colon AR, Stickler GB (1977) Systemic lupus erythematosus in children: the complex problems of diagnosis and treatment encountered in 101 such patients at the Mayo Clinic. Clin Pediatr 16:774
49. Osler W (1904) On the visceral manifestations of the erythema group of skin diseases. Am J Med Sci 127:1
50. Pehrson M (1952) Lupus erythematosus disseminatus treated with ACTH. Acta Paediatr 41:478
51. Ragsdale CG, Petty RE, Cassidy JT, Sullivan DB (1980) The clinical progression of apparent juvenile rheumatoid arthritis to systemic lupus erythematosus. J Rheumatol 7:50
52. Reveille JD (1990) Molecular genetics of systemic lupus erythematosus and Sjögren's syndrome. Curr Opin Rheum 2:733
53. Schaller J (1982) Lupus in childhood. Clin Rheum Dis 8:219
54. Schaller JG, Gilliland BG, Ochs HD, Leddy JP, Agodoa LC, Rosenfeld Si (1977) Severe systemic lupus erythematosus with nephritis in a boy with deficiency of the fourth component of complement. Arthritis Rheum 20:1519
55. Sequeira JH Balean H (1903) Lupus Erythematosus in two sisters. Br J Dermatol 14:367–379
56. Siegel M, Lee SL (1973) The epidemiology of systemic lupus erythematosus. Semin Arthritis Rheum 3:1
57. Stern R, Fishman J. Brusman H, Kunkel HG (1977) Systemicus lupus erythematosus associated with Klinefelter's syndrome. Arthritis Rheum 20:18
58. Stowers JH (1892) Lupus erythematosus in a child. Br J Dermatol 20:236; cited by Stewart CC, Boeckerman WH (1931) Lupus erythematosus disseminatus acutus in a juvenile. Am J Dis Child 42:864
59. Talbot JH (1984) Historical background of discoid and systemic lupus erythematosus. In: Dubois EL (ed) Lupus erythematosus. University of Southern California Press, Los Angeles, p 1

60. Tan EM (1993) Autoantibodies in systemic lupus erythematosus. In: McCarty DJ, Koopman WJ (ed): Arthritis and allied conditions. Lea & Febiger, Philadelphia pp 1179–1184
61. Tan EM, Cohen AS, Fries JF, Masi AT, McShane DJ, Rothfield NF, Schaller JG, Talal N, Winchester RJ (1982) The 1982 revised criteria for the classification of systemic lupus erythematosus. Arthritis Rheum 25:1271
62. Walravens P, Chase HP (1976) The prognosis of childhood systemic lupus erythematosus. Am J Dis Child 130:929
63. Yancey CL, Doughty RA, Athreya BH (1981) Central nervous system involvement in childhood systemic lupus erythematosus. Arthritis Rheum 24:1389
64. Zetterstrom R, Berglund G (1956) Systemic lupus erythematosus in childhood: a clinical study. Acta Paediatr Hung 45:189

Systemic lupus erythematosus – disease management

Mark F. Gourley

National Institutes of Arthritis and Musculoskeletal and Skin Diseases, Building 10, Room 9S210, Bethesda, MD 20982, USA

Introduction

Systemic lupus erythematosus (SLE) is a chronic rheumatic disease in which the etiology is multifactorial. The clinical course of the disease is characterized by relapses and remissions. Therefore, therapy is targeted at both suppression of signs and symptoms of acute illness as well as prevention of future pathology. The role of aggressive therapy is associated with increased risks of toxicities to the patient, requiring that treatment be tailored to the needs of the individual. However, recent advances in our understanding of the immune system may translate into improved outcomes in managing patients with SLE.

General considerations in caring for the patient with SLE

Upon establishing the diagnosis of SLE, initial treatment decisions hinge upon the activity and severity of the disease. For most patients, clinical manifestations are non life-threatening and management is usually conservative, if required at all [80]. Treatment may include simple advice such as avoiding of a stressful lifestyle, avoiding sun exposure, etc. The decision to treat must carefully weigh the risk of the potential untoward effects of therapy against the potential benefits.

As with all antirheumatic drugs, the number of side effects associated with drug therapy agent is respectable. For patients with the most common of complaints – fatigue, myalgias and arthralgias – treatment with salicylates or nonsteroidal anti-inflammatory drugs (NSAIDS) are usually sufficient to provide a satisfactory outcome. Limited skin disease is generally treated topically with corticosteroids. Patients not responding to conservative therapy may benefit from the use of glucocorticoids in low dose (0.15–0.25 mg/kg prednisone equivalent) daily.

When to treat the lupus patient with aggressive therapy remains an issue of controversy. Aggressive therapy with intravenous cyclophosphamide has been shown to slow the progression to endstage renal disease in the patient with glomerulonephritis and may be beneficial in other severe forms of SLE [39]. The problem with aggressive therapy is the increased risk of complications and, therefore, the need for an appropriate balance between efficacy and safety.

Corticosteroids

The use of corticosteroids, most commonly prednisone, remains the mainstay of therapy for the patient with lupus. Corticosteroids should be used in such a way to avoid the large number of side effects known to exist. It is generally recommended that the dose of prednisone be titrated to minimize signs and symptoms with the lowest dose that is practical. To minimize side effects, topical or compartmental (i.e., intra-articular), should be considered first. Systemic administration such as daily or split-dose oral therapy is more toxic than alternate-day therapy which results in less hypothalamic-pituitary-adrenal (HPA) suppression.

Intravenous bolus glucocorticoid therapy in high dose has become widely used to treat acute, severe manifestations of lupus. Indications for pulse therapy have included glomerulonephritis, CNS disease, and thrombocytopenia. One approach used is to infuse 1 gm/m^2 methylprednisolone as bolus therapy. This approach can be used to control disease activity. Concomitantly, the patient is usually started on oral daily prednisone at a dose of 40–60 mg/day for 1 month, then tapered at a rate of 5 mg/week on alternate days. The goal is to get the patient to a low dose (0.15–0.25 mg/kg) every other day as quickly as possible without having an increase in lupus activity. Therapy such as this may provide benefit to some individuals.

When to withdraw corticosteroid treatment in an individual patient who is in remission remains a point of contention. Some authors suggest corticosteroids should be lifelong therapy. The idea is to prevent any possibility of disease reactivation once a remission is achieved. Ideally, with nontoxic therapeutic agents, lifelong therapy to prevent future disease makes sense. Unfortunately, currently existing therapies are not benign.

Cutaneous disease

Treatment of cutaneous lupus begins with prophylaxis against possible exacerbation. Patients should be informed that sun and fluorescent light can be responsible for disease flares (both cutaneous and systemic) [55, 59, 68]. The ill effects of light exposure appear to result from two activities of ultraviolet light: (1) induction of interleukin-1 (IL-1) production by keratinocytes (which augments immunity) [20], and (2) impairment of antigen handling by macrophages [20]. Avoidance of sun exposure through clothing and proper use of sunscreens with a sun-protective factor (SPF) of at least 15 will help protect against ultraviolet irradiation. Avoidance of photosensitizing drugs such as tetracyclines or sulfa drugs should be reinforced.

The drug treatment of cutaneous lupus can vary from topical to intravenous depending upon the type and severity of the skin disease.

Corticosteroid therapy

Trials of topical corticosteroids such as clobetasol propionate, betamethasone diproprionate or fluocinonide are commonly used for well-localized skin manifestations such as malar rash, discoid lesions, or inflanmatory rashes on the trunk and extremities. Generally, ointments transverse the skin better than creams. Adverse events resulting from ointments include cutaneous atrophy, depigmentation, striae and adrenal suppression. Therefore, it is recommended that they not be used for longer than 2 weeks of daily use. After an appropriate period they may be restarted.

Intralesional corticosteroids are effective, particularly with localized discoid disease, but may be impractical in individuals with a large number of lesions. Nevertheless, appropriate lesions may respond to small doses (< 5 mg) of injectable steroid such as triamcinolone acetonide.

Oral corticosteroids are reserved for patients with severe, refractory skin disease. Usually, the patient who requires oral prednisone has failed topical treatment and antimalarials. It is controversial if pulse methylprednisolone has any value in the treatment of chronic cutaneous disease.

Antimalarials

Antimalarials have long been used to treat the cutaneous manifestations of SLE [67]. Hydroxychloroquine, chloroquine and quinacrine hydrochloride are all effective in disease management [14]. These agents are capable of reducing erythema, scaling/hyperkeratosis and dermal inflammation [62]. The mechanism of action in systemic inflammatory disorders remains unclear. Studies suggest that antimalarials may function as immunomodulatory agents. Chloroquine has been shown to impair peripheral blood mononuclear cell response to mitogen [58], alter monocyte/macrophage function [56] and inhibit release of IL-1 by monocytes [63, 64].

When starting antimalarials, higher initial doses allow earlier responses. Initial doses of either hydroxychloroquine 400 mg/day, chloroquine 500 mg/day or quinacrine 100 mg/day are used until a response is observed. Daily maintenance treatment can then be reduced to one-half the initial dose. If a response is not observed within 2 months, the combination of antimalarials provides a synergistic effect.

Toxicities occur with antimalarial therapy but generally are infrequent when used at recommmended doses. Gastrointestinal reactions and rashes are most common; central nervous system (CNS) complications have been rarely reported. Hemolytic reactions occur in individuals with glucose-6-phosphate dehydrogenase (G-6-PD) deficiency. Ocular reactions, such as corneal desposition and retinal toxicity, are among the most serious. Retinopathy is more frequent with chloroquine therapy than hydroxychloroquine [7]. Furthermore, toxicity is related to the daily dose, rather than cumulative dose, and can be minimized by doses less than 6.5 mg/kg per day [50]. The use of antimalarials during pregnancy remains controversials. Of 215 reported pregnancies with chloroquine or hydroxychloroquine exposure, 7 infants with congenital abnormalities were observed [44].

In addition to the benefit to the skin, hydroxychlorochine appears to be useful in long-term management to maintain disease remission. The Canadian Hydroxychloroquine Study found that patients with quiescent disease who were taking hydroxychloroquine were less likey to have a disease flare as compared to those who discontinued hydroxychloroquine [75]. Furthermore, hydroxychloroquine has been shown to possess cholesterol-lowering effects in females with SLE [85]. This effect appeared to be independent of steroid usage. Dapsone, at doses of 100–250 mg/day, has been used for the treatment of vesiculobullous skin disease [67]. The retinoids, isotretinoin, etretinate, and acitretin, appear to have comparable efficacy to hydroxychloroquine [62], although toxicities from these compounds are common. Thalidomide has been used with some success [41], but given the negative public notice of its side effects, its use has been limited. Recent reports suggest that alpha-interferon may have a role in treating lupus skin disease [69]. These successes in treatment by interferon therapy must be tempered against the possible exacerbation of disease [77, 86].

Pulse corticosteroids and cytotoxic agents have a role in the treatment of severe skin disease, but should be reserved for patients in whom conventional therapy has failed. While no randomized clinical trials have examined the use of either pulse methylprednisolone, azathioprine, chlorambucil, methotrexate or cyclophosphamide, anecdotal reports suggest these agents may be efficacious. Since the side effect profile of these agents includes profound immunosuppression and potential risk for malignancy, caution must be exercised before implementation.

Lupus nephritis

The most extensively studied manifestation of SLE by controlled clinical trials is lupus nephritis. Preservation of renal function has a profound impact, not only to the patient but has enormous financial considerations as well. It is projected that the aggressive treatment of lupus nephritis saves an estimated $93 million per annum in the USA alone [53]. Therefore, proper diagnosis, identification of patients with a poor prognosis and treatment interventions are essential in the management of lupus nephritis.

A commonly asked clinical question relates to the role of renal biopsy in a lupus patient with an abnormal urinalysis. In the straightforward case in which both clinical and laboratory parameters favor the diagnosis of lupus nephritis, little may be gained from a renal biopsy. However, when either clinical or laboratory data are ambiguous or nephritis has been altered by previous therapy, a biopsy may be helpful in diagnosis and prognosis and aide therapeutic decisions [65]. It is generally acknowledged that biopsies with World Health Organization classes I and II have a significantly better prognosis than classes III, IV, V, and VI [38, 54]. Furthermore, higher chronicity scores on biopsy have a substantially greater risk of progression to renal failure [1, 57].

Irregardless of findings on renal biopsy, basic elements of therapy begins with renal preservation. Hypertension may precede the onset of nephritis [13] and rigid blood pressure control is essential. The armamentarium available to treat hypertension has grown with effective drugs, such as the calcium channel blockers and angiotensin converting enzyme (ACE) inhibitors, that have few adverse effects. Maintaining the blood pressure within the middle of the normal range is the goal for treatment. Additionally, drugs which diminish renal blood flow, such as aspirin or NSAIDs, should be avoided if possible in the patient with lupus nephritis.

What type of therapy should be used specifically to treat lupus nephritis? The answer to this question is one that must utilize all clinical and laboratory data to provide the patient with the best outcome. Clinical features such as serum creatinine, age, race, hematocrit and C3 complement are associated with an increased probability of doubling the serum creatinine [2]. Additionally, patient concerns require attention. For example, most patients with lupus nephritis are young women of child-bearing potential and aggressive therapy may prevent a desired pregnancy. The risk of cyclophosphamide-induced amenorrhea correlates with increased patient age and duration of drug therapy [10].

Oral corticosteroids have been the mainstay of the treatment of lupus nephritis. In recent years the use of boluses of intravenous methylprednisolone have been adopted by many physicians with the belief that its use is effective and not harmful. While most agree that oral corticosteroids are needed (preferably in alternate-day dosing), the efficacy of intravenous pulse is lacking [10]. Azathioprine in combination with corticosteroids may be efficacious in treating lupus nephritis in a subset of patient with moderate disease activity [15, 71], although in long-term follow-up, the efficacy of azathioprine did not statistically differ from oral prednisone alone [72].

The results of several clinical trials in lupus nephritis point to cyclophosphamide as the drug of choice in severe renal disease [1, 10, 22, 43, 52, 72]. The difficulties in doing studies examining the treatment of lupus nephritis are (i) obtaining a sufficiently large sample size, (ii) defining clinical outcome parameters acceptable by all, and (iii) following patients long enough to detect differences in treatment. The minimum length of follow-up appears to be at least 5 years before significant differences can be determined with cyclophosphamide. Studies have reported that cyclophosphamide is efficacious in controlling active nephritis [1, 10, 22, 43, 52, 72], prevention of renal scarring [4], and reducing the risk of end-stage renal disease [1, 72].

In an ongoing study at NIH, patients with proliferative glomerulonephritis have been treated with monthly pulse cyclophosphamide in combination with prednisone. Cyclophosphamide is given at a dose of 0.5–1 g/m^2 (to achieve a WBC nadir between 1,000 and 3,000/mm^3) and infused over 60 min monthly for six months. Thereafter, cyclophosphamide is infused once every 3 months for a minimum of an additional 2 years. The majority of patients are treated as outpatients and are hydrated with intravenous normal saline at 200 ml/h for 10 h. Antiemetics are given, consisting of one initial 10 mg oral dose of dexamethasone plus ondansetron 4–8 mg, orally or intravenously, every 4 h for three doses beginning 4 h after cyclophosphamide infusion [90]. In addition, patients are given oral prednisone, at a dose of 0.5 mg/kg per day for 4 weeks. At that time, prednisone is tapered at a rate of 5 mg every other day each week to the minimal dose required for control of extrarenal disease. Patients are usually maintained on a minimum of 0.25 mg/kg every other day of prednisone.

Cyclophosphamide has multiple side effects. From a previous and an ongoing lupus nephritis trial at the National Institutes of Health (NIH) [11] women of 25 years of age or less have an incidence of amenorrhea caused by cyclophosphamide of 17%. The mean number of cyclophosphamide pulses before amenorrhea was 20 in this group. The incidence increased to 68% in women of greater than 31 years of age with a mean number of pulses to amenorrhea being 12. Other potential toxicities of cyclophosphamide include alopecia, nausea, vomiting, bone marrow suppression, hemorrhagic cystitis, pulmonary fibrosis and malignancy [27].

Cyclosporine (CSA) has not been extensively studied in lupus nephritis. However, several small studies suggest that CSA may be efficacious in treating kidney disease [25, 26]. The only controlled study examined CSA (3 mg/kg per day) and prednisone versus prednisone (both intravenous and oral) alone [3]. After 1 year of therapy the CSA plus prednisone group had less proteinuria than the prednisone alone group. No change was observed in creatinine clearance in either group. Because of the large number of adverse side effects of CSA, in particular the potential for nephrotoxicity, this drug should reserved for cases refractory to conventional treatment.

Antiphospholipid antibody syndrome

Diagnosis of antiphospholipid antibody syndrome (APS) is facilitated by a high index of suspicion and by improved testing procedures [46]. Lupus anticoagulant tests such as the Russell viper venom time, activated partial thromboplastin time or the platelet neutralization procedure have been shown to have good correlation with thrombosis. ELISA tests for cardiolipin often have false-positives and do not clearly correlate with thrombotic events [46]. Quantitation of these tests are not always precise; therefore, minor changes in titers should not influence clinical decisions.

Individually tailored therapy for each patient optimizes clinical outcome. Considerations for treatment must include the potential for untoward effects of management. Most importantly, a positive test does not warrant treatment without signs of clinical manifestations. Furthermore, any correctable cause must be excluded before the diagnosis of APS can be made. For example, patients with superficial venous thrombosis may be adequately treated with aspirin, but persistence or occurrence of deep venous thrombosis should be managed with long-term warfarin therapy. Arterial thrombosis represents a greater therapeutic dilemma. These patients are likely to have recurrent arterial events and should be initially anticoagulated with heparin followed by long-term warfarin, perhaps for life [46]. Prothrombin times with international normalized ratios (INRs) $\geq$ 2.0 may confer better antithrombotic protection than low- to intermediate-intensity warfarin therapy or aspirin therapy [60]. Some authors recommend adding daily low-dose aspirin to warfarin therapy [29], while others have observed aspirin alone is sufficient [17].

Daily oral prednisone appears not to have a role in the therapy of vascular thrombosis, although anecdotes suggest that the lupus anticoagulant may be steroid responsive. The role of pulse corticosteroids or cytotoxic agents have not been extensively studied. Plasmapheresis in attempts to reduce the level of circulating antiphospholipid antibody has been used, although no clinical trials have examined this approach to therapy.

Antiphospholipid antibody syndrome in pregnancy

The presence of antiphospholipid antibody in the pregnant lupus patient represents a therapeutic quandary. In lupus patients, as many as one-third of the women will have antiphospholipid antibody [47, 48]. The risk of fetal loss correlates with antibody titer [48] and may be as high as 30% in those with high titers. This risk is further increased in women with a previous history of pregnancy loss [48, 61].

Treatment of all pregnancies must include close monitoring. Risk of losing the pregnancy is low for primiparas and treatment consists of observation with or without low-dose (80 mg/day) aspirin [23]. For multiparous women with a history of fetal loss, recommended care includes prednisone (40–60 mg/day) and low-dose aspirin. Although this has been shown to improve survival [12, 49] others studies suggest this therapy induces maternal and fetal morbidity [46, 48]. One small controlled study advocates subcutaneous heparin and aspirin used in a sequential fashion [19]. The authors found better fetal and maternal morbidity outcomes as compared to high-dose prednisone plus aspirin. Another report treated three patients with intravenous immunoglobulin plus aspirin who had favorable outcomes [37].

Hematology

The lupus patient may be anemic for several reasons and all reversible causes should be properly evaluated. Usually the low hemoglobin is explained by the anemia of chronic disease and does not require therapy. In contrast, patients with a hemolytic anemia, if severe, require glucocorticoid therapy in high doses. When a response is observed, the glucocorticoids should be tapered with close monitoring so as to maintain a normal hematocrit. In glucocorticoid-resistant cases, splenectomy and/or immunosuppressive therapy may be beneficial [18].

Similarly, leukopenia is a common problem in the lupus population. Observation without specific treatment is generally the rule. Infection resulting from a low white blood cell count is uncommon. Recombinant human granulocyte-colony-stimulating factor (rhG-CSF) has been shown to be effective in rapidly raising the white blood cell count in chemotherapy-induced leukopenias [20]. Preliminary work suggests rhG-CSF may be useful in cyclic neutropenia [33].

Approximately one-quarter of lupus patients will experience thrombocytopenia during their illness. Specific therapy may not be needed unless the platelet count is profoundly decreased (20,000–50,000 platelets/mm^3). Glucocorticoids at a prednisone dose of 0.25–1.0 g/kg per day will generally raise the platelet count within 2–4 weeks. The addition of intravenous gammaglobulin, 400 mg/kg per day for 5 days, may hasten the response but the relapse rate is similar to that of patients treated with either prednisone or gammaglobulin alone [34]. Failing glucocorticoids and intravenous gammaglobulin commonly results in the patient undergoing splenectomy. The efficacy of splenectomy is arguable. One study found that surgical intervention alone afforded a sustained remission in only 15% of patients [30]. However, in general, splenectomy will provide adequate numbers of platelets for most individuals. Prior to splenectomy, the patient should be vaccinated against *Streptococcus pneumoniae*. Splenectomized children have a lower incidence of pneumococcal infection when vaccinated before splenectomy [41].

Other treatment regimes have been effective in managing immune thrombocytopenia. Danazol, at a dose of 400–800 mg/day may increase platelet counts within 2 weeks but relapses may occur if therapy is given for less than 6 months [88]. Unfortunately, danazol's toxicity profile (virilization, weight gain, rash, hepatitis, etc.) is not acceptable to some patients. For resistant cases, the addition of cytotoxic therapy may be necessary [18, 28, 35]. Agents such as azathioprine, vincristine, daily oral and intermittent intravenous pulse cyclophosphamide have demonstrated efficacy [8]. These agents may be most effective when used in the splenectomized patient [35].

Central nervous system

Establishing the proper diagnosis is the first objective in the management of CNS disease in SLE. Diagnostic tests with a high degree of specificity for CNS SLE do not exist and, therefore, diagnosing CNS lupus is sometimes made by exclusion. CNS manifestations of disease may not be accompanied by a flare of multisystem SLE disease activity [66]. Secondary causes such as hypertension, metabolic disorders, hypoxia, malignancy, and medications should be excluded. Perhaps one of the most difficult dilemmas to diagnosis is the lupus patient with steroid-induced psychosis.

All lupus patients with CNS disease must be evaluated for evidence of hypercoagulability. Although stroke is the most frequent manifestation of APS, antiphospholipid antibodies have been reported to be associated with transverse myelitis, chorea and multiinfarct dementia. The lupus anticoagulant has been found in as many as 40% of SLE patients with CNS manifestations [21]. Treatment for these problems, excluding signs of vasculitis, should consist of anticoagulation. Glucocorticoid or cytotoxic therapy appear not to have a role in therapy [46].

Each specific neurological manifestation should be treated with standard medical care whether more aggressive therapy will be used or not. For example, appropriate anticonvulsive therapy should be used in SLE patient with seizures and antipsychotics in individuals with psychosis. Treatment of the acute event stabilizes the patient and provides time to further investigate the etiology of disease and time to strategize therapy.

There are no randomized trials examining issues of therapy with patients with CNS lupus. Therefore, clinical experience and management issues arise from the findings of controlled trials examining the treatment of other organ involvement. Typically, oral daily steroids at a dose of 1 mg/kg per day are begun, then tapered with clinical improvement. Oral steroids are commonly used in combination with either pulse methylprednisolone or cyclophosphamide. In a retrospective study, seven patients with transverse myelitis were treated with pulse methylprednisolone and/or pulse cyclophosphamide [5]. The patients generally tolerated therapy and stabilized or improved their disease. Boumpas, et al. [9], using cyclophosphamide alone, retrospectively examined nine patients with CNS lupus. Of the nine, seven had focal neurological deficits and/or seizures and two had organic brain syndrome. Antiphospholipid antibodies were present in five of the patients. Cyclophosphamide, 0.75–1.0 g/m^2 was given intravenously for a minimum of 2 months. Eight patients responded with either a full recovery or a recovery with only minor residual dysfunction. Others have noted similar findings [51].

Investigational therapies

Hormonal manipulation

Manipulation of male and female hormones have been extensively studied in murine models of SLE [76]. Androgens reduce and estrogens increase autoantibodies in the NZB model and estrogens cause a marked acceleration of autoimmunity [73]. Agents that posses androgenic activity are able to alleviate some of the signs and symptoms of lupus. One such agent is danazol. Recent studies of dehydroepiandrosterone (DHEA), a weakly androgenic adrenal steroid, have suggested the drug is beneficial in the therapy of premenopausal females with SLE. The result of a preliminary double-blind, placebo controlled, randomized trial examining the efficacy of DHEA in premenopausal women with SLE has been recently reported [81]. An interim analysis, with one-half of the patients completing the 3 months, showed a trend towards lower systemic lupus erythematosus disease activity index (SLEDAI) scores and prednisone doses in the DHEA-treated patients, although the changes did not reach statistical significance. DHEA appeared to be well tolerated; acne was the most common side effect observed. Attempts to alter disease using testosterone derivatives have been examined. In a small, open label, non-controlled study of 4 women and 3 men with clinically active disease, 100 mg of 19-nortestosterone decanoate was administered intramuscularly on a weekly basis. Patients received treatment for up to 24 months. Two men had an increase in SLE activity which was associated with serological changes and the women appeared clinically stable despite the persistence of high titer anti-DNA antibodies [42].

Monoclonal antibodies

Animal data suggests targeted treatment with monoclonal antibodies has potential in treating autoimmune disease [36, 86, 89]. Monoclonal antibodies have been humanized, conjugated and targeted to a number of specific cellular molecules or cytokines thought to mediate the disease process.

Several studies have examined the use of monoclonal antibody therapy in patients with lupus nephritis. A total of eight patients with active glomerulonephritis and two patients with thrombocytopenia have been treated with anti-CD5 ricin A chain immunoconjugate (CD5 PLUS) [70, 83]. CD5 is a molecule on the surface of T cells and a subpopulation of B cells. CD5 PLUS was administered at a dose of 0.1 mg/kg intravenously for 5 consecutive days. The patients with thrombocytopenia did not respond to treatment. Five of the eight patients with glomerulonephritis improved in both urine and laboratory parameters and this improvement persisted for a minimum of 4 to 15 months. T cell counts dropped and appeared to be diminished 6 months after treatment [70]. B cell changes were not consistent. Treatment with anti-CD5 appeared to be well tolerated with minimal side effects observed. Human anti-monoclonal antibody (HAMA) production was investigated in four patients, all with positive results.

Several animal studies have examined the effects of anti-CD4 antibodies in murine models of lupus [24, 89] Studies in lupus patients, however, suggest that the clinical effect of anti-CD4 may be limited [31, 32]. Five patients with severe disease were treated with 0.3 mg/day for 7 consecutive days with anti-CD4 MAX.16H5. Three patients entered a remission but only after receiving a methylprednisolone pulse in addition to the anti-CD4. Anti-CD4 may perhaps have a role in the care of the severely affected patient.

The number of potential targets for monoclonal antibody therapy are abundant. Such targets include specific T cell and cytokine receptors, adhesion molecules and other surface markers which are capable of delivering signals to other cells. Long-term effects of this form of treatment are unknown.

Apheresis

The removal of pathogenic autoantibodies via plasmapheresis in treating SLE, in theory, makes sense. Unfortunately, the theory has not been convincingly established by clinical results and, as a result, apheresis has not gained a spotlight in treating SLE. Most physicians reserve this form of therapy for those patients who have either failed conventional treatment or have life-threatening disease. To improve the efficiency of antibody removal, the technique of immunoadsorption has been added to plasmapheresis. This technique has been examined in patients with lupus nephritis [74], where anti-DNA antibodies were targeted, and with the APS [84], where anti-DNA and antiphospholipid antibodies were marked for removal.

Plasmapheresis has been advocated for the treatment of lupus nephritis because the procedure reduces circulating antibody, immune complexes, and other circulating inflammatory mediators. A study conducted by the Lupus Nephritis Collaborative Study Group compared the effect of plasmapheresis, plus a standard regimen of prednisone and oral cyclophosphamide therapy, to the standard regime alone. The findings of the trial indicated that the nephritis did not improve with the addition of plasmapheresis [45]. A randomized multicenter trial of plasmapheresis and subsequent intravenous pulse cyclophosphamide versus pulse cyclophosphamide alone in severe lupus is underway by the Lupus Plasmapheresis Study Group (LPSG) [16].

Another modification of apheresis, photophoresis, is based on the premise that ultraviolet light influences the immune system. Photopheresis uses low-energy ultraviolet A irradiation of leukocytes following the injection of the photoactivatable drug, 8-methoxypsoralen (8-MOP). Studies in animal models have shown that photophoresis suppresses T cell proliferation [6] and production of tumor necrosis factor α (TNF-α) [82]. In an open trial, photopheresis was used to treat 10 patients with mild to moderate lupus that flared when maintenance corticosteroid therapy was reduced or eliminated [40]. In this study, patients underwent photopheresis on 2 consecutive days for 6 months followed by photopheresis every 3 months. Of the eight patients who completed the trial, seven improved clinically.

Purine analogues

Newer agents found to be immunosuppressive continue to make their way into clinical trials. Most of these drugs come from the oncology field. Two new adenosine-deaminase (ADA) resistant purine analogues, 2-Chloro-deoxyadenosine (CdA) and fludarabine, have found there way into clinical trials involving autoimmune disease. Compared to other purine analogues, these drugs offer the advantages of increased specificity for lymphoid cells and fewer adverse effects.

Future directions in therapy

Immune oral tolerance has been the subject of ongoing studies in rheumatoid arthritis (RA) [87] and multiple sclerosis [79]. It is believed a tolerant state to the implicated antigen can be achieved by oral administration of antigen. Type II chicken collagen has been used in RA and bovine myelin in multiple sclerosis. Preliminary data support the theory. While the offending antigen(s) remains unknown in SLE, candidates such as DNA or ribonuclear proteins may be potential antigens for studies of oral tolerance in the future.

Gene therapy of immunological disorders is based upon the premise that circulating levels of peptide hormones and cytokines can be manipulated. Animal studies support this premise. Manipulation has been achieved either by direct intramuscular injection of a cDNA expression vector or transfection of the cDNA into cultured cells originally removed from, then reintroduced back into the animal. For example, the cDNA may be a immunostimulatory or immunosuppressive cytokine, such as IL-2 or transforming growth factor-β-1, respectively, or a receptor antagonist such as the IL-I receptor antagonist protein (IRAP). By directly influencing the expressing of cytokines at the genetic level, it is possible to alter the functional circulating level either at a localized compartment (joint) or in the systemic circulation. Although the number of abnormally expressed cytokines and/or receptors in the lupus patient is large, these abnormalities can be methodically dissected to implicate the major participants of disease. Armed with this knowledge, directed gene therapy may have the potential to correct the genetic defects.

References

1. Austin HA, Klippel JH, Balow, JE, le Riche NG, Steinberg AD, Plotz PH, Decker JL (1986) Therapy of lupus nephritis. Controlled trial of prednisone and cytotoxic drugs. N Engl J Med 314:614
2. Austin HA III, Boumpas DT, Vaughan EM, Balow JE (1994) Predicting renal outcomes in severe lupus nephritis: contributions of clinical and histologic data. Kidney Int 45:544
3. Balletta M, Sabella D, Magri P, Sepe V, Stanziale P, Di Luccio R, Colucci G, Fuiano G (1992) Ciclosporin plus steroids versus steroids alone in the treatment of lupus nephritis. Contrib Nephrol 99:129
4. Balow JE, Austin HA, Muenz LR, Joyce KM, Antonovych TT, Klippel JH, Steinberg AD, Plotz PH, Decker JL (1984) Effect of treatment on the evolution of renal abnormalities in lupus nephritis. N Engl J Med 311:491
5. Barile L, Lavalle C (1992) Transverse myelitis in systemic lupus erythematosus – the effect of IV pulse methylprednisolone and cyclophosphamide. J Rheumatol 10:370
6. Berger CL, Perez M, Laroche L, Edelson R (1990) Inhibition of autoimmune disease in a murine model of systemic lupus erythematosus induced by exposure to syngeneic photoinactivated lymphocytes. J Invest Dermatol 94:52
7. Bernstein HN (1983) Ophthalmalogic considerations and testing in patients receiving long-term antimalarial therapy. Am J Med 75:25
8. Boumpas DT, Barez S, Klippel JH, Balow JE (1990) Intermittent cyclophosphamide for the treatment of autoimmune thrombocytopenia in systemic lupus erythematosus. Ann Intern Med 112:674
9. Boumpas DT, Yamada H, Patronas NJ, Scott D, Klippel JH, Balow JE (1991) Pulse cyclophosphamide for severe neuropsychiatric lupus. Q J Med 81:975
10. Boumpas DT, Austin Liii Vaughan EM, Klippel JH, Steinberg AD, Yarboro CH, Balow JE (1992) Controlled trial of pulse methylprednisolone versus two reimens of pulse cyclophosphamide in severe lupus nephritis. Lancet 340:741
11. Boumpas DT, Austin HA III, Vaughan EM, Yarboro CH, Klippel JH, Balow JE (1993) Risk for sustained amenorrhea in patients with systemic lupus erythematosus receiving intermittent pulse cyclophosphamide therapy. Ann Intern Med 119:366
12. Branch DW, Scott JR, Kochenour NK, Hershgold E (1985) obstetric complications associated with the lupus anticoagulant. N Engl J Med 313:1322
13. Budman D and Steinberg AD (1976) Relationship between hypertension and renal disease in systemic lupus erythematosus. Arch Intern Med 136:1003
14. Callen JP (1990) Treatment of cutaneous lesions in patients with lupus erythematosus. Dermatol Clin 8:355

15. Carette S, Klippel JH, Decker JL, Austin III HA, Plotz PH, Steinberg AD, Balow JE (1983) Controlled studies of oral immunosuppressive drugs in lupus nephritis. A long-term follow-up. Ann Intern Med 99:1
16. Clark WF, Dau PC, Euler HH, Guillevin L, Hasford J. Heer AH, Jones JV, Kashgarian M, Knatterud G, Lockwood CM (1991) Plasmapheresis and subsequent pulse cyclophosphamide versus pulse cyclophosphamide alone in severe lupus: design of the LPSG trial. Lupus Plasmapheresis Study Group (LPSG). J Clin Apheresis 6:40
17. Cohen MG, Lui SF (1992) Multiple complications of the antiphospholipid syndrome with apparent response to aspirin therapy. J Rheumatol 19:803
18. Coon WW (1988) Splenectomy for cytopenias associated with systemic lupus erythematosus. Am J Surg 155:391
19. Cowchock FS, Reece EA, Balaban D, Branch DW, Plouffe L (1992) Repeated fetal losses associated with antiphospholipid antibodies: a collaborative randomized trial comparing prednisone with low-dose heparin treatment. Am J Obstet Gynecol 166:1318
20. Crawford J, Ozer H, Stoller R, Johnson D, Lyman G, Tabbara I, Kris M, Grous J. Picozzi V. Rausch G (1991) Reduction by granulocyte colony-stimulating factor of fever and neutropenia induced by chemotherapy in patients with small-cell lung cancer. N Engl J Med 325:164
21. Derksen RH, Bouma BN, Kater L (1986) The association between the lupus anticoagulant and cerebral infarction in systemic lupus erythematosus. Scand J Rheumatol 15:179
22. Donadio JV Jr, Holley KE, Ferguson RH, Ilstrup DM (1978) Treatment of diffuse proliferative lupus nephritis with prednisone and combined prednisone and cyclophosphamide. N Engl J Med 299:1151
23. Druzin ML, Lockshin M, Edersheim TG, Hutson JM, Krauss AL, Kogut E (1987) Second-trimester fetal monitoring and preterm delivery in pregnancies with systemic lupus erythematosus and/or circulating anticoagulant. Am J Obstet Gynecol 157:1503
24. Ermak TH, Steger HJ, Wofsy D (1989) Treatment of murine lupus with monoclonal antibody to L3T4. II. Effects on immunohistopathology of thymus, spleen, and lymph node. Lab Invest 61:447
25. Favre H, Miescher PA, Huang YP, Chatelanat F, Mihatsch MJ (1989) Cyclosporin in the treatment of lupus nephritis. Am J Nephrol 9 [Suppl 1]:57
26. Feutren G, Querin S, Tron F, Noel LH, Chatenoud L, Lesavre P, Bach JF (1986) The effects of cyclosporine in patients with systemic lupus. Transplant Proc 18:643
27. Gourley MF, Seldin MF, Steinberg AD (1992) Immunoregulatory agents. In: Gallin JI, Goldstein IM, Synderman R (eds) Inflammation: basic principles and clinical correlates. Raven Press, New York, pp 1103–1126
28. Gruenberg JC, VanSlyck EJ, Abraham JP (1986) Splenectomy in systemic lupus erythematosus. Am Surg 52:366
29. Hahn BH (1993) Management of systemic lupus erythematosus. In: Kelley WN, Harris ED, Ruddy S, Sledge CB (eds) Textbook of Rheumatology. Saunders, Philadelphia, pp 1043–1056
30. Hall S, McCormick JL, Greipp PR, Michet CJ, McKenna CH (1985) Splenectomy does not cure the thrombocytopenia of systemic lupus erythematosus. Ann Intern Med 102:325
31. Hiepe F, Volk HD, Apostoloff E, von Baehr R, Emmrich F (1991) Treatment of severe systemic lupus erythematosus with anti-CD4 monoclonal antibody. Lancet 338:1529
32. Hiepe F, Thiele B, Brink I, Volk HD, Emmrich F (1993) Investigations on the treatment of systemic lupus (SLE) with the monoclonal anti-CD4 antibody MAX.16H5. Arthritis Rheum 36:S227
33. Hirashima K, Yoshida Y, Asano S, Takaku F, Omine M, Furusawa S, Abe T, Dohy H, Tajiri M (1991) Clinical effect of recombinant human granulocyte colony-stimulating factor (rhG-CSF) on various types of neutropenia including cyclic neutropenia. Biotherapy 3:297
34. Jacobs P, Wood L (1989) The comparison of gammaglobulin to steroids in treating adult immune thrombocytopenia. An interim analysis. Blut 59:92
35. Jacobs P, Wood L, Dent DM (1986) Results of treatment in immune thrombocytopenia. Q J Med 58:153
36. Janson CH (1993) Biology of monoclonal antibodies in tumor therapy. Med Oncol Tumor Pharmacother 10:21
37. Kaaja R, Julkunen H, Ammala P, Palosuo T, Kurki P (1993) Intravenous immunoglobulin treatment of pregnant patients with recurrent pregnancy losses associated with antiphospholipid antibodies. Acta Obstet Gynecol Scand 72:63
38. Kater L, Derksen RH, Heneë RJ (1991) Treatment of systemic lupus erythematosus: which options do we have for therapy regimens? Rheumatol Int 11:137

39. Klippel JH (1993) Is aggressive therapy effective for lupus? Rheum Dis Clin North Am 19:249
40. Knobler RM, Graninger W, Lindmaier A, Trautinger F, Smolen JS (1992) Extracorporeal photochemotherapy for the treatment of systemic lupus erythematosus. A pilot study. Arthritis Rheum 35:319
41. Konradsen HB, Henrichsen J (1991) Pneumococcal infections in splenectomized children are preventable. Acta Paediatr Scand 80:423
42. Lahita RG, Cheng CY, Monder C, Bardin CW (1992) Experience with 19-nortestosterone in the therapy of systemic lupus erythematosus: worsened disease after treatment with 19-nortestosterone in men and lack of improvement in women. J Rheumatol 19:547
43. Lehman TJA (1991) Long-term outcome of systemic lupus erythematosus in childhood. Rheum Dis Clin North Am 17:921
44. Levy M, Buskila D, Gladman DD, Urowitz MB, Koren G (1991) Pregnancy outcome following first trimester exposure to chloroquine. Am J Perinatol 8:174
45. Lewis EJ, Hunsicker LG, Lan SP, Rohde RD, Lachin JM (1992) A controlled trial of plasmapheresis therapy in severe lupus nephritis. The Lupus Nephritis Collaborative Study Group. N Engl J Med 326:1373
46. Lockshin MD (1993) Which patients with antiphospholipid antibody should be treated and how? Rheum Dis Clin North Am 19:235
47. Lockshin MD, Qamar T, Druzin ML, Goei S (1987) Antibody to cardiolipin, lupus anticoagulant, and fetal death. J Rheumatol 14:259
48. Lockshin MD, Druzin ML, Qamar T (1989) Prednisone does not prevent recurrent fetal death in women with antiphospholipid antibody. Am J Obstet Gynecol 160:439
49. Lubbe WF, Butler WS, Palmer SJ, Liggins GC (1983) Fetal survival after prednisone suppression of maternal lupus-anticoagulant. Lancet I:1361
50. Mackenzie AH (1983) Dose refinements in long-term antimalarial therapy. Am J Med 75:40
51. McCune WJ, Friedman AW (1993) Immunosuppressive drug therapy for rheumatic desease. Curr Opin Rheumatol 5:282
52. McCune WJ, Golbus J. Zeldes W, Bohlke P, Dunne R, Fox DA (1988) Clinical and immunologic effects of monthly administration of intravenous cyclophosphamide in severe systemic lupus erythematosus. N Engl J Med 318:1423
53. McInnes PM, Schuttinga JA, Sanslone WR, Stark SP, Klippel JH (1993) The economic impact of treatment of severe lupus nephritis with prednisone plus intravenous cyclophosphamide. Arthritis Rheum 36:S65
54. McLaughlin J. Gladman DD, Urowitz MB, Farewell VT, Cole E (1991) Kidney biopsy in systemic lupus erythematosus. II. Survival analysis according to biopsy results. Arthritis Rheum 24:1268
55. Nived O, Johansen PB, Sturfelt G (1993) Standardized ultraviolet-A exposure provokes skin reaction in systemic lupus erythematosus. Lupus 2:247
56. Norris DA, Weston WL, Sams WM (1977) The effect of immunosuppressive and anti-inflammatory drugs on monocyte function in vitro. J Lab Clin Med 90:569
57. Nossent HC, Henzen-Logmans SC, Vroom TM, Berden JH, Swaak TJ (1990) Contribution of renal biopsy data in predicting outcome in lupus nephritis. Analysis of 116 patients. Arthritis Rheum 33:970
58. Panayi GS, Neille WA, Duthie JJR, McCormick JN (1973) Action of chloroquine phosphate in rheumatoid arthritis. I. Immunosuppressive effect. Ann Rheum Dis 32:316
59. Rihner M, McGrath H Jr (1992) Fluorescent light photosensitivity in patients with systemic lupus erythematosus. Arthritis Rheum 35:949
60. Rosove MH Brewer PM (1992) Antiphospholipid thrombosis: clinical course after the first thrombotic event in 70 patients. Ann Intern Med 117:303
61. Rosove MH, Tabsh K, Wasserstrum N, Howard P, Hahn BH, Kalunian KC (1990) Heparin therapy for pregnant women with lupus anticoagulant or anticardiolipin antibodies. Obstet Gynecol 75:630
62. Ruzicka T, Sommerburg C, Goerz G, Kind P, Mensing H (1992) Treatment of cutaneous lupus erythematosus with acitretin and hydroxychloroquine. Br J Dermatol 127:513
63. Salmeron G, Lipsky PE (1983) The immunosuppressive potential of antimalarials. Am J Med 75:19
64. Scala G, Oppenheim JJ (1983) Antigen presentation by human monocytes: evidence for stimulant processing and requirement for interleukin 1. J Immunol 131:1160
65. Schwartz MM, Lan SP, Bernstein J. Hill GS, Holley K, Lewis EJ (1992) Role of pathology indices in the management of severe lupus glomerulonephritis. Lupus Nephritis Collaborative Study Group. Kidney Int 42:743

66. Sibley JT, Olszynski WP, Decoteau WE, Sundaram MB (1992) The incidence and prognosis of central nervous system disease in systemic lupus erythematosus. J Rheumatol 19:47
67. Sontheimer RD (1988) Lupus erythematosus. In: Provost TT, Farmer ER (eds) Current therapy in dermatology, vol. 2. Decker, Philadelphia, pp 123–128
68. Sontheimer RD (1993) Fluorescent light photosensitivity in patients with systemic lupus erythematosus. Arthritis Rheum 36:428
69. Stadler R, Ruszczak Z (1993) Interferons. New additions and indications for use. Dermatol Clin 11:187
70. Stafford FJ, Fleisher TA, Brown M, Lee G, Austin HA III, Balow JE, Klippel JH (1993) Clinical and biological effects of anti-CD5 ricin A chain immunoconjugate in systemic lupus erythematosus (SLE). Arthritis Rheum 36:S227
71. Steinberg AD (1986) The treatment of lupus nephritis. Kidney Int 30:769
72. Steinberg AD, Steinberg SC (1991) Long-term preservation of renal function in patients with lupus nephritis receiving treatment that includes cyclophosphamide versus those treated with prednisone only. Arthritis Rheum 34:945
73. Steinberg AD, Melez KA, Raveche ES, Reeves JP, Boeger WA, Smathers PA, Taurog JD, Weinlein L, Duvic M (1979) Approach to the study of the role of sex hormones in autoimmunity. Arthritis Rheum 22:1170
74. Suzuki K, Hara M, Harigai M, Ishizuka T, Hirose T, Matsuki Y, Kawaguchi Y, Kitani A, Kawagoe M, amd Makamura H (1991) Continuous removal of anti-DNA antibody, using a new extracorporeal immunadsorption system, in patients with systemic lupus erythematosus. Arthritis Rheum 34:1546
75. The Canadian Hydroxychloroquine Group (1991) A randomized study of the effect of withdrawing hydroxychloroquine sulfate in systemic lupus erythematosus. N Engl J Med 324:150
76. Theofilopoulos AN) aed Dixon FJ (1985) Murine models of systemic lupus erythematosus. Adv Immunol 37:269
77. Tolaymat A, Leventhal B, Sakarcan A, Kashima H, Monteiro C (1992) Systemic lupus erythematosus in a child receiving long-term interferon therapy. J Pediatr 120:429
78. Reference deleted
79. Trentham DE, Dynesius-Trentham RA, Orav EJ, Combitchi D, Lorenzo C, Sewell KL, Hafler DA, Weiner HL (1993) Effects of oral adminstration of type II collagen on rheumatoid arthritis. Science 271:1727
80. Urowitz MB (1992) Is "aggressive" therapy necessary for systemic lupus erythemathosus? Rheum Dis Clin North Am 19:263
81. van Hollenhoven RF, Engleman EG, Elaine Lambert R, Lynda Lee YS, McGuire JL (1993) Treatment of systemic lupus erythematosus with dehydroepiandrosterone. Interim analysis of a double-blinded, randomized, placebo-controlled, clinical trial. Arthritis Rheum 36:S92
82. Vowel BR, Cassin M, Boufal MH, Walsh LJ, Rook AH (1992) Extracorporal photochemotherapy induces the production of tumor necrosis factor-α: implications for the treatment of cutaneous T-cell lymphoma and systemic sclerosis. J Invest Dermatol 98:686
83. Wacholtz MC, Lipsky PE (1992) Treatment of lupus nephritis with CD5 PLUS, and immunoconjugate of an anti-CD5 monoclonal antibody and ricin A chain. Arthritis Rheum 35:837
84. Waldmann TA (1991) Lymphokine receptor-directed therapy: a model for immune intervention in leukemia, autoimmunity and immunodeficiency. dlin Immunol Immunopathol 61:S37
85. Wallace DJ, Metzger AL, Stecher VJ, Trunbull BA, Kern PA (1990) Cholesterol-lowering effect of hydroxychloroquine in patients with rheumatic disease: reversal of deleterious effects of steroids on lipids. Am J Med 32289:322
86. Wandl UB, Nagel-Hiemke M, May D, Kreuzfelder E, Kloke O, Kranzhoff M, Seeber S, Niederle N (1992) Lupus-like autoimmune disease induced by interferon therapy for myeloproliferative disorders. Clin Immunol Immunopathol 64:70
87. Weiner HL, Mackin GA, Matsui M, Orav EJ, Khoury SJ, Dawson DM, Hafler DA (1993) Double-blind pilot trial of oral tolerization with myelin antigens in multiple sclerosis. Science 259:1321
88. West SG, Johnson SC (1988) Danazol for the treatment of refractroy autoimmune thrombocytopenia in systemic lupus erythematosus. Ann Intern 108:703
89. Wofsy D (1993) Treatment of murine lupus with anti-CD4 monoclonal antibodies. Immunol Ser 59:221
90. Yarboro CH, Pacino F, Wesley R, Klippel JH, Amantea M (1993): Antiemetic efficacy of oral dexamethasome (DMT) and ondansetron (OND) in lupus nephritis (LN) patients. Arthritis Rheum 36:S228

Drug combination therapy of systemic lupus erythematosus

Peter A. Miescher[1], Hervé Favre[2], Robert Lemoine[3], You-Peng Huang[1]

[1] Division of Haematology, Geneva University Hospital, CH-1211 Geneva 4, Switzerland
[2] Division of Nephrology, Geneva University Hospital, CH-1211 Geneva 4, Switzerland
[3] Institute of Clinical Pathology, Geneva University Hospital, CH-1211 Geneva 4, Switzerland

Introduction

During the past few decades, the survival of systemic lupus erythematosus (SLE) patients has steadily improved, so much so that it has become a minor issue with a mortality rate of approximately 1–2% per annum [2, 11]. The main problem today for lupus patients concerns their quality of life and the risk of loss of kidney function. Indeed, too many patients still lose this function (9% after 5 years of disease, 17% after 10 years) [2]. The aim of today's management of SLE is thus centred on allowing patients a good quality of life in both professional and personal terms, including the possibility of having children.

SLE has a wide spectrum of disease expression, from very mild to most severe forms. In the mild cases, it is easy to offer patients a good quality of life with small doses of steroids given on an alternate-day schedule, possibly in association with antimetabolites. This report deals only with the more severe forms of SLE not responding to the association of steroids and antimetabolites.

The introduction of cyclophosphamide (Cy)-pulse therapy has been very beneficial for the treatment of high-risk patients [16]. However, this drug may produce quite serious side effects, particularly with regard to the ovaries. Since many SLE patients are young girls, the ovary toxicity, which would compromise future pregnancies, constitutes a major problem.

Cyclosporin (CsA) has provided a new approach to the treatment of autoimmune diseases. However, clinicians are aware of the risk of CsA-associated kidney toxicity and, for this reason, there has been much hesitation to use this drug in a disease where the kidneys represent a major target of pathology [4]. CsA was initially administered to patients suffering from autoimmune diseases at a dose of 10 mg/kg per day, a dose which proved definitely toxic for the kidneys. Because of this nephrotoxicity, it was thought that CsA would increase the rate of kidney function loss in patients with lupus nephritis [4].

Correspondence to: P.A. Miescher

Nevertheless, in 1982 we introduced CsA for patients with very severe SLE who had not responded to the association of steroids and antimetabolites. Because of the potential renal toxicity of this drug, from the beginning we limited the dose to 5 mg/kg lean bodyweight (l.b.w.) per day. In fact, the first SLE patient to receive CsA medication, a 14 year-old girl, after 1 week of treatment, refused the proposed dose of 10 mg/kg, finally taking half of this amount (5 mg/kg). Subsequently, 5 mg/kg l.b.w. per day became the standard dose for our patients. It is interesting that this first patient, who is still on CsA medication, showed no signs of CsA-associated kidney toxicity on two kidney biopsies performed 4 and 8 years after initiation of CsA medication.

Here, we report on 73 patients (66 females and 7 males) with severe SLE who were on long-term CsA combination therapy with the aim of controlling disease activity with a minimum of overall side effects. All 73 patients agreed to undergo kidney biopsy to assess the degree of CsA-associated toxicity. One hundred kidney biopsies were performed in 69 patients. Two patients were on continuous anti-coagulant treatment which precluded kidney biopsy. Prior biopsy revealed type IV glomerulonephritis (GN) for the first, type V for the second patient. Two patients, who had initially agreed to this procedure, refused the kidney biopsy (one patient with type II GN, the other with type IV).

Patient selection and methods

For this study, all SLE patients on CsA medication for more than 18 months within the period 1 January 1981 to 30 December 1990 and who had accepted to undergo kidney biopsy, were included. Subsequently, these patients were followed until 1 May 1994. The aim of the study was to assess the overall treatment efficacy in terms of mortality, maintenance of kidney function, and quality of life, and to assess the nephrotoxicity of this treatment. CsA was given to patients not responding well to a steroid-antimetabolite therapy, i.e. to patients with a disease activity score [12] of more than 10/24, or steroid requirement above 150 mg prednisone/week. In these patients, antimetabolites were replaced by CsA at a dose of 5 mg/kg l.b.w. per day. From 1 January 1981 to 30 December 1990 we followed 246 patients with SLE (Table 1). Of these, 124 patients were well controlled with steroids plus antimetabolites (methotrexate, azathioprine); in 46 patients, it was possible to discontinue CsA (tapered gradually) after 4–6 months; 3 patients did not tolerate CsA. These 173 patients represent group A of Table 1. The remaining 73 patients (66 females, 7 males) met the requirements set for this study (group B of Table 1). Assuming that mild forms of SLE require a less intensive treatment, this study group concerns patients with a more severe form of SLE than those in group A. This is also reflected in the mortality rate and loss of kidney function rate in the two groups (Table 2). The causes of death are listed in Table 3.

This report summarises the results of the study after an average observation period of 7.1 ± 1.91 years for patients under long-term CsA medication. Age at the end of the study was 37 ± 9 years. The average observation period in Geneva for these patients was 9.25 ± 3.16 years. In 19 patients, the combination of steroids/CsA was sufficient to control disease activity. In 24 patients, i.m. or i.v. methotrexate (MTX) had to be added. In 30 patients, a quadruple combination therapy with steroids/CsA/MTX/Cy was necessary to control disease activity.

Table 1. SLE patients during period 1 January 1981 to 30 September 1990

Treatment	No. of patients		Mean observation period (years)
Group A			
Steroids + antimet.	124	173	6.5
Short-term (< 18 M)	46		
CsA medication			
CsA intolerance	3		
Group B			
Long term (< 18 M) CsA medication	73		7.1
Total no. of patients	246		

Antimet., Antimetabolites; M, months; CsA, cyclosporin A

Patients included in the present analysis had to meet the following criteria: (1) diagnosis of SLE as defined by the American Rheumatism Association; (2) participation in a long-term therapeutic trial with one or more kidney biopsies; and (3) informed consent with regard to kidney biopsies.

Table 2. Mortality and loss of kidney function rate in 246 SLE patients (groups A and B according to Table 1)

	Mortality (% per annum)	Loss of kidney function (% per annum)
Group A (173 patients)	0.44	0.27
Group B (73 patients)	0.58	0.39

Table 3. Cause of death in patients from groups A and B (according to Table 1)

Group A:	Myocardial infarction	2
	Post-surgery septicaemia (trans-vaginal hysterectomy)	1
	Tuberculosis-meningitis	1
	Cerebral SLE (Cachexia)	1
Group B:	Cerebral aneurism	1
	Septicaemia	1
	Encephalomeningitis	1

Patients with a creatinine value exceeding 1.4 mg/100 ml were excluded. However, once the creatinine level dropped to below 1.3 mg, they entered the study. In 4 out of 5 patients, an initially high creatinine level could be reduced with a pulse therapy including dexamethasone (DXM) + Cy as in the case of a 20-year-old female shown in Fig. 1. At the first consultation, this patient presented with a most severe nephrotic syndrome and a creatinine level of over 3 mg/100 ml. During the first 10 days, she received 6×40 mg dexamethasone boli and large doses of furosemide. CsA was only given when the creatinine level reached 1.2 mg/100 ml.

Prior to entry into the study, for a period of 4.6 ± 2.7 years all 73 patients had received a treatment with high-dose steroids plus antimetabolites (MTX and azathioprine) with unsatisfactory results (proteinuria above 2 g/l, persistence of disease

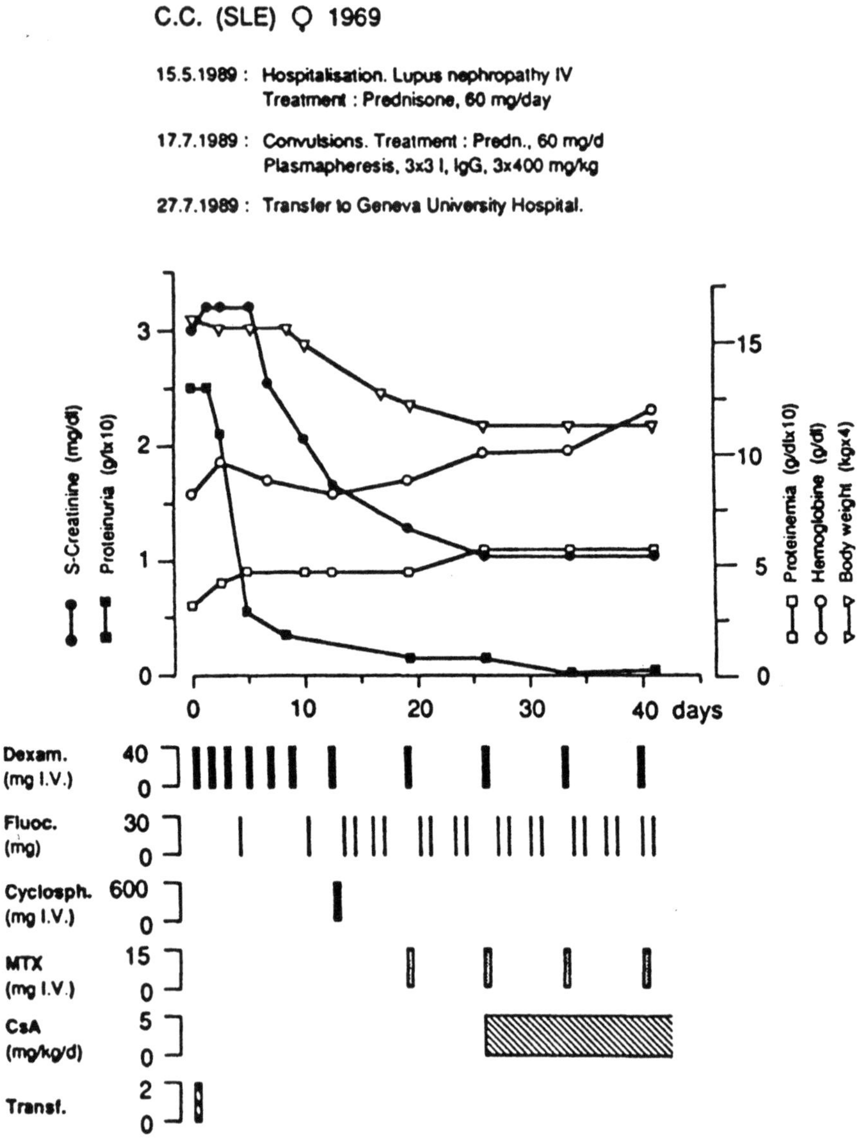

Fig. 1. Response to drug combination therapy of patient C.C. Dexan, dexamethasone; Fluoc, fluocortolone; Cy, cyclophosphamide; MTX, methotrexate; CsA, cyclosporin; Transf, transfusion

activity under treatment, unacceptable side effects). Antimetabolites were replaced by CsA at a dose of 5 mg/kg l.b.w. per day, 6 days/week. Steroid medication was adjusted to the disease activity and given only 5 days/week to limit steroid-induced side effects [1]. The short-acting steroids fluocortolone and cloprednol were used since these preparations produce the least Cushingoid features and do not cause water retention. If the result of the steroid/CsA therapy was unsatisfactory after 2 months, with a disease activity score of more than 7/24, MTX was added at a rate of one injection of 15 mg/week, 4 weeks out of 6 (24 patients). In 30 patients, even after the addition of MTX, disease activity remained above the index of 7/24. For these patients, i.v. Cy pulses were added during the MTX-free weeks at a dose of 500 mg every 6 weeks until the index dropped to 7/24.

Cell separation and culture

Peripheral blood lymphocytes (PBL) from venous blood were prepared by Ficoll-Hypaque density gradient centrifugation. T cells were obtained as the cells forming rosettes with SRBC as described [8]. All cell cultures were performed at 37°C, 5% CO_2 in RPMI 1640 medium supplemented with 10% heat-inactivated, non-mitogenic FCS, 2 mM L-glutamic acid, 25 mM HEPES buffer, 100 U/ml penicillin, and 100 μg/ml streptomycin (all reagents from Gibco Europe, Switzerland).

Assay for IgG secretion

Duplicate cultures of 1 ml were set up with 10^6 PBL in 24-well plates. After 9 days, the culture supernatants were collected and the IgG levels were quantitated by an ELISA as described [7].

Assay for interleukin-2 secretion

Triplicate cultures of 200 μl were set up with 10^5 PBL in 96-well flat-bottom microplates in the presence of 5 μg/ml PHA and 10 ng/ml PMA (Sigma Chemical Co., St. Louis, Mo.). After 30 h, the culture supernatants were collected and stored at −20°C until the assay for IL-2 activity. The IL-2 biological activity was determined by CTLL proliferation assay [5].

Assays for IL-2 and IL-2 receptor in serum

The serum IL-2 concentration was measured by a commercial ELISA (Intertest 2; Genzyme Corp., Boston, Mass.). We confirmed that in the case of fresh recombinant IL-2, 1 ELISA unit (U) corresponds to about 0.8 to 1.2 U defined by the CTLL assay. Serum IL-2 receptor (R) was also measured by a commercial ELISA (Cell-free IL-2R test kit; T Cell Sciences, Cambridge, Mass.) [15].

Serum anti-double-stranded (ds) DNA antibodies were quantitated by a modified Farr assay as described [10]. Complement activity was determined by the method of Perrin et al. [14]. The lymphocyte activity score represents the logarithm of the ratio of spontaneous IgG secretion (ng/μl)/IL-2 secretion (U/μl) [13].

Renal survey

Renal survey consisted of measuring serum creatinine and 24-h proteinuria. After 4.6 ± 1.4 years on the protocol, all patients had a complete renal evaluation, including renal function tests using EDTA ^{51}Cr and Hippuran ^{125}I with a single-shot technique

[3] and renal biopsy tissue examination. In the sub-group of patients exhibiting severe SLE nephropathy, renal evaluation was done 2 and 5 years after initiation of CsA medication. One kidney biopsy was performed in 69 patients; a second biopsy in 24 patients, and a third in 7 patients. Two patients refused the biopsy; two others were on continuous anticoagulation because of a severe antiphospholipid antibody syndrome and, therefore, could not undergo biopsy.

Results

Clinical data

All 73 patients were followed from the beginning to the end-point (1 May 1994) of this study. In 19 patients the disease was well controlled with the steroid/CsA combination. In 24 patients, MTX injections were necessary for disease control. In 30 patients, quadruple drug therapy was necessary, using steroids, CsA, MTX and Cy. Conditions for the addition of Cy were as follows: (1) insufficient control of kidney parameters in 20 patients (creatinine $>$ 1.4 mg/100 ml, proteinuria above 3 g/l); (2) pericarditis in 5 patients; and (3) uncontrollable fever plus arthritis in 5 patients.

Three patients died: a 50-year-old female from acute meningoencephalitis, and a second 50-year-old female, with severe anti-phospholipid syndrome and class III lupus nephropathy, from septicaemia. The latter patient had very deep ulcers on her legs which penetrated as far as the periosteum. Furthermore, she did not comply with the discontinuous steroid schedule and took 20 mg/day of fluocortolone, a treatment which certainly increased the risk of septicaemia. The third deceased patient was a 26-year-old female with class Va nephropathy. She repeatedly contracted β-haemolytic type A streptococci infections from her fiancé. During a period of well-being, she suddenly succumbed to an acute sub-arachnoid haemorrhage caused by rupture of a congenital or mycotic aneurysm.

Two patients lost their kidney function. The first was a 26-year-old female suffering from class IV lupus nephritis with minimal extrarenal symptoms. Despite our recommendation that MTX and Cy be added to the steroid/CsA treatment, her local nephrologist under-estimated the gravity of her condition and continued with the original treatment until the kidney damage became irreparable, leading to end-stage kidney. The second patient, a 34-year-old female with class IV nephropathy, was doing very well on the steroid/CsA regimen. However, she had an aversion to the oily CsA solution and, without informing us, stopped taking it. Three months later, she developed a rapidly progressive kidney failure which could not be arrested, even with massive intervention (plasmapheresis, steroid boli, Cy boli). Six months later, she underwent kidney transplantation and is again doing very well on a combined low-dose steroid (80 mg/week given on 5 days)/CsA/MTX regimen.

During the 7-year observation period, 6 patients with a class III or IV lupus nephritis showed a slow increase in serum creatinine levels to a maximum of 2.5 mg/100 ml, with no concomitant rise in antibody titres to dsDNA and with normal levels of C3/C4 complement component levels in 3 patients. We applied the following protocol to these 6 patients: (1) discontinuation of CsA medication when creatinine exceeded 1.4 mg/100 ml; (2) addition of i.v. methylprednisolone injections at a rate of 125 mg twice per week; and (3) i.v. Cy (400 mg), alternating weekly with i.v. MTX (10 mg).

As soon as the creatinine level fell to < 1.4 mg/100 ml, CsA was resumed at a dose of 3.5 mg/kg l.b.w. per day, 5 days/week. It should be mentioned that the gradual rise in creatinine did not reflect CsA toxicity. In fact, when we stopped CsA medication in two patients, creatinine rose at a faster rate, only returning to normal levels when i.v. injections of methylprednisolone + Cy + MTX were administered. In all 6 patients, CsA medication could be resumed at a dose of 3.5 mg/kg l.b.w. per day, 5 days/week.

Of the 70 surviving patients, 66 live a normal life (in business, studying, or as housewives). During the observation period, 7 patients in remission had successful pregnancies under the following medication: fluocortolone, 10 mg every day except Thursday and Sunday; CsA, 4.5 mg/kg l.b.w. per day on an alternate-week schedule with azathioprine 100 mg/day; aspiria (ASA) 100 mg/day. In one of the 7 patients, several i.v. injections of 125 mg methylprednisolone were necessary in the last 3 months of pregnancy because of a platelet number below 20 000/mm^3. Two patients can be considered as invalid because of severe depression; a third patient is invalid because of deep vein thrombosis; one patient is on haemodialysis. None of the 70 surviving patients suffers from Cushing-type steroid side reactions. Two patients previously on daily steroid medication developed a mild form of aseptic necrosis of the femur head.

During the observation period, 12 patients had severe relapses. In 10 patients, full recovery was obtained; 2 patients lost their kidney function (see Table 4). Table 5 summarises the overall results in terms of activity index, serum creatinine and prednisone equivalent requirements (fluocortolone, 1:1; cloprednol, 10 mg corresponds to 15 mg of prednisone).

Table 4. Relapses during 7-year observation period

No. of patients	Cause	Complication	Recovery	Loss of kidney function
6	Non-compliance	NS with increase in creatinine	4	2
3	Sun exposure	NS, pericarditis NS; rise in creat: 1.6 mg/100 ml NS, rise in creat: 2.5 mg/200 ml	3	0
2	Influenza	Rise in creat: 2.0 mg/100 ml NS, rise in creat: 2.85 mg/100 ml	2	0
1	Psychological trauma	Lymph node + skin involvement with rise in anti-dsDNA	1	0

NS, Nephrotic syndrome; creat: serum creatinine; ds, double-stranded

Table 5. Activity index, serum creatinine and prednisone-equivalence requirement before CsA medication (A) and at the end of the observation period (B)

Activity index score (0–24)		Creatinine (mg/100 ml)		Prednisone equivalence (mg/week)	
A	B	A	B	A	B
10.13 ± 3.4	2.65 ± 0.9	1.01 ± 0.43	0.98 ± 0.2	192.8 ± 118.9	45.8 ± 19.1

All data are mean values

At the end of the study, 60 patients had a creatinine level below 1.19 mg/100 ml, 10 patients had a higher creatinine level but still below 1.9 mg/100 ml (Table 6). Table 7 summarises the drug requirements during and at the end of the study. In 29 patients,

Table 6. Serum creatinine levels at the end of the observation period

Creatinine (mg/100 ml)	No. of patients
< 1.19	60
1.2–1.39	5
1.4–1.59	4
1.6–1.8	1

Table 7. Number of patients requiring drugs during and at the end of the observation period

Drug requirement	During observation period	At end of observation period
No drugs	0	1 (1.4%)
St + CsA	19 (26%)	35 (50%)
St + CsA + MTX	24 (32.9%)	31 (44.3%)
St + CsA + MTX + Cy	30 (41.1%)	3 (4.3%)

St, Steroids; MTX, methotrexate; Cy, cyclophosphamide

CsA was finally given only every 2nd week, 6 out of 7 days, at a dose of 4 mg/kg l.b.w. The only patient receiving no treatment had a type V nephropathy. Initially she did not tolerate CsA at a dose of 5 mg/kg l.b.w. per day because of a rise in serum creatinine to above 1.5 mg/100 ml. After 2 months of treatment with only 3 mg/kg l.b.w., she tolerated 4.5 mg/kg per day , 6/7 days.

CsA-induced side effects

Mild hypertrichosis occurred in 63 patients, mostly during the first 6 months. Two patients suffered from gingival hyperplasia. This complication was reduced to a minimum by prophylactic massage of the gingiva after each meal. Blood pressure was controlled with diuretics given singly or in combination with inhibitors of the angiotensin converting enzyme, or with calcium antagonists (nifedipine). Since CsA leads to water retention, diuretics were given first preference. Blood pressure was monitored with the aim of keeping the diastolic pressure below 90 mmHg. Four patients complained of mild gastrointestinal (GI) symptoms (in addition to the 3 patients who did not tolerate CsA because of GI symptoms).

The overall side effects of the treatment were minimal in most cases. At the end of the study, no patient exhibited Cushing-type symptoms and signs. i.v. Cy pulses frequently produced slight nausea. For this reason, we started to protect patients with a prior injection of 3 mg of granisetrol. Mild hyperacidity in two-thirds of the patients required the use of gastro-protective measures (H2 receptor antagonists or the local gastroprotective compound, sucralfate).

Lymphocyte function studies

Table 8 summarises the results of the studies on lymphocyte function. The increased levels of serum IL-2 and IL-2R indicate in vivo T cell activation. The difference between serum levels of IL-2 and IL-2R in blood donors and SLE patients is highly significant (P = 0.0005 for IL-2, 0.0001 for IL-2R). The difference between the respective values before and after CsA-drug combination therapy is also significant (P = 0.001 for IL-2, P = 0.005 for IL-2R). The diminished lectin-induced IL-2 secretion is probably also the consequence of in vivo activation of the T cells, since the IL-2 secretion defect of CD4 cells is reversible in vitro [7, 8], and since a similar secretion defect is inducible in vivo by vaccine immunisation [9]. The increased spontaneous IgG secretion reflects the well-known polyclonal B cell activation of SLE. The difference between the IgG production by PBMC from blood donors and from SLE patients with active disease is statistically significant with a P value of 0.0001. The diminution of spontaneous IgG production between the beginning and the end of the study is also significant (P = 0.003), as is the diminution of the antibody titre to dsDNA (P = 0.004). The lymphocyte activity score, which measures the overall T and B cell activity, correlates well with the standard activity score with a correlation coefficient of 0.723, r^2 of 0.522, resulting in a P value of 0.0001 (Fig. 2).

Table 8. Effect of a combined drug therapy on T cell-IL-2 and B cell activity in SLE

	Normal control blod donors	SLE patients after CsA drug combination therapy		
		Before CsA	6 months–1 year	2–5 years
Serum IL-2 (IU/ml)	3.5 ± 3.3[a](12)	19 ± 18(18)	6.3 ± 2.9(16)	5.3 ± 1.4(4)
Serum IL-2R (U/ml)	878.3 ± 289.8(23)	3245 ± 8823(17)	–	1221 ± 437.4(27)
IL-2 secretion (U/ml) (response to PHA + PMA)	396.5 ± 159(20)	15 ± 36.2(42)	70.8 ± 95.8(38)	213.4 ± 144.3(41)
Spontaneous IgG secretion (mg/ml)	450 ± 260(12)	3448 ± 1798(34)	2332 ± 2029(39)	700.5 ± 425(34)
Anti-dsDNA antibodies (binding activity)	1.5 ± 2.3(20)	17.2 ± 19.1(73)	12.5 ± 18.4(20)	6.4 ± 11.7(70)
Lymphocyte activity score	0.88 ± 0.60(20)	3.5 ± 0.94(41)	2.5 ± 0.97(42)	0.82 ± 0.77(42)
Clinical activity score	0	10.1 ± 3.4(73)		2.65 ± 0.9(70)

IL, interleukin; PHA, phytohemagglutinin; PMA, phorbol 12-myristate 13-acetate
[a] Arithmetic mean ±1 SD, number of cases in parentheses

Renal evaluation

Patients were first divided into four classes according to the histological classification of renal lesions proposed by WHO. Of the patients 28% met the criteria of class I or II lupus nephropathy, 27% belonged to class III, 25% had characteristics of class IV and 20% those of class V. In a second step, the patients were separated into two groups (Table 9). Group 1 consisted of patients with class I or II lupus nephropathy who differed from patients of the other classes because of highly statistically significant lower histological activity and chronicity indices. These patients also had a lower standard activity score and better renal function. Patients from WHO classes III, IV and V were grouped together since they presented a similar chronicity index as well as identical standard activity scores and glomerular filtration rate (GFR).

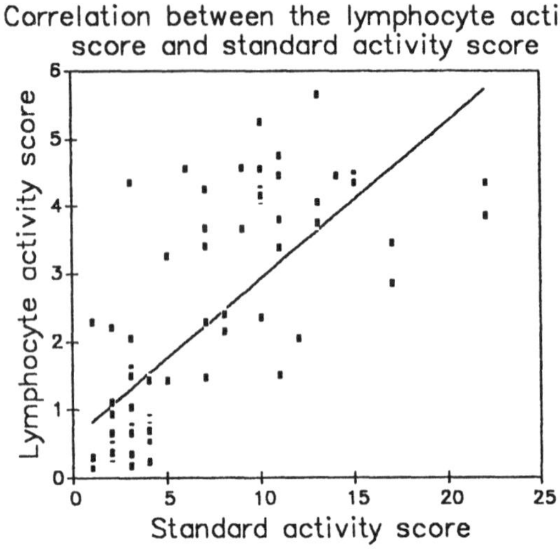

Fig. 2. Correlation between standard activity score and lymphocyte activity score

However, it has to be noted that patients belonging to class IV had a significantly higher histological activity index than patients from classes III and V. Altogether, after 4.7 years of CsA combined therapy, patients from group 2 had a greater residual lupus activity than those from group 1 (Table 9). The higher standard activity score in group 2 compared to group 1 reflects a need for more therapy in patients with a severe lupus nephropathy. These patients had severer histological damage in terms of activity and chronicity indices as well as of reduced renal function with a mean GFR of 93 ± 22 ml/min. The capacity of this selected CsA combination therapy to control the renal expression of the disease in the long-term is illustrated in Fig. 3. This figure compares standard activity score, GFR and renal plasma flow (RPF) as well as histological features in patients from group 2 after 2 and 5 years of treatment. There are no significant differences in any of these parameters. Among the biological markers of the lupus disease, the hemolytic complement level (CH_{50}), measured before starting the combined CsA treatment, was low in those patients who required three or four drugs, whereas a normal CH_{50} level was observed in patients who finally had been treated with prednisone and CsA alone. Complement level was the only parameter which predicted the severity of the disease and the need for adjunction of cytotoxic agents. Low complement levels were observed only in patients with severe nephropathy which was in agreement with the fact that only 18.5% of the patients in this group had been treated by prednisone and CsA alone. By contrast, 47.4% of patients from group I could be controlled by treatment with these two drugs (Table 10).

Membranous lupus nephropathy is a special category which deserves separate comment. Seven such patients who had been treated by steroids and cytotoxic agents were enrolled in the study. Before entering the protocol and despite important immunosuppressive treatment, all these patients presented a nephrotic range proteinuria and a high standard activity score. They also had low CH_{50} and high levels of ds-DNA. Thus, these patients had a very serious renal disease which contrasts to the accepted opinion that membranous glomerulonephritis is rather a benign lesion. It has to be noted that introduction of CsA in combination with other drugs – steroids

Table 9. Comparison of global evaluation of the disease activity, renal function and renal histology between patients with a minor renal involvement and those with a severe lupus nephropathy after 4.7 years of CsA combined therapy

	Group 1 (minor renal involvement)	Group 2 (severe lupus nephropathy)		
Renal morphology				
WHO class	I–II	III	IV	V
Activity index	2.2 ± 0.4	6.02 ± 0.6	9.5 ± 1.7	6.25 ± 1.1
Chronicity index	1.81 ± 0.5	5.6 ± 0.7	6.3 ± 0.7	5.0 ± 0.6
Global evaluation				
Standard activity score	3.4 ± 1.2		6.2 ± 2.2	
Renal function				
GFR ml/min	110 ± 23		93 ± 22	
RPF ml/min	535 ± 176		466 ± 130	

Values are means ±SD. All values from group 1 differ significantly from those of group 2 (Wilcoxon $P < 0.05$). For the morphological data, activity and chronicity indices from group 1 were significantly lower than those from group 2 (Mann-Whitney $P < 0.001$). In group 2, there was no difference in chronicity indices from classes III, IV and V, whereas the activity score of class IV was higher than that of classes III and V ($P = 0.023$)
GFR, Glomerular filtration rate; RPF, renal plasma flow

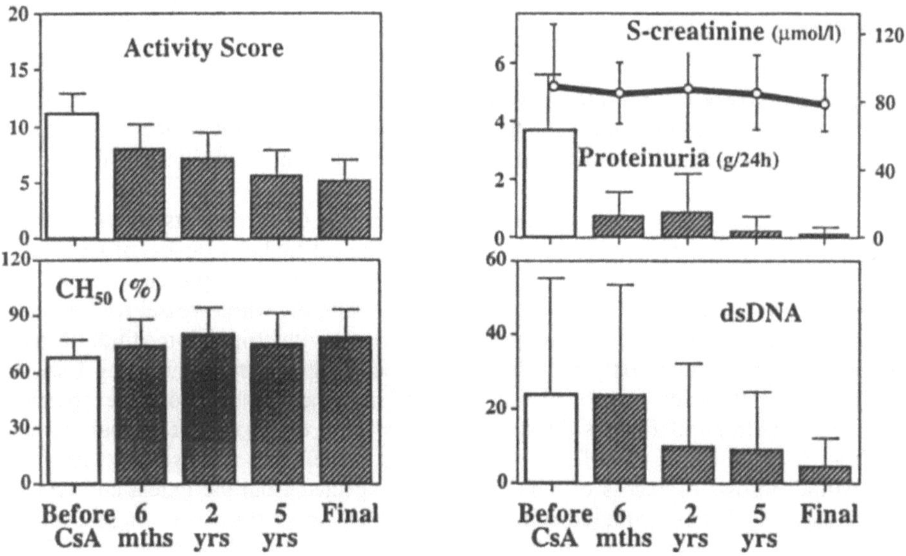

Fig. 3. Comparison of standard activity score, glomerular filtration rate (GFR) and renal plasma flow (RPF), histological activity and chronicity indices, after 2 and 5 years of cyclosporin A (CsA) combined therapy. *Light hatched bar*: 2 years of treatment; *dark hatched bar*: 5 years of treatment. Data are means ±SD

and cytotoxic agents – given as triple or quadruple therapy permitted normalisation of proteinuria by month 6, at a time when dsDNA and CH_{50} had not yet been corrected. Complete normalisation was observed at the final evaluation after more than 5 years of treatment. In those patients who had two renal biopsies, it was interesting to observe that, in most cases, the subepithelial deposits present at the first biopsy

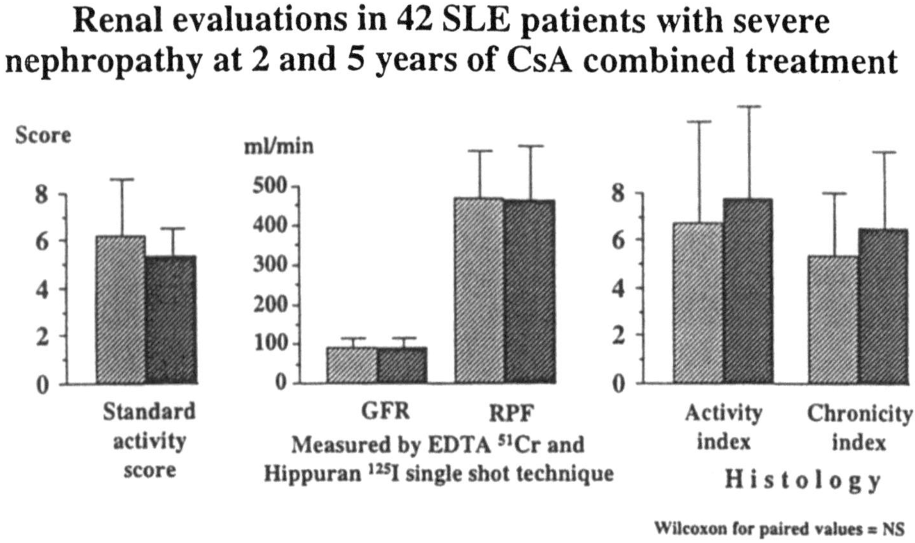

Fig. 4. Evolution of membranous lupus glomerulonephritis on CsA combined treatment. *Open bar*: data before entering the protocol. *Hatched bar*: data at 6 months, 2 and 5 years and final. Data are means ±SD. S-Creatinine, serum creatinine

were progressively incorporated into the basement membrane where they were fully or partially resorbed. Abolition of the proteinuria and digestion of the deposits are exceptional with classic immunotherapy and may represent a specific benefit of CsA (Fig. 4).

Nephrotoxicity is a major concern when CsA is used in patients suffering from diseases which already involve the kidney. Histological findings typical of CsA toxicity were found in 20.5% of the patients. Half of these patients presented with CsA arteriolopathy with proteinaceous depositions involving the whole vessel wall, including the media, while the remaining patients presented with striped interstitial fibrosis. These two lesions were only seen in patients receiving treatment including CsA. In addition, in this series, we found other lesions in equal numbers to those observed in patients with similar lupus disease but treated with cytotoxic agents and steroids without CsA. Thus, 26.1% of our patients in the present series presented with focal interstitial fibrosis in excess of what was to be expected from the extent and type of the glomerular lesions simultaneously present in the same specimen. In 38% of the patients, the lesions were clearly SLE-related. Finally, 7.4% of the patients exhibited normal renal biopsies. It is relevant to note that the incidence of CsA nephrotoxicity was dependent on the type of treatment the patients received. Of the patients treated with steroids and CsA alone 14% had CsA-related renal lesions compared to 23% of those receiving steroids, CsA and MTX and 36% of those receiving steroids, CsA, MTX and Cy. There were no statistically significant differences in GFR, RPF and histological activity index between the patients exhibiting CsA nephrotoxicity and those who did not. However, the histological chronicity index was significantly higher in those patients with histological evidence of CsA nephrotoxicity (with nephrotoxicity versus without nephrotoxicity: 6.9 vs 4.0, $P < 0.001$). However, this difference in chronicity index was not reflected in GFR and/or serum creatinine level which were identical at the final evaluation after a mean period of 7.5 years whether CsA lesions

Table 10. Drug requirements during the observation period

Drug requirements	GN 0-II	GN III-V, TIN
ST + CsA	9 (47.4%)	10 (18.5%)
ST + CsA + MTX	8 (42.1%)	16 (29.6%)
ST + CsA + MTX + Cy	2 (10.5%)	28 (51.9%)

GN, Glomerulonephritis; TIN, tubulointerstitial nephritis

were present or not. It appears that the renal tissue is sensitised to CsA effect by cytotoxic agents as already noted during bone marrow transplantation.

The global renal evaluation clearly shows that CsA when combined with other drugs is able to preserve the renal function over a long period of time in patients suffering from severe SLE nephropathy who are not controlled by a time-limited therapy based on cytotoxic agents and prednisone. CsA is well tolerated and, when present, the renal lesions related to its prescription were most often of grade I, exceptionally of grade II, and never of grade III. In none of the cases were we obliged to stop CsA, and second biopsy or survey of the renal function provided arguments for a non-progression of the lesions. However, it must be emphasised that, at low doses, CsA alone does not control lupus nephropathy as it does, in experimental murine models, at a nephrotoxic range prescription of 17 mg/kg per day. We rely then on polychemotherapy, 18.5% of the patients from group 2 receiving steroids and CsA, 29.6% steroids, CsA and MTX, and 51.9% steroids, CsA, MTX and Cy (Table 10).

General discussion

Although tremendous progress has been achieved in the management of SLE during the past 40 years, morbidity and fatality remain a serious problem for the patient and his physician. Steroids have revolutionised the outcome of SLE, but the price paid in side reactions has been very high, compromising the overall quality of life. Furthermore, steroids alone do not prevent progression of lupus nephropathy.

During the past 15 years, we have tried to improve the management of SLE while keeping side reactions to a minimum. For this purpose, it seemed reasonable to use a drug combination therapy with drugs known to affect disease activity at different levels, and each drug with different side effects, so that the combination should permit an increase in treatment intensity according to the degree of disease activity, without concomitant increase in drug toxicity (Fig. 5).

SLE patients are referred to us when therapy poses a problem. Consequently, we have very few patients with mild SLE and doing well on conventional treatment. In the past, in addition to steroids, we used antimetabolites and Cy for drug combination therapy. With the advent of CsA, the therapeutic potential of drug combination increased, since it acts quite differently on the immune response. To build up the intensity of treatment, we use the following protocol, schematically represented in Fig. 5: A, low-dose steroids for very mild cases; B, steroids + CsA, if treatment A proves insufficient; C, addition of i.v. MTX; D, addition of i.v. Cy. Cy is not given priority in drug combination therapy because of its cumulative toxicity as an alkylating agent.

Today, treatment evaluation requires a long period of time, especially with regard to loss of kidney function. The 73 patients reported here have been under our observation for a mean period of 9.25 years, 7.1 years under CsA medication. This period

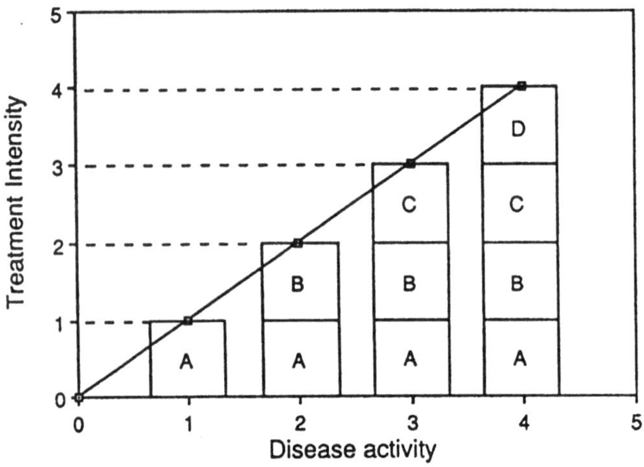

Fig. 5. Principle of drug combination therapy with four drugs, all active as immunosuppressive or immunomodulating agents, yet with different mechanisms of action. *A, B, C, D*: Drugs all known to affect disease activity, each with different side reaction(s)

seems sufficiently long for assessment of the overall validity of this drug combination treatment strategy.

The 73 patients represent a selection from 246 patients whom we followed in the 10-year period 1981–1990. The other 173 patients did well on the steroid-antimetabolite regimen, or required CsA for a period of less than 18 months. The latter group thus represents a milder form of SLE, which is reflected in the slightly lower mortality and loss of kidney function rate (Table 2). Myocardial infarction has become a relevant cause of death with the increasing length of survival of lupus patients (Table 3), a development which warrants ASA prophylaxis in all lupus patients. Mortality has to be compared with that of an age- and sex-matched control population (Table 11). The data for the control population were obtained from the Swiss Federal Statistics Bureau. For all SLE patients of the present series (on long-term CsA medication), mortality is three times as high as for the control population. If patients under 49 years are analysed separately, the ratio is 3.5 (difference not significant). However, this ratio increases to 6 if patients with lupus nephritis type III to V are analysed. This confirms the observation that type III to V nephropathy represents a more serious type of SLE. This fact is also reflected in the treatment requirement, keeping in mind that treatment intensity was set up according to disease activity measured by the standard activity index, and not according to the histology report. Patients with type 0 to II GN required significantly less treatment than patients with type III to V and tubulointerstitital nephritis (Table 10). Kidney toxicity has been relatively mild. Grade I CsA toxicity, exceptionally grade II, was present in only 20.5% of the patients. The combination of CsA with MTX and Cy does slightly increase the nephrotoxicity (14% in patients under CsA-steroid combination, 23% under CsA-steroid-MTX, 36% with all four drugs). However, loss of kidney function is very low in this series. Furthermore, kidney function loss in the two patients was not due to drug toxicity, but to non-compliance with treatment. It thus appears that CsA-drug combination therapy permits preservation of the renal function over a long period of time in patients suffering from severe SLE nephropathy.

Table 11. Mortality of patients during the 7-year CsA medication period. Separate listing of patients under 49 years of age and patients with class III, IV, V, GN or tubulointerstitial nephritis (TIN) (patients at risk)

	Age (yrs)	No. of SLE patients	Mortality % per annum	
			SLE patients	Age- and sex-matched control population
All SLE	14–63	73	0.58	0.19
Patients < 49 years	14–48	51	0.28	0.08
Lupus nephritis III, IV, V and TIN	19–55	54	0.78	0.13

Table 12. Correlation between Δ dsDNA fixation and C4 values (highest levels of anti-dsDNA titres, lowest values of C4, during observation period under CsA medication)

dsDNA	No. of patients	ΔdsDNA fixation	ΔC4
≥ 20	22	38.6 ± 19	29 ± 23
			$P < 0.01$
< 20	44	6.5 ± 4.3	48 ± 25.3

C4 values are expressed as % of a pool of blood donors. dsDNA levels are determined using a modified Farr method (see [10]). Δ dsDNA fixation = DNA fixation of patient serum minus DNA fixation of pooled blood donor serum (normal controls show less than 3% dsDNA fixation). Data are expressed as mean values $\pm$ SD

Table 13. Correlation between C4 values and Δ dsDNA fixation

C4 range	No. of patients	ΔC4 (% C4)	ΔdsDNA fixation (%)
0–10	7	3.9 ± 4.16	35 ± 26
			$P < 0.01$
11–25	10	19.7 ± 3.6	16 ± 10.2

Data are expressed as mean values $\pm$ SD

In the surveillance of SLE patients, much attention is paid to changes in complement serum levels and antibody titres to dsDNA. In statistical terms, there exists a significant correlation between these two parameters (Tables 12, 13). However, this correlation does not always apply to individual cases. Indeed, kidney function would have been lost in six patients with type III and IV nephropathy if treatment had been oriented towards these parameters. In these patients, the creatinine level increased slowly without changes in complement and anti-dsDNA titre. In fact, in three of the patients the complement levels of C3 and C4 were normal, and in two patients no antibodies to dsDNA could be detected at the time of deterioration of the kidney function. In all six patients, creatinine returned to levels below 1.8 mg/100 ml upon moderate intensification of therapy (125 mg methylprednisolone i.v., twice per week, 400 mg Cy i.v. alternating weekly with 10 mg MTX).

Appropriate surveillance certainly adds to the success of treatment and is particularly important in dealing with exacerbations of disease (Table 4). Early intervention is essential to bring the disease process under control again.

For young female patients, the question of pregnancy is important. Of the 73 patients 7 had a successful pregnancy, carefully planned once disease activity had been controlled with a mild pregnancy-compatible treatment (low-dose steroids, CsA and azathioprine, with 100 mg ASA daily, and supplementation with iron and folic acid).

In several patients, we assessed the T and B cell activity in terms of serum levels of IL-2 and IL-2R, as well as by lectin-induced IL-2 production in vitro and spontaneous IgG secretion. The results (Table 8) suggest that active SLE involves in vivo hyperactivation of T cells and a hyperreactive T cell-IL-2 system. Indeed, expression of the genes encoding IL-2Rα and the IL-2 ligand are undetectable in resting T cells, but are efficiently induced upon T cell activation [17]. It has also been shown that soluble IL-2R are released from activated human lymphoid cells including T and B cells in vitro [15]. It thus appears that T cells are engaged in active SLE with the hyperproduction of IL-2 in vivo. The diminished response of these T cells to lectin stimulation in vitro has to be interpreted as the consequence of this T cell activation in vivo, and not as being the consequence of a lupus-predisposing dysfunction of T cells. With regard to the spontaneous IgG production of B cells, the increase reflects the polyclonal B cell hyperstimulation in lupus patients. We have previously shown a negative correlation to the lectin-induced IL-2 secretion [8]. Moreover, there is a significant positive correlation between the serum IL-2 level and B cell IgG secretion. Also, the IL-2 responsiveness of B cells is increased in SLE [8].

In the follow-up of our patients, there is a concomitant trend to normalisation of all activity parameters, i.e. diminution of IL-2 and IL-2R serum levels, normalisation of in vitro lectin-induced IL-2 production, diminution of spontaneous IgG secretion in vitro, and improvement of the combined lymphocyte activity and standard activity scores (Table 8, Fig. 2).

Conclusion

This long-term study on 73 patients with severe SLE has shown that drug combination therapy with steroids, CsA, MTX and Cy permits a control of disease activity and maintenance of kidney function with very few side effects and, to a large extent, allows patients a good quality of life in both professional and personal terms. In particular, it has been possible to drastically reduce steroid medication (Table 5). The mortality rate is now well under 1% per year, but is still three to four times higher than in an age- and sex-matched control population. Further efforts are necessary to improve the management of SLE. The investigation of the cytokine network might lead to the introduction of new agents [6]. There is also hope that CsA analogues, devoid of or with less toxicity, will be developed.

Acknowledgement. This work has been supported by the Geneva Hematology Research Foundation.

References

1. Beris P, Burger A, Favre L, Riondel A, Miescher PA (1986) Adrenocortical responsiveness after discontinuous corticosteroid therapy. Klin Wochenschr 64: 70
2. Esdaile JM (1994) Prognosis in systemic lupus erythematosus. Springer Semin Immunopathol 16: 337
3. Favre H (1973) Détermination des fonctions rénales par la technique de l'injection unique. Analyse statistique de modèle bicompartimental proposé par Sapirstein. J Urol Nephrol 79: 1007

4. Feutren G, Querin S, Tron F, Noel LH, Chatenoud L, Lesavre P, Bach JF (1986) The effects of cyclosporine in patients with systemic lupus. Transplant Proc 18: 643 factor: parameters of production and a quantitative microassay for activity. J Immunol 120: 2027
6. Horwitz DA, Jacob CO (1994) The role of cytokines in the pathogenesis of systemic lupus erythematosus. Springer Semin Immunopathol 16: 181
7. Huang YP, Miescher PA, Zubler RH (1986) The interleukin 2 secretion defect in vitro in systemic lupus erythematosus is reversible in rested cultured T cells. J Immunol 137: 3515
8. Huang YP, Perrin LH, Miescher PA, Zubler RH (1988) Correlation of T and B cell activities in vitro and serum IL-2 levels in systemic lupus erythematosus. J Immunol 141: 827
9. Huang YP, Pechere JC, Michel M, Gauthey L, Loreto M, Curran JA, Michel JP (1992) In vivo T cell activation, in vitro defective IL-2 secretion, and response to influenza vaccination in elderly women. J Immunol 148: 715
10. Izui S, Lambert PH, Miescher PA (1976) Determination of anti-DNA antibodies by a modified 125I-labelled DNA-binding test. Elimination of non-specific binding of DNA to non-immunoglobulin basic proteins by using an anionic detergent. Clin Exp Immunol 26: 423
11. McLaughlin J, Gladman DD, Urowitz MB, Bombardier C, Farewell VT, Cole E (1991) Kidney biopsy in systemic lupus erythematosus. II. Survival analyses according to biopsy results. Arthritis Rheum 34: 1268
12. Miescher PA, Favre H, Chatelanat F, Mihatsch MJ (1987) Combined steroid-cyclosporin treatment of chronic autoimmune diseases. Klin Wochenschr 65: 727
13. Miescher PA, Huang YP, Zubler RH (1988) New approaches to the treatment of RA. Springer Semin Immunopathol 10: 251
14. Perrin LH, Lambert PH, Nydegger U, Miescher PA (1973) Quantitation of C3PA and other complement components in diseases associated with a low C3 level. Clin Immunol Immunopathol 2: 16
15. Rubin LA, Kurman CC, Fritz ME, Biddison WE, Boutin B, Yarchoan R, Nelson DL (1985) Soluble interleukin 2 receptors are released from activated human lymphoid cells in vitro. J Immunol 135: 3172
16. Steinberg AD, Steinberg S (1991) Long-term preservation of renal function in patients with lupus nephritis receiving treatment that includes cyclophosphamide versus those treated with prednisone only. Arthritis Rheum 34: 945
17. Waldmann TA (1993) The IL-2/IL-2 receptor system: a target for rational immune intervention. Immunol Today 14: 264

Central nervous system involvement in systemic lupus erythematosus: a new therapeutic approach with intrathecal dexamethasone and methotrexate

G. Valesini[1], R. Priori[1], A. Francia[2], G. Balestrieri[3], A. Tincani[3], P. Airo[3], R. Cattaneo[3], A. Zambruni[3], B. Troianello[4], M. Chofflon[5], P.A. Miescher[5]

[1]Clinica Medica I, Università "La Sapienza", Viale del Policlinico, I-00161 Rome, Italy
[2] III Clinica Neurologica, Università "La Sapienza", Rome, Italy
[3] Servizio di Immunologia Clinica, Ospedali Civile, Brescia, Italy
[4] I Divisione Neurologia, Ospedali Civile, Brescia, Italy
[5] Hôpital Cantonal Universitaire, Genève, Switzerland

Summary. In systemic lupus erythematosus (SLE), neurological involvement has been reported to occur with frequencies ranging from 14% (severe cases) to 83% (mild forms included). In spite of early diagnosis and aggressive treatment, neuropsychiatric SLE may represent a serious problem of management. We describe three cases, one with acute transverse myelitis, one with hemiparesis, and one with signs of focal and diffuse cerebral dysfunction, in whom improvement following intrathecal therapy with methotrexate and dexamethasone was observed.

Introduction

Central nervous system (CNS) involvement represents a common complication in systemic lupus erythematosus (SLE), occurring in 14–83% of cases [1, 12, 13, 28]. Such involvement includes: non-focal cerebral dysfunction (organic brain disease, psychosis, affective disorders), seizures, focal deficit (strokes, transverse myelitis, cranial neuropathies), peripheral neuropathies, and movement disorders, etc. [19, 24, 29]. Neurological symptoms in SLE may appear during exacerbations of the illness but may also constitute the first manifestation of disease [2, 9, 35, 37].

Diagnosis and therapy of neurological disease represent a challenge in the management of SLE with severe CNS involvement. In these cases, in spite of early diagnosis and aggressive therapy, CNS complications are still associated, in the long term, with a poor prognosis [24, 31, 33].

We describe three women with SLE and severe CNS involvement who improved considerably following intrathecal (IT) therapy with methotrexate (MTX) and dexamethasone (DXM).

Correspondence to: G. Valesini

Case 1

An 18 year-old woman, born in 1967, presenting in Rome with hemolytic anemia, leukopenia, arthritis, Raynaud's phenomenon and both antinuclear antibodies (ANA) and anti-dsDNA antibodies, was diagnosed as having SLE and was treated with oral steroids and occasionally hydroxychloroquine. Six years later, she complained of mild but progressive leg numbness and sphincter disturbance. Despite increase of prednisone medication to 25 mg/day, she developed a flaccid paralysis of her lower extremities, sensory deficit at T7, and sphincter incontinence.

Investigations at admission revealed the following: peripheral white blood cells 1,900/ml, lymphocytes 209/ml, red blood cells 3.7×10^6/ml, Hb 11 g/100 ml, C3 low at 59 mg/100 ml (normal values, nv 70–170), C4 17 mg/100 ml (nv 16–45). ANA (determined by IIF (indirect immunofluorescence) on HEp2 cells) and anti-DNA antibodies (determined by IIF (indirect immunofluorescence) on *Crithidia luciliae*) were both present as well as IgG and IgA anticardiolipin antibodies at a low titer [23].

Magnetic resonance imaging (MRI) of brain and spinal cord did not show any abnormalities except for a discrete cortical atrophy. Lumbar puncture yielded cerebrospinal fluid (CSF) with a white cell count of 2/ml (nv < 5), protein 2.03 g/l (nv < 0.5), glucose 0.44 g/l (nv 0.4–0.7).

Cortisone medication was increased to 80 mg/day of prednisolone, without improvement. On the contrary, general and neurological conditions worsened and, at the beginning of the 5th week from onset of symptoms, the patient became tetraplegic. In this critical situation, 10 mg MTX and 20 mg DXM were administered IT by lumbar infusion. Her neurological status improved dramatically. Within a few days, sensitivity returned, as well as arm and leg movement. Only a mild hyposthenia of the lower extremities and sphincter disturbance persisted. A second bolus of IT MTX and DXM was repeated 2 weeks later. The patient was discharged with no neurological deficit except a mild sphincter incontinence.

There has been no further neurological deterioration after 11 months on mild maintenance therapy (oral steroids +2.5 mg MTX, 3 times per week, 4 weeks out of 6).

Case 2

This female patient, born in 1971, was diagnosed in Brescia as having SLE at the age of 15, when she presented with fever, skin rash, alopecia, lymphadenopathy, splenomegaly, hemorrhage, hypocomplementemia, ANA, high titer anti-dsDNA, anti-Sm, and false-positive VDRL, Veneral Disease Research Laboratory (anticardiolipin antibodies and lupus anticoagulant were absent). Partial remission was obtained with pulse methylprednisolone and cyclophosphamide (Cy). However, in the following years, despite treatment with high-dose oral steroids and immunosuppressive drugs (azathioprine or MTX), SLE continued to be active, as indicated by the persistence of mild fever, arthralgia and positive serology. Moreover, systemic hypertension and thrombophlebitis were observed.

Since the age of 18, she has suffered very frequent (almost daily) episodes of transient neurological deficit (motor aphasia, migrant hyposthenia) lasting a few hours. Six months after the first symptoms, she suddenly developed a short-term memory loss which improved slowly after intravenous (IV) DXM and MTX, followed by pulse Cy (600 mg every 3 weeks). Nevertheless, despite continuous treatment with Cy (reduced to 500 mg every 4 weeks), she also developed mild kidney involvement with 0.5 g/l proteinuria and a creatinine level of 1.5 mg/100 ml. At the age of 19, pulmonary hypertension was noted and therapy with oral anticoagulant was started. Eleven months later, she abruptly presented a right hemiparesis. At that time, she was receiving steroids (fluocortolone 30 mg/day for 5 non-consecutive days per week), Cy 500 mg IV every 4 weeks, nifedipine 60 mg/day, atenolol (100 mg/day), enalapril (20 mg/day), ranitidine (150 mg/day), and oral anticoagulants. No abnormalities were observed on CT scan and MRI of the CNS. EEG showed diffuse slow waves, without signs of lateralization. Examination of the CSF showed 14 white cells/ml (nv < 5) and 1.8 g/l protein (nv < 0.6). Anti-dsDNA was 202 IU (nv < 7), CH50 390 U/ml (nv > 950), C3 38 mg/100 ml and C4 9 mg/100 ml.

On days 2, 3 and 4 after admission, DXM 40 mg IV was administered. Since no benefit was observed, 20 mg DXM and 10 mg MTX were administered IT by lumbar puncture on day 6. This was followed within 24 h by a dramatic improvement of her neurological signs. On day 10, she was given 40 mg DXM plus 400 mg Cy IV. Finally, on day 20, she was given a second IT treatment with 20 mg DXM plus 10 mg MTX. After discharge, the neurological improvement continued during the following months with progressive reduction in the frequency of transient deficit until it completely disappeared.

After 15 months, she is in good condition receiving IV Cy pulses (400 mg) every 6 weeks, and steroids, anticoagulant and antihypertensive drugs as described above.

Case 3

Between 1970 and 1980 this female patient, born in 1946, presented with a variety of allergic reactions (attacks of urticaria, allergic rhinitis with asthmatic attacks). In 1981, she suffered from angioedema-type episodes. At that time, an IgG level of 2,064 mg/100 ml was found. In December 1982, she developed CNS symptoms for the first time with equilibrium problems and loss of memory. An EEG showed slightly abnormal delta waves. In the autumn of 1983, she developed fever with a recurrence of the same CNS symptoms. There was also joint involvement. With positive results for lupus serology, SLE was diagnosed and high-dose steroid treatment initiated. Because of the side effects, the patient discontinued this treatment in July 1984.

The CNS complications gradually worsened. She developed increasingly frequent fever spikes, finally with daily peaks of 39°–40°C. In the following months, her condition gradually deteriorated with loss of equilibrium, development of slurred speech and hallucinations. Furthermore, she had hypoesthesia, mostly of the lower extremities. In March 1985, she came to Geneva for evaluation of her condition. Clinical examination revealed arthralgia of the wrists. There was a slight butterfly rash on the face. Multiple ecchymoses reflected the frequent falls due to lack of equilibrium. Lupus parameters were positive in the peripheral blood (positive LE cell phenomenon; ANA 1:64; anti-dsDNA, Δ 1.6% fixation of ds DNA in a modified Farr test [10]; positive Latex 1: 320; low complement level of C3 and C4, presence of IgG anti-phospholipid antibodies). There was a high level of antibodies to dsDNA in the cerebrospinal fluid (Δ 15.2% fixation). Otherwise the CSF proved normal with 0.36 g/l protein (IgG 41 mg/ml, albumin 191 mg/l); 1 WBC/ml (90% lymphocytes). No oligoclonal bands were found on isoelectric focusing.

With a positive biology for SLE, she was placed on IV pulse treatment with DXM + MTX but with no beneficial effect. On 24 April 1985 she was admitted to hospital in a comatose state. She did not react to acoustic signals nor to painful stimulation. Tendon reflexes were strong with a positive Hoffmann sign on both sides. There was also a positive Babinski sign on the right side. MRI showed no abnormality. An electroencephalogram was characterized by dysrhythmia of the slow and rapid high-amplitude waves. There was an intermittent rhythmic delta activity and a frontal intermittent rhythmic delta activity. When systemic treatment failed, we decided on IT medication with intralumbar administration of 10 mg of MTX + 50 mg of methlyprednisolone.

The result of the IT treatment was dramatic. After less than 48 h, the entire CNS symptomatology subsided. The day following the injection, she complained of moderate cephalia.

The patient was subsequently placed on low-dose steroids, 15 mg fluocortolone 5 days/week + cyclosporin A (CsA) 5 mg/kg per day. She remained in remission for 2 months, when she developed an allergy to the oily solution of CSA, with generalized erythematous skin rash and increased transaminases to an ALAT level of 600 U/l. CSA was replaced by azathioprine. Two months later, there was a sudden recurrence of the CNS symptoms requiring a second IT injection, producing the same positive result. One month later, she has another recurrence but with only mild CNS symptoms. It was decided to start a new trial with the oily CSA solution but this produced the same allergic manifestations as the first time. Subsequently, the disease was characterized by monthly recurrences of the CNS symptoms, each time with a positive response to IT treatment requiring a hospital stay of 4 days.

After the fifth course of IT treatment in December 1985, we decided to replace azathioprine by the lipotropic immunosuppressant, thalidomide, at a dose of 100 mg/day. With this treatment, she remained in remission for over 16 months. She relapsed in April 1987, requiring a further course of IT treatment. Despite continuation of the thalidomide medication, the course of her disease was characterized by increasingly frequent relapses, every 1–2 months. In July 1987, after the 8th course of treatment, we tried CSA in capsule form which was well tolerated (the allergy was thus due to the vehicle and not to the CSA). On a maintenance therapy with a combination of fluocortolone, CSA and thalidomide, the rate of relapses slowed. However, she still required treatment every 2–3 months.

In 1988, methylprednisolone was replaced by DXM (20 mg). Thalidomide was discontinued for 2 years. Relapses still occurred about every 2 months. We finally resumed thalidomide in April 1990, alternating this drug on a weekly basis with CSA. With this regimen, she only relapsed twice in 3 years. All in all, the patient received 20 courses of IT treatment.

Initially, a hysterical behavior was suspected, the same scenario being repeated each time, going from a comatose state to full remission. It should be mentioned that only the initial CSF had a high antibody titer to dsDNA, with negative results in all subsequent episodes. During a further relapse, to test the hypothesis of hysteria, physiological saline was injected at the site of the intra-lumbar puncture instead of the IT DXM/MTX, letting the patient believe it was the normal IT treatment. Her condition did not improve; on the contrary, it deteriorated. 24 h later, she received the proper IT treatment and improved rapidly within 48 h. On three occasions an EEG was performed before and 3 days after the IT treatment. Each time, at the moment of relapse, a diffuse CNS involvement was seen with intermittent rhythmic delta

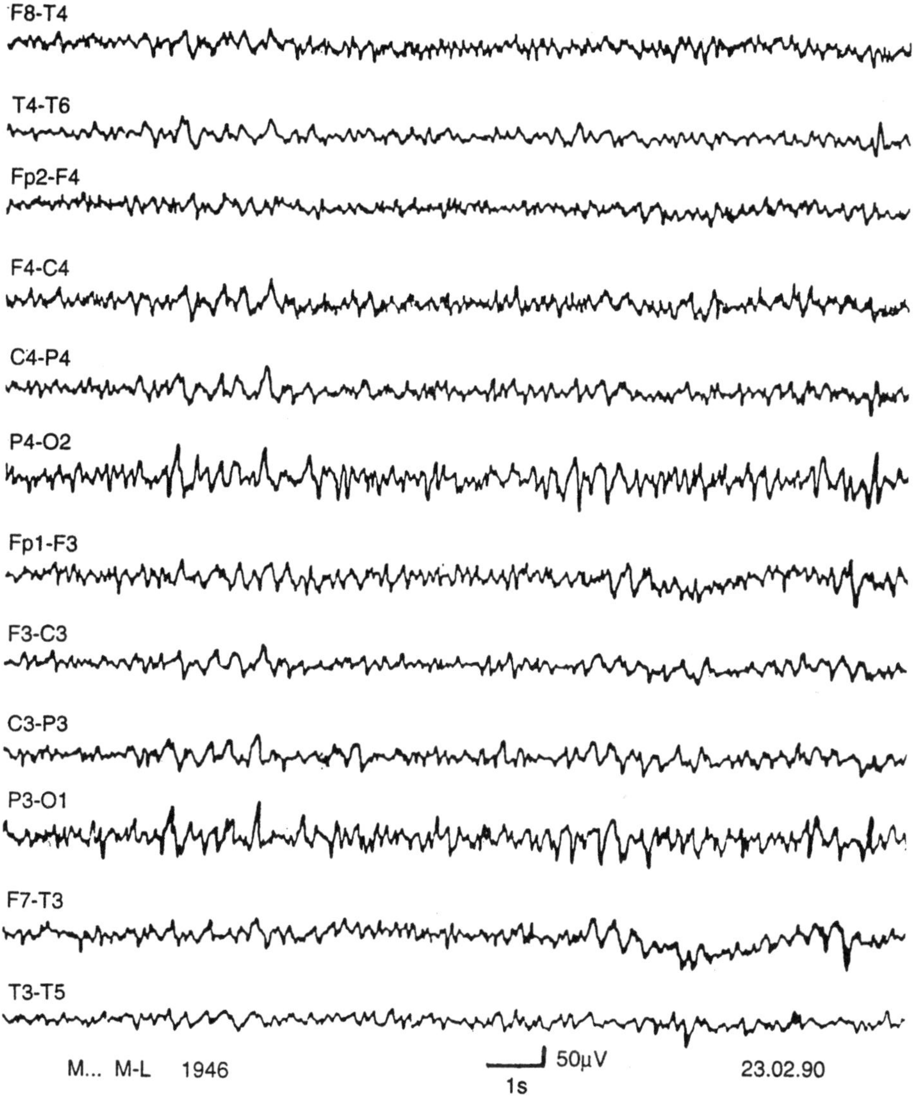

Fig. 1A. On three occasions, an EEG was performed prior to and 3 days after intrathecal therapy. Each time, at the moment of relapse, a diffuse CNS involvement was seen with intermittent rhythmic delta activity and frontal intermitten rhythmic delta activity

activity and frontal intermittent rhythmic delta activity. Each time, the EEG became completely normal 3 days after treatment (see Fig. 1).

This patient is presently doing well on the following maintenance therapy: fluocortolone, 10 mg/day, 5 days/week; CsA, 4 mg/kg per day alternating weekly with thalidomide 100 mg/day.

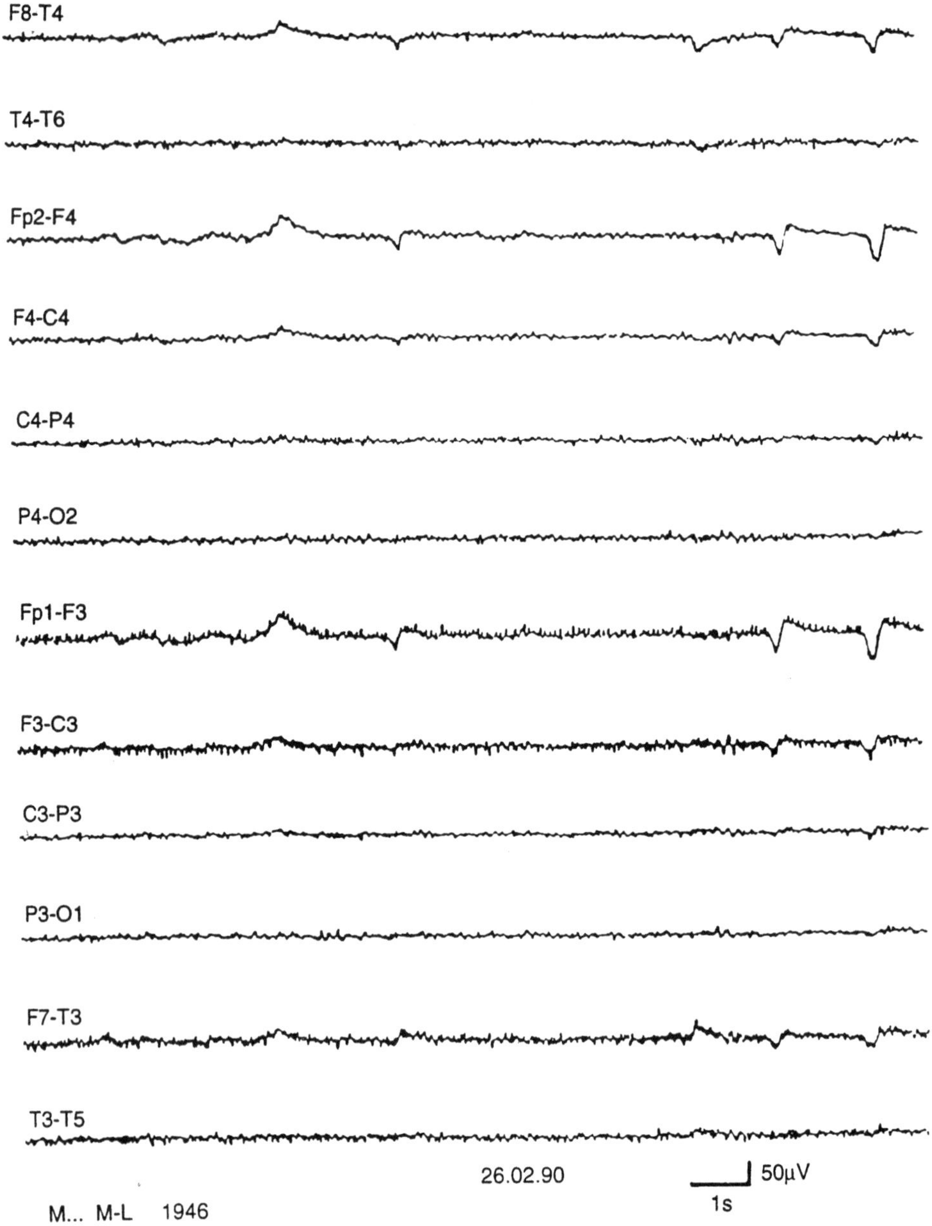

Fig. 1B. Each time, the EEG became completely normal 3 days after treatment

Discussion

Different mechanisms are operational in CNS involvement of SLE, with a wide spectrum of clinical manifestations [20, 34, 36]. Depending on the gravity of the neurological complications, the prognosis becomes poor, despite aggressive therapeutic approaches [15, 16, 24, 31, 33].

Various regimens have been proposed for the treatment of CNS manifestations, including high-dose oral prednisone, bolus IV methylprednisolone, bolus IV Cy plus steroids, and plasmapheresis [2, 14, 24, 30, 32]. In cases with a secondary antiphospholid antibody (aPL) syndrome with cerebrovascular disease, anticoagulants have been used [3, 4].

Among the various types of cerebral lupus, acute transverse myelitis (ATM) is a rare, often devastating, complication of SLE, reported in less than 1–4% of cases [1, 12, 13, 28]. Recently, a close relationship has been shown to exist between ATM, as well as other neurological manifestations, and the presence of aPL [17]. A direct involvement of these antibodies via a thrombotic vascular occlusion, or via direct interaction with spinal cord phospholipids has been suggested [22]. Indeed, it seems unlikely that aPL are secondary to the primary damage (i.e., antigen driven), since other forms of transverse myelitis are not accompanied by such antibodies [25]. However, the pathogenic significance of aPL in SLE remains uncertain. If there is evidence of a thrombotic process, as in the "classical" aPL syndrome, systemic anticoagulation is certainly mandatory.

In the three cases described, there was no evidence of thrombosis within the CNS. In the second case, anticoagulation was given in view of deep vein thrombophlebitis and severe pulmonary hypertension.

Case 1 represents a typical ATM, with no signs of vasculitis on MRI, but with an increase of protein in the CSF and a slight rise in the cell count. The second case is characterized by hemiparesis, again with no objective evidence of vasculitis, but with an increase of protein in the CSF. In such severe forms of cerebral lupus, steroid monotherapy has not proved beneficial [11, 18]. More encouraging results have been published with high-dose steroids associated with IV Cy boli [8, 26, 30, 32, 39], although still with a quite poor long-term prognosis.

Assuming that ATM represents a parenchymal involvement of the CNS, inaccessible to IV medication with Cy and MTX because of the brain-blood barrier, and in view of the resistance to intensive conventional therapy, we applied MTX in association with DXM via the IT route. In this way, high DXM and MTX concentrations in the CNS are obtained, with minimal systemic exposure, thus avoiding general MTX toxicity [6, 27].

In the second case, the clinical expression consisted of transient episodes of motor-aphasia and memory loss which was partially controlled with IV pulses of steroids and Cy. Despite this medication, within a few days the patient became hemiparetic, not responding to IV DXM. Subsequently, she also received IT treatment.

The third patient presents a rare case of parenchymal CNS lupus, totally resistant to aggressive systemic treatment with negative findings upon MRI and in the CSF, but with a pathological EEG. To once more circumvent the brain-blood barrier, IT treatment was given.

In the first two cases, the therapeutic effect was very rapid. In view of the resistance to prior treatment and the chronological relationship between the IT injection and the clinical improvement, a cause and effect relationship seems most probable. In the third case, such a relationship is evidenced by the fact that there was the same result each time the patient relapsed (20 times in 9 years). It is interesting to note that, on 3 occasions, the EEG became normal 3 to 4 days after IT treatment, a further proof of the direct relationship between this therapeutic approach and the clinical response.

MTX has been shown to be a potent immunosuppressive drug both in experimental animal models and in human disease, mostly SLE and rheumatoid arthritis [38]. If administered orally, it only has an immunosuppressant effect. When injected IV or intramuscularly in a dose of 15–20 mg, it exerts a strong anti-inflammatory effect on immunologically induced inflammation, which lasts about 1 week. However, MTX does not penetrate the CNS. Thus, it seems logical to administer this drug IT, as in the treatment of leukemia with CNS involvement. In this latter indication, neurotoxic reactions following MTX-IT injections have been described [7, 21]. With the doses used in our three patients, no signs of delayed toxicity were observed. In case no. 3, the patient usually complained of cephalia for 1–3 days. With regard to the choice of steroids, we gave preference to DXM, a long-acting steroid with very low local toxicity and excellent penetration into the CNS [5].

In conclusion, we propose the use of IT treatment with MTX and DXM for severe CNS lupus, refractory to conventional therapy, particularly in the case of ATM and parenchymal CNS involvement.

References

1. Abel T, Gladman DD, Urowitz MB (1980) Neuropsychiatric lupus. J Rheumatol 7: 325
2. Adelman DC, Saltiel E, Klineberg JR (1986) Neuropsychiatric manifestations of systemic lupus erythematosus: an overview. Semin Arthritis Rheum 15: 185
3. Asherson RA, Mercey D, Phillips G, Sheehan N, Gharavi AE, Harris EN, Hughes GRV (1987) Recurrent stroke and multiinfarct dementia in systemic lupus erythematosus: association with antiphospholipid antibodies. Ann Rheum Dis 46: 605
4. Asherson RA, Khamashta MA, Gil A, Vaquez JJ, Chan O, Baguley E, Hughes GRV (1989) Cerebrovascular disease and antiphospholipid antibodies in systemic lupus erythematosus, lupus-like disease and the primary antiphospholipid antibody syndrome. Am J Med 86: 391
5. Balis FM, Lester CM, Chrousos GP, Heidman RL (1987) Differences in cerebrospinal fluid penetration of corticosteroid: possible relationship to the prevention of meningeal leukemia. J Clin Oncol 5: 5202
6. Blaney SM, Balis FM, Poplak DG (1991) Current pharmacological treatment approaches to central nervous system leukemia. Drugs 41: 702
7. Bleyer WA (1981) Neurologic sequelae of methotrexate and ionizing radiation: a new classification. Cancer Treat Rep 65 [Suppl 1]: 89
8. Boumpas DT, Patronas NJ, Dalakas MR, Hakin CA, Klippel JH, Balow JE (1990)Acute transverse myelitis in systemic lupus erythematosus: magnetic resonance imaging and review of the literature. J Rheumatol 17: 89
9. Brinciotti M, Ferrucci G, Trasatti G, Priori R, Squilloni E, Valesini G (1993) Case report: reflex seizures as initial manifestation of systemic lupus erythematosus in childhood. Lupus 2: 281
10. Creighton WD, Lambert PH, Miescher PA (1973) Detection of antibodies and soluble antigen-antibody complexes by precipitation with polyethylene glycol. J Immunol 111: 1219
11. Dubois EL, Wallace DJ (1987) Clinical and laboratory manifestations of SLE. In: Wallace DJ, Dubois EL (eds) SLE, 3rd edn, Lea and Fabiger, Philadelphia, pp 385–403
12. Ellis SG, Verity MA (1979) Central nervous system involvement in systemic lupus erythematosus. A review of neuropathologic findings in 57 cases, 1955–1977. Semin Arthitis Rheum 8: 212
13. Feinglass EJ, Arnett FC, Dorsch CA, Zizic T, Stevens MB (1976) Neuropsychiatric manifestations in systemic lupus erythematosus: diagnosis, clinical spectrum and the relationship to other features of the disease. Medicine 55: 323
14. Fruchter L, Gauthier B, Marino F (1983) The use of plasmapheresis in a patient with systemic lupus erythematosus and necrotizing cutaneous ulcers. J Rheumatol 10: 341
15. Ginzler EM, Shorn K (1988) Outcome and prognosis in systemic lupus erythematosus. Rheum Dis Clin North Am 14: 67
16. Gladman DD (1991) Prognosis of systemic lupus erythematosus and the factors that affect it. Curr Opin Rheumatol 3: 789

17. Goldstein M, Meyer O, Bourgeois P, Palazzo E, Nicaise P, Labarre C, Kahn MF (1993) Neurological manifestations of systemic lupus erythematosus: role of antiphospholipid antibodies. Clin Exp Rheumatol 11: 373
18. Hachen HJ, Chantraine A (1979) Spinal cord involvement in SLE. Paraplegia 17: 337
19. Hanly JG (1992) Nervous system involvement in systemic lupus erythematosus. Transfus Sci 13: 145
20. Hay EM, Isemberg DA (1993) Autoantibodies in central nervous system lupus. Br J Rheumatol 32: 329
21. Kaplan RS, Wirnik PH (1982) Neurotoxicity of antineoplastic drugs. Semin Oncol 9: 103
22. Lavalle C, Pizzarro S, Drenkard C, Sanchez Guerrero J, Alarcon Segovia D (1990) Transverse myelitis: a manifestation of systemic lupus erythematosus associated with antiphospholipid antibodies. J Rheumatol 17: 34
23. Loizou S, McCrea JD, Rudge AC, Reynolds R, Boyle CC, Harris EN (1985) Measurement of anticardiolipin antibodies by enzyme-linked immunoabsorbent assay (ELISA): standardization and quantitation of results. Clin Exp Immunol 62: 738
24. McCune JW, Golbus J (1988) Neuropsychiatric lupus. Rheum Dis Clin North Am 14: 149
25. Medina Rodriguez F, Garcia E, Frago A (1990) Transverse myelitis and antiphospholipid antibodies. J Rheumatol 17: 1250
26. Misteli LM, Conen D (1991) Acute Transverse myelitis in systemic lupus erythematosus: successful therapy with cyclophosphamide and prednisone. Ter Arkh 63: 77
27. Olsen EA (1991) The pharmacology of methotrexate. J Am Acad Dermatol 25: 306
28. Omdal R, Mellgren SI, Husby G (1988) Clinical neuropsychiatric and neuromuscular manifestations in systemic lupus erythematosus. Scand J Rheumatol 17: 113
29. Priori R, Llitta A, Valesini G (1990) Manifestazioni neurologiche e psichiatriche nel lupus eritematoso sistemico. Folia Allergol Immunol Clin 4: 187
30. Propper DJ, Bucknall RC (1989) Acute transverse myelitis complicating systemic lupus erythematosus. Ann Rheum Dis 48: 512
31. Rosner G, Ginzler EM, Diamond HS et al (1985) A multicenter study of outcome in systemic lupus erythematosus. II. Causes of death. Arthitis Rheum 25: 612
32. Sands ML, Ryczak M, Brown RB (1988) Recurrent aseptic meningitis followed by transverse myelitis as a presentation of systemic lupus erythematosus. J Rheumatol 15: 862
33. Swaak AJG, Nossent JC, Bronsveld W, van Rooyen A, Nieuwenhuys EJ, Theuns L, Smeenk TJT (1989) Systemic lupus erythematosus. I. Outcome and survival: Dutch experience with 110 patients studied prospectively. Ann Rheum Dis 48: 447
34. Teh LS, Hay M, Amos N, Huddy A, Creed F, Bernstein RM, Holt PJL, Williams BD (1993) Anti-P antibodies are associated with psychiatric and focal cerebral disorders in patients with systemic lupus erythematosus. Br J Rheumatol 32: 287
35. Tola MR, Granieri E, Caniatti L, Paolino E, Monetti C, Dovigo L, Scolozzi R, De Bastiani P, Carreras M (1992) Systemic lupus erythematosus presenting with neurological disorders. J Neurol 239: 61
36. van Dam AP (1991) Diagnosis and pathogenesis of CNS lupus. Rheumatol Int 11: 1
37. van der Kaaden AJ, Kamphuis DJ, Nossent JC, Rico RE (1993) Longstanding isolated cerebral systemic lupus erythematosus in an eight year-old Black girl. Clin Neurol Neurosurg 95: 241
38. Wilke WS, Krall PL, Scheetz RJ, Babiak T, Danao T, Mazanec DJ, Segal AM, Clough JD (1991) Methotrexate for systemic lupus erythematosus: a retrospective analysis of 17 unselected cases. Clin Exp Rheumatol 9: 581
39. Zerbini CAF, Fidelix TSA, Rabello GD (1986) Recovery from transverse myelitis of systemic lupus erythematosus with steroid therapy. J Neurol 233: 188

Extracorporeal photochemotherapy for the treatment of lupus erythematosus: preliminary observations

Robert M. Knobler

Division of Special and Environmental Dermatology, Department of Dermatology, University of Vienna General Hospital, Währinger Gürtel 18–20, A-1090 Vienna, Austria

Systemic lupus erythematosus (SLE) is a T cell-mediated disease for which a highly specific therapy is not available [1, 5, 14, 15]; thus, nonspecific immunosuppressive therapy including corticosteroids and/or cytotoxic drugs is repeatedly required to control the disease. As is well known these drugs can lead to limiting side effects and complications [5, 7]. In the past few years extracorporeal photochemotherapy (ECP) of circulating blood leukocytes was described as a new and seemingly effective method of immunomodulation [2, 4, 6, 9, 11, 18, 19, 20]. Under ECP, low-energy ultraviolet A (UVA) irradiation of peripheral blood leukocytes takes place after addition of the photoactivatable drug 8-methoxypsoralen (8-MOP). Subsequent reinfusion of such photomodified leukocytes is considered to initiate a modulation of the immune system. Even though the exact mechanisms underlying the clinical responses reported with ECP have not been unraveled, encouraging clinical effects with ECP have been documented in treating human cutaneous T cell lymphoma [6, 10, 11], pemphigus vulgaris [20], progressive systemic sclerosis [19], AIDS-related complex [4], and cardiac transplant patients in an acute and chronic rejection phase (on-going multicenter clinical trials). As reported [12, 13] an open 2-year clinical trial on ten patients was performed to evaluate the safety, feasibility and efficacy of ECP in the management and treatment of SLE.

Ten patients who satisfied the criteria of the American Rheumatism Association for SLE were entered into a 2-year open clinical trial. For this particular study patients were included if their systemic involvement was not life threatening in the short run and if they had: (1) mild-to-moderate disease activity adequately controlled with conventional treatment, including nonsteroidal anti-inflammatory drugs, low-dose steroids, chloroquin, oral azathioprine and or oral cyclophosphamide; and (2) flare of disease activity upon attempted reduction and/or elimination of these drugs within 3 months prior to inclusion.

Results

Eight of the ten patients completed the trial. In seven of the eight, there was a significant reponse to the treatment, with no or minor and easily controllable side effects such as hypotension. The clinical activity score, which was determined using the SLE activity index scoring system (SIS) as previously described [21], decreased from a median of 7 (range 4–9) to a median of 1 (range 0–5) ($P < 0.05$). The utilized score (SIS) has been validated in other studies and against other indices such as SLAM, SLEDAI, and BILAG [3, 8, 16, 17, 22]. The laboratory abnormalities did not change significantly but were mild at the outset.

Discussion

The reported results demonstrate the feasibility and safety of ECP therapy in the treatment of SLE; they provide encouraging results with respect to clinical improvement, particulary with regard to the arthritic and cutaneous manifestations of SLE. This is the first observation that this form of therapy can be used in patients with known photosensitivity without exacerbating the disease. The efficacy of this therapeutic approach should be studied further in controlled clinical trials before final recommendations can be made.

References

1. Balow JE, Tskokos GC (1984) T and B lymphocyte function in patients with lupus nephritis: correlation with renal pathology. Clin Nephrol 21:93
2. Berger CL, Perez M, Laroche L, Edelson R (1990) Inhibition of autoimmune disease in a murine model of systemic lupus erythematosis induced by exposure to syngeneic photoinactivated lymphocytes. J Invest Dermatol 94:52
3. BILAG: British Isles Lupus Assessment Group (1986) A comparison of disease activity scores in SLE. Br J Rheumatol 25:16
4. Bissacia E, Berger C, Klainer AS (1990) Extracorporeal photopheresis in the treatment of AIDS-related complex: a pilot study. Ann Intern Med 113:270
5. Blaese RM, Grayson J, Steinberg AD (1980) Increased immunoglobulinsecreting cells in the blood of patients with systemic lupus erythematosus. Am J Med 69:345
6. Edelson R, Berger C, Gasparro F, et al (1987) Treatment of cutaneous T cell-lymphoma by extracorporeal photochemotherapy. N Engl J Med 316:297
7. Eisenberg D, Schönfeld Y, Schwartz RS (1987) The importance of the study of monoclonal antibodies. In: Smolen JS, Zielinski CC (eds) Systemic lupus erythematosus, clinical and experimental aspects. Springer Verlag, Berlin Heidelberg New York, pp 88–104
8. French Cooperative Study Group (1985) Activity criteria count. A randomized trial of plasma exchange in severe acute SLE. Plasma Ther Trans Technol 6:535
9. Heald PW, Edelson R (1988) Photopheresis for T cell mediated diseases. Adv Dermatol 3:25
10. Knobler RM (1987) Photopheresis – extracorporeal irradiation of 8-MOP containing blood – a new therapeutic modality. Blut 54:247
11. Knobler RM, Edelson R (1986) Cutaneous T cell lymphoma. Med Clin North Am 70:109
12. Knobler RM, Graninger M, Lindmaier A, Trautinger F (1991) Photopheresis for the treatment of lupus erythematosus. Ann NY Acad Sci 636:340
13. Knobler RM, Graninger W, Graninger W, Lindmaier A, Trautinger F, Smolen JS (1992) Extracorporeal photochemotherapy for the treatment of systemic lupus erythematosus. Arthritis Rheum 35:319
14. Koffler D, Schur P, Kunkel H (1967) Immunohistochemical studies on the nephritis of lupus erythematosus. J Exp Med 126:617

15. Morrow WJ, Younion P, Isenberg DA, Smith ML, (1983) Systemic lupus erythematosus: 25 years of treatment related to immunopathology. Lancet II:206
16. Liang MH, Stern S, Esdaile JM (1988) Towards an operational definition of SLE activity for research. Rheum Dis Clin 14:57
17. Liang MH, Scoher SA, Larson MG, Schur PH (1989) Reliability and validity of six systems for the clinical assessment of disease activity of systemic lupus erythematosus. Arithitis Rheum 32:1107
18. Perez M, Edelson R, Laroche L, Berger C, (1989) Inhibition of antiskin allograft immunity by infusions with syngeneic photoinactivated effector lymphocytes. J Invest Dermatol 92:669
19. Rook AH, Freundlich B, Nahass G, Washko R, Macelis B,Skolnicki M, Bromley P, Witmer WK, Jegasothy BV (1989) Treatment of autoimmune disease with extracorporeal photochemotherapy: progressive systemic sclerosis. Yale J Biolog Med 62:639
20. Rook HL, Jegasothy BV, Heald P, Nahass GT, Ditre C, Witmer WK, Lazarus GS, Edelson R (1990) Extracorporeal photochemotherapy for drug-resistant pemphigus vulgaris. Ann Intern Med 112:303
21. Smolen JS (1987) Clinical and serological features: incidence and diagnostic approach. In: Smolen JS, Zielinski CC (eds) Systemic lupus erythematosus: clinical and experimental aspects. Springer, New York Berlin Heidelberg, pp 170–196
22. Urowitz MB, Gladman DD, Tozman ECS (1984) The lupus activity criteria count LACC. J Rheumatol 11:783

Immunological intervention reveals reciprocal roles for tumor necrosis factor-α and interleukin-10 in rheumatoid arthritis and systemic lupus erythematosus

Ravinder N. Maini, Michael J. Elliott, Peter J. Charles, Marc Feldmann

Kennedy Institute of Rheumatology, 6 Bute Gardens, London W6 7DW, UK and Academic Department of Rheumatology, Charing Cross and Westminster Medical School, London W6 8RP

Introduction

Current concepts of the immunopathogenesis of autoimmune diseases such as rheumatoid arthritis (RA), systemic lupus erythematosus (SLE), and multiple sclerosis (MS) have encouraged anticipation that immunological intervention with biological agents will prove to be beneficial. Since the role of autoimmunity in SLE is more firmly established than in many other disorders, one might have expected this disorder to feature in the vanguard of clinical trials with biological agents. However, there is a surprising paucity of such trials, in contrast to the evolving scene in the treatment of RA and MS. Thus, despite the promise of therapy with anti-HLA class II and anti-CD4 antibodies in experimental models of lupus [1, 30] the toxicity of anti-HLA antibodies in primates has prevented their use in man, and there are only anecdotal accounts of the benefit of anti-CD4 antibodies in SLE patients [20].

There may be many good reasons underlying the relatively slow development of biologicals agents for treatment of SLE. Firstly, treatment with corticosteroids and immunosuppressive agents appears to have made a real impact on the long-term outcome of SLE, in contrast to existing therapies for RA and MS. Secondly, the chronic disability and suffering from RA and MS affect a larger population than severe SLE and, therefore, attracts greater interest from investigators and investment by the pharmaceutical industry, and for less common diseases the cost of long-term clinical trials may, thus, be impossible to recoup. Thirdly, for ethical reasons, it is more difficult to justify withholding established treatment in severe cases of SLE, in which events proceed at a very rapid pace, than it is in RA and MS, in which the failure of therapy can be readily documented over months.

Our experience in exploring the role of cytokines in RA has revealed the power of the pharmacological approach to gain insight into the pathogenesis of disease and to chart novel developments in targeting molecules for therapeutic purposes. Here we discuss how these studies have not only pinpointed tumor necrosis factor-α (TNF-α)

Correspondence to: R.N. Maini

as a critical molecule in RA, but have, quite unexpectedly, given new insights into the role of TNF-α and interleukin-10 in SLE.

The biological and clinical role of TNF-α

As the name implies, interest in TNF-α began at the end of the last century when William Coley noted that bacterial infections sometimes caused hemorrhagic necrosis and regression of tumors and tried to mimic this effect with Coley's toxin [4]. The fact that an endogenously produced protein was responsible for this activity was only discovered more than half a century later. In the 70s and 80s it became apparent that TNF-α was not only the active principle induced by bacterial endotoxins which was responsible for necrosis of tumors, but that it was also responsible for a wide range of biological activities such as fever, cachexia, and septicemic shock.

Early hints that TNF-α may be involved in the pathogenesis of RA arose from observations of its similarity and synergy of action with IL-1 in inducing prostaglandin and collagenase production and promoting degradation of cartilage and bone in vitro [3, 12, 28]. The molecular characterization of TNF-α and its two (p55 and p75) receptors in the past few years has provided powerful probes for their detection, measurement, and assessment of function in health and disease. The realization that naturally occurring specific inhibitors of TNF-α are, in fact, shed (soluble) TNF receptors has further complemented our understanding of a bio-feedback system which operates under physiological conditions [10]. Thus, a biological response initiated by the ligation of its receptors by TNF-α can be terminated by neutralization of the ligand by soluble TNF receptors. These concepts provide a framework for analyzing the role of TNF-α in chronic inflammatory diseases such as RA.

Establishing a role for TNF-α in RA

Our studies in RA began almost 10 years ago by developing systems for studying the production and regulation of cytokines in the rheumatoid joint. These observations soon revealed the complexity of the situation, namely, that many (almost all) cytokines appeared to be locally produced, as judged by the expression of their mRNA in rheumatoid joints. Although most of these cytokines were also detectable at protein level, some were abundant [IL-1α, IL-1β, TNF-α, granulocyte/macrophage colony-stimulating factor (GM-CSF), IL-8, and IL-10] [6, 9, 18, 24], whereas others appeared to be present in relatively small amounts [IL-2, interferon-γ (IFN-γ, IL-4] [8, 26]. Using specific antibodies directed against cytokines, it was possible to visualize the site at which cytokines and their cognate receptors were being expressed in diseased joints, and this gave important insight into the dynamics of the disease process and cellular interactions that were likely to be taking place. Indeed, we observed that TNF-α and the p55 and p75 TNF receptors were present in the lining layer of synovium, in macrophages in deeper cellular aggregates, in vascular endothelium, and in the invasive zone of pannus [13].

However, real progress depended on the recognition that TNF-α was capable of initiating the inflammatory cascade by regulating other pro-inflammatory cytokines, such as IL-1 and subsequently IL-8, and GM-CSF in vitro, (reviewed in [7]). The resulting hypothesis that TNF might be an attractive target for blockade in RA was substantiated by studies on animal models. By early 1992 we had enough confidence on the predictive value of our research to undertake a trial with monoclonal anti-TNF-α antibody in patients [25].

Clinical trials with anti-TNF-α in RA

Our initial experience in an open-label study of 20 long-standing RA patients refractory to treatments with disease-modifying drugs, such as gold, hydroxychloroquine, methotrexate, and salazopyrin, produced encouraging results [14]. These may be summarized as follows:

1. Within days following the infusion of a large dose of a 'chimeric' anti-TNF-α (with the variable domains of mouse anti-TNF-α bioengineered onto a backbone of constant domains of light and heavy chains of human IgG_1) we saw a marked reduction of clinical signs of inflammation, as evidenced by joint swelling, joint tenderness, joint pain, duration of morning stiffness, and ability to perform tasks, as well as a dramatic reduction in C-reactive protein and serum amyloid A protein and a lesser, but still impressive, fall in erythrocyte sedimentation rate.

2. The improvement from baseline was large, and of an order previously seen only with large doses of corticosteroids reminiscent of the seminal observation by Philip Hench of the effect of cortisone in the 1950s [19].

3. The duration of benefit lasted a median of about 12 weeks, with a range of 8–22 weeks, following the initial cycle of infusions which were given over the first fortnight in either two or four boluses, with a constant total dose of 20 mg/kg.

4. In all patients treated, the acute rheumatoid disease activity seemed well controlled only for a finite period, with loss of efficacy of the infusion in all patients, suggesting that the drug was controlling the disease process rather than curing it.

5. The duration of response was at least partly accountable for by the surprisingly long life of the injected antibody in the circulation, with significant amounts being detectable up to 40–50 days following the last injection, thus validating the expectation that chimerizing the murine antibody would be associated with a prolonged persistence of the immunoglobulin in patients. In this initial cycle of therapy, no detectable antiglobulin responses were apparent, suggesting that the intravenously injected antibody was not very immunogenic.

6. In the short period of the clinical trial, at least, it seemed that administration of anti-TNF antibody was well tolerated and not associated with any significant clinical side effects.

Encouraged by these data from the preliminary trial, we proceeded to gain further experience in two further clinical trials. In the first of these, a selected group of patients from the open-label study volunteered for further infusions of the anti-TNF antibody. The protocol demanded that the antibody only be re-injected when disease relapse occurred and, therefore, after the initial infusion, seven patients were able to receive up to three further infusions over a period of many months [15]. This trial clearly demonstrated that each infusion was accompanied by the same level of clinical benefit as was observed with the initial treatment. However, in a proportion of patients, the duration of the response appeared to be diminished compared to the first, although only half the initial dose had been used. This could, in part, be related to the induction of an anti-idiotype antibody response. In a few of the retreated patients, side effects were observed, but none were serious. We concluded from this study that anti-TNF antibodies may be usable in the long-term control of the disease. If our experiments in the collagen-induced arthritis model [29] could be extrapolated to man, prolonged therapy may be associated not only with suppression of inflammation but also with arrest of the erosive disease process.

The performance of a randomized double-blind placebo-controlled trial seemed mandatory to confirm the initial clinical impression and has been undertaken [16]. Seventy-three patients with refractory RA were included in a multi-center trial undertaken in our hospital and in the university hospitals of Erlangen, Vienna, and Leiden. This trial has vindicated our open-label experience and has conclusively shown that anti-TNF-α antibodies reduce disease activity in the short term, and the indications are that control is more rapid in onset, more consistent and more effective than that seen with currently used disease-modifying agents.

TNF-α: evidence for a reciprocal role in RA and SLE

We have previously noted that the concentrations of soluble TNF receptor generated by cells in RA joints are high, but insufficient to neutralize TNF-α and terminate the inflammatory cascade. However, levels of soluble TNF receptor in the blood of RA patients are also higher than in normal individuals and could indirectly reflect the overproduction of TNF-α in joints, which in turn controls the increased production and release of soluble TNF receptors, which overspill into blood. We might speculate from our findings that the high blood levels of soluble TNF receptors in active SLE, which exceed levels observed in RA, similarly reflect increased TNF-α production in diseased tissues [2]. Inaccessibility of tissue samples other than blood in SLE has hindered investigation of this possibility. Studies of animal models have raised paradoxical findings, on the one hand suggesting that a genetically determined TNF-α deficiency (discussed later) predisposes to SLE, and on the other, suggesting that TNF-α potentiates established disease [5].

Unexpected clues about the role of TNF-α in SLE have come from observations on patients with RA who received monoclonal anti-TNF-α antibody in our therapeutic trials. In the open-label trial, we were monitoring rheumatoid factor titers and due to a long-standing interest in anti-nuclear antibodies (ANA) these were also measured While we noted a general trend in reduction of rheumatoid factor even in the 8-week period following the first infusion, we had not anticipated the result we observed in 2 of the 20 patients who developed anti-double-stranded DNA (dsDNA) antibodies as described below.

Case histories

Patient A was a 47-year-old female with a 12-year history of seropositive, nodular, erosive RA. Previous disease-modifying therapy included sulfasalazine, cyclophosphamide, and methotrexate, but at trial entry, anti-rheumatic therapy was limited to paracetamol only. Before treatment, clinical and laboratory assessment confirmed moderately active disease and knee arthropscopy revealed marked synovial hypertrophy, villous change, and hyperemia, with visible pannus extending onto the femoral cartilage surface. Although there was a history of thinning of the hair (while taking methotrexate) and of intermittently decreased peripheral blood lymphocyte counts and

C3 and C4 complement levels, there were no other features to suggest SLE. The tissue type was HLA DR3, 4.

A weakly positive fluorescence ANA test (FANA) prior to commencement of therapy, together with an anti-dsDNA of 4 U/ml (normal range < 7) and anti-cardiolipin of 12 U/ml (normal range < 15) – a serological profile in up to 30% of classical chronic RA. These indices remained unchanged when tested at 4 weeks post-infusion. However, on testing at 6 weeks after treatment, her FANA had become strongly positive and antibodies to both dsDNA and cardiolipin were detected. These peaked at 8 weeks after treatment, then fell before a secondary rise following a further cycle of anti-TNF-α. Associated with the development of these antibodies, total serum IgG rose from a pretreatment level of 13.3 g/l (normal range 5.5–14.5 g/l) to 19.4 g/l, IgM from 2.9–4.0 g/l (normal range 0.5–3.1 g/l) and C4 fell from 0.14 to 0.08 g/l (normal range 0.13–0.43 g/l). Circulating immune complexes containing activated C3 fragments were detected by ELISA concurrent with the appearance of the antibodies. The lupus-associated serological abnormalities reverted to normality in the subsequent 9 months.

Table 1. The induction of lupus serology in two patients with rheumatoid arthritis treated with anti-tumor necrosis factor-α (TNF-α) therapy

	HLA-DR	FANA	Anti-dsDNA (U/ml)	Anti-cardiolipin (U/ml)	IgG (g/l)	IgM (g/l)	C4 (g/l)
Normal		–	< 7	< 15	5.5–14.5	0.5–3.1	0.13–0.43
Patient A	3,4	pre +	4	12	13.3	2.9	0.14
		peak ++++	86	58	19.4	4.0	0.08
Patient B	1,6	pre +	0	< 10	11.5	1.7	0.25
		peak ++++	53	< 10	11.5	2.6	0.16

FANA; fluorescence test for anti-nuclear antigen antibodies; ds, double-stranded; –, negative; +, weak; ++++, strongly positive

Patient B was a 48-year-old female with a 14-year history of seronegative RA without significant extra-articular disease. X-rays of hands and feet showed erosive change. Previous disease-modifying therapy included myocrisin, methotrexate, D-penicillamine, sulfasalazine, auranofin, and azathioprine. At trial entry, anti-rheumatic therapy included low-dose prednisolone, indomethacin, and paracetamol. Before treatment, clinical and laboratory assessment showed moderately active disease and knee arthroscopy showed synovial hypertrophy, with clubbed villi and hyperemia. There were no clinical features to suggest other autoimmune disease. The tissue type was HLA DR 1, 6.

This patient at entry to the trial had a weakly positive FANA prior to treatment without detectable anti-dsDNA or anti-cardiolipin antibodies (0 U/ml and < 10 U/ml respectively). The autoantibodies were unchanged when tested at 2 and 4 weeks, but by 6 weeks following the last cycle of anti-TNF-α she had developed antibodies to dsDNA. The peak level of anti-dsDNA was 53 U/ml, but the anti-cardiolipin remained negative. This patient's total circulating IgG remained steady, but IgM rose from 1.7 to 2.6 g/l, and C4 fell from 0.25 to 0.16 g/l. The anti-dsDNA remained detectable for 6 months following immunotherapy.

The magnitude and duration of beneficial response of these two patients to anti-TNF-α therapy was within the same range observed in the other 18 patients in the open-label trial [14]. The remarkable development of dsDNA antibodies in two treated patients and anticardiolipin antibodies in one of these two was clearly related to the therapy, since levels of these antibodies fell following cessation of therapy, and one patient showed a transitory rise following re-treatment. In neither patient did clinical symptoms of SLE develop, but it is possible that the duration of the raised concentration of anti-DNA antibody was too short for clinical manifestations to become apparent. Evidence of complement activation and the presence of circulating immune complexes further supports the possibility that the immunological abnormalities might have heralded ultimate clinical expression.

The role of TNF-α and IL-10 in SLE

The unexpected transient occurrence of anti-DNA antibodies and other serological abnormalities in 2 out of 20 RA patients (an incidence of 10%) is interesting and merits an explanation in terms of cellular and molecular mechanisms. Leaving aside the possibility of a fortuitous development of SLE in a case of RA, which the rapidity of induction and reversibility of the autoantibodies argue against, we reasoned that the lupus antibodies observed were likely to be related to the deficiency of TNF-α created by neutralization of excess TNF-α present in patients, by the administered anti-TNF-α antibody. A possible explanation lay in experimental studies which have shed an intriguing light on the role that TNF-α deficiency plays in one of the murine models of SLE, the NZB/W F_1 hybrid mouse.

In the NZB/W F_1 mouse a genetic polymorphism of an allele of the TNF-α gene, which lies within the class III region of the MHC complex in the vicinity of C4 and C2 genes, correlates with the production of low levels of TNF-α. A cause and effect relationship between TNF-α deficiency and SLE has been strongly suggested by the retardation of onset and reduced severity of immune complex nephritis in NZB/W mice by the regular administration of TNF-α by systemic injection from birth [22]. These observations could conceivably provide a rational explanation for the development of lupus-associated autoantibodies and serological abnormalities in the two RA patients, in whom depletion of TNF-α would have resulted from administration of anti-TNF-α antibody. It is tempting to speculate that the atypical response of a minority of treated RA patients might be associated with a combined genetic predisposition to SLE and RA. The co-occurrence of HLA DR3 and 4 (the former being linked to SLE) in one of the two patients described is relevant to this concept. An increased frequency of drug-induced disorders including a lupus syndrome following disease modifying drugs in a proportion of RA patients is well documented and has been attributed to underlying genetic factors peculiar to a subpopulation of RA patients [27]. Whether genomic analysis of the RA patients who develop lupus serology would reveal TNF-α polymorphism associated with a low producer phenotype has not been investigated, and if proven would be problematical, since we have argued for a pivotal position for overproduction of TNF-α in all RA patients.

Deficiency of TNF-α by itself does not offer an explanation for the development of autoimmunity and B cell hyperactivity in lupus. Recent published work suggests that anti-IL-10 antibodies injected into NZB/W Fl mice provide disease protection [21]. In this study it was found that regular administration of anti-IL-10 to NZB/W F_1 mice (but not BALB/c mice) decreases anti-DNA antibody production as well as severity of the renal disease, slows onset of proteinuria, and substantially enhances survival (increased from 10% to 80% at 9 months in treated mice). Significantly, anti-IL-10 therapy resulted in increased serum levels of TNF-α. In mice protected by anti-IL-10, the simultaneous injection of neutralizing anti-TNF-α rapidly brought on lupus and they showed a marked increase in mortality, findings which support the concept that TNF-α is protective in this model. The role of IL-10 in disease acceleration was confirmed by the effect of regular injections of recombinant IL-10.

The situation in murine models has a parallel in the results we obtain in RA. In active RA joints we readily detect IL-10 production, predominantly by macrophages, despite the excess production of TNF-α [24]. The addition of anti-IL-10 antibodies to cultured mononuclear cells from RA synovium significantly increased TNF-α production, suggesting that the negative feedback inhibition produced by IL-10 is operational but insufficient to switch off TNF-α production. Conversely, we find that the addition of recombinant IL-10 to RA mononuclear cells from joints lowers TNF-α production. In established collagen II-induced arthritis in DBA/1 mice, IL-10 partially inhibits disease expression (Katsikis et al., unpublished results). Taken together, we interpret our data to signify that the amount of IL-10 produced in RA joints is insufficient to exert its maximal inhibitory effect on TNF-α overproduction. Addition of exogenous IL-10 could, therefore, be beneficial in suppressing rheumatoid inflammation but potentiate lupus. Similarly, while anti-TNF-α ameliorates RA, it may not only induce lupus in genetically susceptible RA patients but could also exacerbate SLE in man by accentuating TNF-α depletion. These findings and our conclusions are summarized in Table 2.

Table 2. The reciprocal response to TNF-α and IL-10 and their respective antibodies in RA (collagen II-induced arthritis) and SLE (or NZB/W lupus)

		Effect in vivo or in vitro		
Disease model	Anti-TNF-α	TNF-α	Anti-IL-10	IL-10
RA	Suppresses inflammation (in vivo)	Pro-inflammatory: regulates IL-1, GM-CSF, IL-8 ... (in vitro)	Augments TNF-α and IL-1: pro-inflammatory (in vitro)	Decreases TNF-α and IL-1: anti-inflammatory (in vitro)
CIA	Suppresses Inflammation and erosions (in vivo)	Accelerates inflammation	Accelerates? (in vivo)	Suppresses disease (in vivo)
SLE	Induced in RA: 5–10% (in vivo)	Not known	Not known	Not known
NZB/W F_1	Accelerates disease in anti-IL-10-treated mice (in vivo)	Replacement protects (in vivo)	Protective (in vivo)	Accelerates (in vivo)

CIA, Collagen induced arthritis; NZB/W F_1, New Zealand Black/White F_1 hybrid mice; GM-CSF, granulocyte/macrophage colony-stimulating factor

Conclusion

In RA (and in collagen-induced arthritis in DBA/l mice) experimental evidence has convincingly demonstrated the therapeutic benefit of anti-TNF-α antibodies, whereas anti-TNF-α also induces lupus-associated DNA antibodies in a minority of presumably genetically susceptible individuals, and accelerates SLE nephritis in NZB/W mice whose disease is suppressed by anti-IL-10. Conversely, TNF-α replacement protects NZB/W F_1 mice from developing SLE, as does anti-IL-10 therapy, by inducing TNF-α. Likewise, IL-10 accelerates lupus and production of DNA antibodies in NZB/W F_1 mice but is partially protective in collagen II-induced arthritis and may ameliorate RA by reducing TNF-α production.

The discussion would be incomplete without reference to the observation that IFN-γ treatment has occasionally induced SLE in RA patients [17]. Paradoxically it has been noted that monoclonal anti-IFN-γ accelerates autoimmunity in NZB/W F_1 mice [23]. These conflicting findings do not allow a firm conclusion on the role of IFN-γ in SLE, but in RA at least, exogenous (excess) IFN-γ appears to occasionally promote the development of SLE. It is likely that the restored lymphocyte response we have observed in RA patients treated with anti-TNF-α is associated with normalization of IFN-γ production [11]. This restoration of IFN-γ production by activated T cells using anti-TNF-α therapy could additionally contribute to the induction of lupus in the patients in our study, although this is difficult to rationalize with current immunological ideas.

In extrapolating these emerging concepts from trials of immunotherapy, we hypothesize inverse roles for the cytokines TNF-α and IL-10 (to which IL-4 could also be theoretically added) in RA and SLE. We would speculate that whereas blockade of TNF-α is beneficial in RA, it may prove harmful in SLE. Similarly, anti-IL-10 antibodies may be a logical therapy in SLE but could be harmful in RA. Exogenous administration of IL-10 (and IL-4), it might be argued, could be beneficial in RA but harmful in SLE. These predictions can initially be tested in animal model systems, but can ultimately only be proven by experimental interventions in man. Such interventions might support our contention that, as far as cytokine pharmacology is concerned, what is good for RA is not necessarily good for SLE.

Acknowledgement. The work of the Kennedy Institute of Rheumatology is funded by the Arthritis and Rheumatism Council of Great Britain.

References

1. Adelman NE, Watling DL, McDevitt HO (1983) Treatment of (NZB×NZW)F_1 disease with anti-I-A monoclonal antibodies. J Exp Med 158:1350
2. Aderka D, Wysenbeek A, Engelmann H, Cope AP, Brennan FM, Molad FY, Hornick V, Levo Y, Maini RN, Feldmann M, Wallach D (1993) Correlation between serum levels of soluble tumor necrosis factor receptor and disease activity in systemic lupus erythematosus. Arthritis Rheum 36:1111
3. Bertolini DR, Newdin GE, Bringmann TS, Smith DD, Mundy GR (1988) Stimulation of bone resorption and inhibition of bone formation in vitro by human tumor necrosis factor. Nature 319: 516
4. Beutler B, Cerami A (1989) The biology of cachectin/TNF – A primary mediator of the host response. Annu Rev Immunol 7:625–655
5. Brennan DC, Yui MA, Wuthrich RP, Kelley VE (1989) Tumor necrosis factor and IL-1 in New Zealand black/white mice: enhanced gene expression and acceleration of renal injury. J Immunol 143: 3470

6. Brennan FM, Zachariae CO, Chantry D, Larsen CG, Turner M, Maini RN, Matsushima K, Feldmann M (1990) Detection of interleukin-8 biological activity in synovial fluids from patients with rheumatoid arthritis and production of interleukin-8 mRNA by isolated synovial cells. Eur J Immunol 20:2141
7. Brennan FM, Maini RN, Feldmann M (1992) TNF-α: a pivotal role in rheumatoid arthritis?. Br J Rheumatol 31:293
8. Buchan G, Barrett K, Fujita T, Taniguchi T, Maini RN, Feldmann M (1988) Detection of activated T cell products in the rheumatoid joint using cDNA probes to Interleukin-2 (IL-2) receptor and IFN-γ. Clin Exp Immunol 71:295
9. Buchan G, Barrett K, Turner M, Chantry D, Maini RN, Feldmann M (1988) Interleukin-1 and tumor necrosis factor mRNA expression in rheumatoid arthritis: prolonged production of IL-1 alpha. Clin Exp Immunol 73:449
10. Cope A, Aderka D, Doherty M, Engelmann H, Gibbons D, Jones Ac, Brennan FM, Maini RN, Wallach D, Feldmann M (1992) Increased levels of soluble tumor necrosis factor (TNF) receptors in the sera and synovial fluids of patients with rheumatic diseases. Arthritis Rheum 35:1160
11. Cope AP, Londei M, Chu NR, Cohen SBA, Elliott MJ, Brennan FM, Maini RN, Feldmann M (1994) Chronic exposure to tumor necrosis factor (TNF) in vitro impairs the activation of T cells through the T cell receptor/CD3 complex; reversal in vivo by anti-TNF antibodies in patients with rheumatoid arthritis. J Clin Invest 94:749
12. Dayer J-M, Beutler B, Cerami A (1985) Cachectin/tumor necrosis factor stimulates collagenase and prostaglandin E2 production by human synovial cellls and dermal fibroblasts. J Exp Med 162: 2163
13. Deleuran BW, Chu CQ, Field M, Brennan FM, Mitchell T, Feldmann M, Maini RN (1992) Localization of tumour necrosis factor receptors in the synovial tissue and cartilage/pannus junction in rheumatoid arthritis: implication for local actions of TNF-α. Arthritis Rheum 35:1170
14. Elliott MJ, Maini RN, Feldmann M, Long-Fox A, Charles P, Katsikis P, Brennan FM, Walker J, Bijl H, Ghrayeb J, Woody J (1993) Treatment of rheumatoid arthritis with chimeric monoclonal antibodies to tumor necrosis factor α. Arthritis Rheum 36:1681
15. Elliott MJ, Maini RN, Feldmann M, Long-Fox A, Bijl H, Woody JN (1994) Repeated therapy with a monoclonal antibody to tumor necrosis factor α in patients with rheumatoid arthritis. Lancet 344:1125
16. Elliott MJ, Maini RN, Feldmann M, Kalden JR, Antoni C, Smolen JS, Leeb B, Breedveld FC, Macfarlane JD, Bijl H, Woody JN (1994)Treatment with a chimæric monoclonal antibody to tumor necrosis factorα suppresses disease activity in rheumatoid arthritis. Lancet 344:1105
17. Graninger WB, Hassfeld W, Pesau BB, Machold KP, Zielinski C, Smolen JS (1991) Induction of systemic lupus erythematosus by interferon-γ in a patient with rheumatoid arthritis. J Rheumatol 18:1621
18. Haworth C, Brennan FM, Chantry D, Turner M, Maini RN, Feldmann M (1991) Expression of granulocyte-macrophage colony-stimulating factor in rheumatoid arthritis: regulation by tumor necrosis factor-α. Eur J Immunol 21:2575
19. Hench PS, Kendall EC, Slocomb CH, Polley HF (1949) Effect of a hormone of the adrenal cortex and of pituitary adrenocorticotropic hormone on rheumatoid arthritis. Mayo Clin Proc 24:181
20. Hiepe F, Volk H-D, Apostoloff E, Baehr Rv (1991) Treatment of severe systemic lupus erythematosus with anti-CD4 monoclonal antibody. Lancet 338:1529
21. Ishida H, Muchamuel T, Sakaguchi S, Andrade S, Menon S, Howard M (1994) Continuous administration of anti-interleukin 10 antibodies delays onset of autoimmunity in NZB/W F_1 mice. J Exp Med 179:305
22. Jacob CH, McDevitt HO (1988) Tumor necrosis factor-a in murine autoimmune lupus nephritis.Nature 331:356
23. Jacob CO, van der Meide PH, McDevitt HO (1987) In vivo treatment of (NZB$\times$NZW)F_1 lupus-like nephritis with monoclonal antibody to γ interferon. J Exp Med 166:798
24. Katsikis P, Chu CQ, Brennan FM, Maini RN, Feldmann M (1993) Immunoregulatory role of interleukin-10 (IL-10) in rheumatoid arthritis. J Exp Med 179: 1517
25. Maini RN, Brennan FM, Williams R, Chu CQ, Cope AP, Gibbons D, Elliott, Feldmann M (1993) TNF-α in rheumatoid arthritis and prospects of anti-TNF therapy. Clin Exp Rheumatol 11: S173
26. Moissec P, Naviliat M, D'angeac AD, Sany J, Banchereau J (1990) Low levels of interleukin 4 and high levels of transforming growth factor β in rheumatoid synovium. Arthritis Rheum 33:1180
27. Panayi GS, Wooley P, Batchelor JR (1978) Genetic basis of rheumatic disease: HLA antigens, disease manifestations and toxic reactions to drugs. Br Med J 2:1326

28. Saklatava J (1986) Tumour necrosis factor α stimulates resorption and inhibits synthesis of proteoglycan in cartilage. Nature 322:547
29. Williams RO, Feldmann M, Maini RN (1992) Anti-tumor necrosis factor ameliorates joint disease in murine collagen-induced arthritis. Proc Natl Acad Sci USA 89:9784
30. Wofsy D, Carteron NL (1990) CD4 antibody therapy in systemic lupus erythematosus. Semin Immunol 2:419

Prognosis in systemic lupus erythematosus

John M. Esdaile

Divisions of Rheumatology and Clinical Epidemiology, and the Centre for the Analysis of Cost-Effective Care, Department of Medicine, Montreal General Hospital and McGill University, Montreal, Canada

Introduction

Knowledge about prognosis assists physicians in informing patients about possible outcomes and in determining treatment. New subsets of patients with distinct prognoses that merit further evaluation or special therapy can be identified. Fortunately, the prognosis for an individual with newly diagnosed systemic lupus erythematosus (SLE) has improved markedly over the past several decades [34, 66, 77]. With the extent that new treatment regimens have been developed or will be developed in the future, the predictive markers of the past may not be the predictive markers of today or tomorrow.

Sound evaluation of prognosis requires long-term studies of inception cohorts. These studies require teams of physicians to devote years to meticulous data collection with the knowledge that a major advance in treatment may render much of the information collected obsolete. Thus, studies of prognosis are costly but not glamorous.

Because single center studies may not provide large enough groups of patients, multi-center evaluations are needed. Multi-center studies create additional problems for accurate data collection. Studies of specific therapy are an excellent basis for studies of prognosis. The studies by the National Institutes of Health and the Lupus Nephritis Collaborative Study Group are two recent examples of therapeutic studies that have provided valuable data on prognosis. Much of the debate about choosing the appropriate therapy for an individual patient might be resolved if better information on prognosis was available.

The present review will focus on selected topics and work that has been reported recently.

Correspondence to: J.M. Esdaile, 1650 Cedar Avenue, Montreal, Quebec, Canada H3G 1A4

Prognosis for what?

A host of questions concerning prognosis might be asked by a patient with SLE. Among them are: Will I be able to finish school? Will I have a normal social life? Will I be able to have children? Will my children develop SLE? Will I have the energy to bring up my children? Will I be able to keep working. What will having SLE cost in financial terms? Will I develop kidney or brain involvement? Will I require dialysis? Will I die? Answers to only a few of these questions are available in sufficient detail to satisfy patients and physicians. Not surprisingly, the predictive markers may vary depending on the specific outcome or question.

Death in general. Most studies of prognosis have evaluated death as the outcome. In this respect the improvement in the prognosis for patients with SLE has been dramatic. Three decades ago the majority of patients were dead within 4 or 5 years. Currently, the 5-year and 10-year patient survival rates exceed 90% and 85%, respectively.

Renal involvement is the major predictor of overall fatality [27, 66, 71, 76]. Neuropsychiatric involvement [27, 34, 67, 76], hypertension [67, 68], mouth ulcers [71, 76], thrombocytopenia [66, 67, 71], anemia [27, 67, 71] and hypocomplementemia [71] are lesser predictors of an increased likelihood of death. The prognostic importance of certain sociodemographic markers are discussed in detail below.

Vascular morbidity and mortality. While active SLE and infection remain important correlates of fatality, morbidity and fatality due to vascular disease have become notable outcomes in a number of studies. Vascular thrombosis and vasculopathy can affect the coronary, cerebral and peripheral vascular systems, sometimes in a catastrophic manner. This is unexpected given that most SLE patients are young women who would normally be expected to be protected from such events.

Proposed risk factors for vascular disease in SLE have included circulating immune complexes, antiphospholipid antibodies, lupus anticoagulants, corticosteroids, and nephrotic syndrome. Also, the conventional risk factors such as age, sex, smoking, hypertension, hypercholesterolemia, left ventricular hypertrophy, and diabetes mellitus, some of which may be aggravated by the SLE process or by its treatment, are relevant [2, 26, 28, 34, 50, 63, 64, 68, 75].

Coronary artery disease is the most common cause of hospitalization after active SLE [60]. Overall, the risk of coronary disease is increased ninefold in SLE [34]. Coronary disease has been associated with age [28, 64], disease duration [34, 64, 68], diabetes [28], hyperlipidemia [28, 64], hypertension [28, 64], and treatment with corticosteroids [75]. In the only multivariate evaluation, Petri et al. [64] reported a statistical model for coronary disease in SLE that included as significant risk factors, age at diagnosis, duration of prednisone use, requirement for antihypertensive treatment, maximum cholesterol level and obesity.

Peripheral vascular disease occurs in approximiately 2% of SLE patients. Risk factors include longer duration of SLE and longer treatment with prednisone [50]. Stroke has been reported in 3–20% of SLE patients [20, 23, 72]. While both lupus anticoagulants and antiphospholipid antibodies have been linked to vascular disease in SLE in many studies, the association may be especially important for cerebrovascular disease, particularly transient ischemic attacks and stroke [32].

As survival in SLE improves because of better therapy, vascular disease will play an increasingly important role in determining outcome. The importance of cumulative lupus activity, antiphospholipid antibodies and lupus anticoagulants, treatment with corticosteroids, co-morbid disease, and conventional risk factors, have been suggested as being important. The present decade will see increased attention to this topic.

Pregnancy. This subject is reviewed in detail elsewhere in this issue [47].

Costs. There has been little attention to the financial costs of SLE. A recent study in Canada reported that the average annual cost for health care (direct costs) for patients with SLE followed at one center in 1990 was $6,023 Canadian dollars [10]. The best predictors of the health care costs were serum creatinine and a poorer level of physical function. This attests to the importance of renal involvement for this outcome. It suggests that direct costs arise from organic complications which induce physical disability.

Although only 44% of the patients were fully employed, indirect costs (wages foregone due to illness and charges for housekeeping services) were on average $7,071 per year. Had the costs due to premature death been included in the estimate of the indirect costs, the mean cost would have increased from $7,071 to $15,169 per year. The best predictors of the indirect costs included a lower level of well-being, a combination of education and employment status, and a weaker level of social support. These effects are potentially amenable to psychological or social interventions [9, 10].

A study of a lupus cohort from the United States has reported, average health care costs of $6,634 per year (US dollars) [21]. Predictors of the direct costs included black race, female sex, and the presence of hypertension. This study found that both disease activity and damage indices predicted direct health care costs. The Canadian study reported that a damage index was a significant predictor of both direct and indirect costs [40].

Major prognostic subsets

Sociodemographic markers

The markers age, sex, race and socioeconomic status have attracted considerable recent attention. In general, interpretation of these factors as predictive markers is confounded by inter-relationships between the variables. For example, men tend to be older and blacks tend to be of lower socioeconomic status. Also, these variables are sometimes surrogates for different frequencies of major organ system involvement, in which case it is likely that the prognostic importance of the sociodemographic marker is determined partially by the underlying organ involvement.

Age. Patients under the age of 20 years may have a poorer prognosis than older patients (generally those over age 50 or 60) [66, 84, 91]. Younger patients have a higher frequency of malar rash [33, 84], renal involvement [33, 66, 91], seizures [66, 84], vasculitis [33], proteinuria [66, 84], thrombocytopenia [84], elevated DNA antibodies [84, 91], and hypocomplementemia [84, 91]. Many of these variables are independent markers of a poorer outcome.

Older patients have a greater frequency of rheumatoid factor seropositivity and subcutaneous nodules [91]. A number of studies [35], but not all [79], have found a negative association of the presence of rheumatoid factor and the severity of lupus arthritis with the development of lupus nephritis. If some older patients are protected against developing lupus nephritis, this would improve the prognosis for the group as a whole.

Both younger and older lupus patients may have a greater risk of dying than those between age 20 to 50 years [67]. The younger group die from severe SLE and the older group from co-morbid disease.

Sex. Men with SLE have been reported to have a poorer prognosis than women in some [38, 66, 76, 85], but not all studies [53, 67, 74]. Men appear to be more likely to develop nephritis [34, 38, 66, 85]. Thrombocytopenia [38] and seizures [85] may also be more common in men. Others have found no clinically important associations of sex with specific clinical manifestations [22, 33]. Overall, the sex of the patient does not appear to be a powerful predictor of outcome in SLE.

Race and socioeconomic status. The importance of race (particularly black race) and socioeconomic status as prognostic factors in SLE have been evaluated most extensively in the United States. A major review of this topic has recently been published [46]. Black race is closely associated with low socioeconomic status, and both are linked to poor outcomes in almost all studies [33, 46, 62, 67, 83]. The close association of race and socioeconomic status in individual patients makes it difficult to disentangle the separate effects of these factors on outcome. Furthermore. while socioeconomic status seems a conceptually simple concept it is difficult to quantify. Studies have used formal education, income, occupation, and source of medical funding as proxy variables for socioeconomic status. Nonetheless, the majority of studies have demonstrated that once socioeconomic status (assessed by these surrogate measures) is taken into account in the analysis, the link of black race to poor outcome is no longer statistically significant [46]. Confirmation of this comes from a study of SLE patients followed in a large private rheumatology practice. The patients were mainly middle class and few received social assistance. Blacks, hispanics and whites had similar outcomes [66].

The mechanisms by which low socioeconomic status influences outcome are unclear. Limited access to quality health care, lack of educational programs that enhance understanding of SLE, non-adherence to medical regimens, and lack of self-confidence and social support, are all likely important [46, 62].

While socioeconomic status is clearly a major explanation for the prognostic impact of black race, there remains the belief that blacks with SLE have an earlier disease onset and more severe disease manifestations [46]. When age, sex and socioeconomic status are accounted for, proteinuria, and in selected subgroups, psychosis, serositis and urinary cellular casts, are more common in blacks [83]. Thus, race may have some impact on outcome because of distinct organ involvement.

A study of US death certificates noted a significantly higher mortality rate from SLE for Asian Americans (Chinese, Japanese, and Filipinos) than for whites [37]. This could arise from a higher incidence of SLE, from a more severe disease with a higher case fatality rate, or a combination of both. Other studies have suggested that Asian Americans have a more severe disease, with a higher frequency of renal involvement [66] and more severe renal involvement [43].

Limited disease

The focus of most reports on the prognosis of SLE is adverse outcomes. Markers for good outcomes are rare. Limited forms of the disease, which are in fact not truly SLE, are important to identify.

Pre-lupus. A not uncommon cause for consultation is the patient with selected features of SLE, but insufficient manifestations to be labelled as definite SLE. Frequently, these persons have only one or two of the American College of Rheumatology (ACR) criteria for SLE. The condition has been referred to as "pre-lupus", "latent lupus", "incipient lupus", or "incomplete lupus" [25, 59]. The features tend to be the more nonspecific ones such as photosensitivity, mucosal ulcers, serositis, Raynaud's phenomenon, cytopenia, and positive antinuclear antigen (ANA) tests. The more pathognomonic findings such as malar rash, renal or neuropsychiatric involvement, and an elevated DNA binding are uncommon. The minority evolve into SLE over 5 years. Markers for those that will develop SLE have unfortunately not been identified. Nonetheless, the short-term prognosis for these individuals is excellent [25, 59].

Discoid lupus. Cutaneous lupus erythematosus, particularly discoid lupus, exists with mild systemic features and serological abnormalities, but without definite SLE, sufficiently frequently to justify close attention. In discoid lupus, arthritis or arthralgia, and a positive ANA each occur in one half of patients; and, photosensitivity, malar rash, alopecia, leukopenia, antiphospholipid antibodies, and a high sedimentation rate each occur in one quarter to one third. Organ-threatening disease is rare. Only 5–8% evolve to SLE, and those that do, usually do so within the first 2 years after diagnosis [82].

Subacute cutaneous lupus erythematosus. Recently a new subset of cutaneous lupus has been recognized. Subacute cutaneous LE occurs in 5–10% of SLE cases. Rarely, it occurs in patients with Sjogren's syndrome or rheumatoid arthrittis, or is provoked by drugs such as hydrochlorthiazide. Almost all patients with subacute cutaneous LE initially have papulosquamous lesions that promptly evolve into psoriasiform or annular lesions. The absence of follicular plugging, adherent scale, and skin atrophy helps distinguish subacute cutaneous LE from discoid lupus.

In subacute cutaneous LE, photosensitivity occurs in three quarters, anti-Ro antibodies and elevated sedimentation rates in one half, mucous membrane lesions in one third, and reduced complement levels and leukopenia each in one fifth. Antibodies to Sm are rare, but anti-dsDNA antibodies are detected in 10–20%. Approximately one half meet the ACR criteria for SLE and it is among these patients that renal and neuropsychiatric involvement are noted. Unfortunately, predictors for which patients will develop severe SLE manifestations have not been identified [73].

Both discoid lupus and subacute cutaneous LE have a good prognosis overall. This has implications for therapy. Most patients respond to topical corticosteroids or antimalarials [73, 82].

Lupus nephritis

The prognosis for lupus nephritis has attracted considerable recent study. Studies have evaluated clinical and biopsy markers for both short-term and long-term outcomes. Renal involvement in SLE is the major marker for a potentially poor outcome (Fig. 1). A recent study of patients that had largely been treated with immunosuppressive drugs noted patient survival at 5, 10, and 20 years of 84%, 72% and 52%, respectively [18].

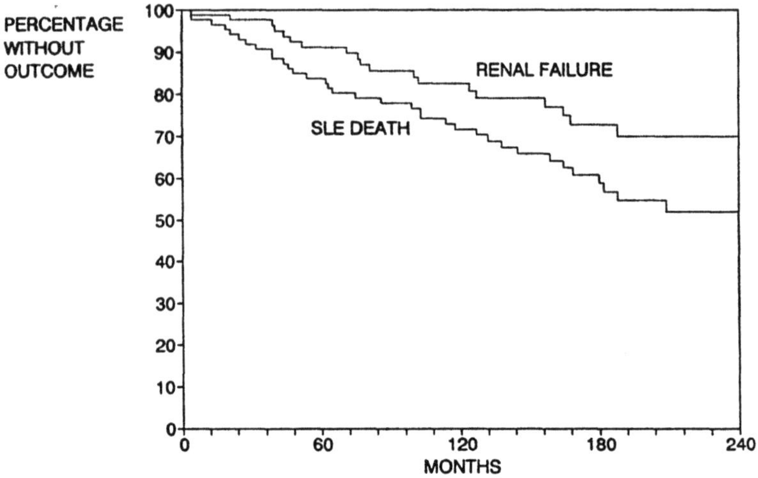

OUTCOME	NUMBER OF PATIENTS AT RISK				
RENAL FAILURE	87	69	48	29	8
SLE DEATH	87	72	54	31	8

Fig. 1. Life-table of lupus nephritis patients (n = 87) who do not develop renal failure requiring dialysis or renal transplantation over a 20-year observation period following first renal biopsy. A separate curve depicts overall survival. The patients are described further in [18]

Long-term prognosis

Clinical predictors. The single most consistent baseline (usually pre-therapy) predictor for long-term outcome has been serum creatinine (Fig. 2). Patients with an abnormal serum creatinine are more likely to develop renal failure or die than those with normal values [3, 12–14, 18, 31, 42, 44, 48, 49, 55]. Serum creatinine is a powerful predictor, likely because it is a marker of irreversible damage. However, it is important to note that serum creatinine and creatinine clearance can remain within the normal range even though there is ongoing loss of renal function [61].

Marked proteinuria has been identified as a marker of progressive renal disease in some studies [1, 3, 18]. Marked proteinuria probably reflects the activity of the nephritis more than serum creatinine. In a similar fashion, immunological activity, as assessed by low levels of serum complement or elevated anti-dsDNA levels, as well as thrombocytopenia, have been noted in some studies to predict end-stage renal disease. The lack of consistent results for these variables as predictive markers may reflect the ability of conventional therapy to alter the level of the test in many patients.

Several studies have noted that younger persons (generally those $<$ 23 years) have a greater likelihood of developing renal failure, although their risk of death is not increased [3, 14, 41]. Whether this results from more severe disease, delayed detection, lower compliance with therapy, or from the need for a better knowledge about management in younger persons, is unknown.

A number of studies suggest that men with nephritis are more likely to develop renal failure than are women [3, 12, 14, 85].

Non-renal clinical markers. Markers such as serum creatinine or other laboratory tests at presentation are linked to the disease process and thereby to the prognosis of lupus nephritis. Modification of the outcome requires treatment of the underlying

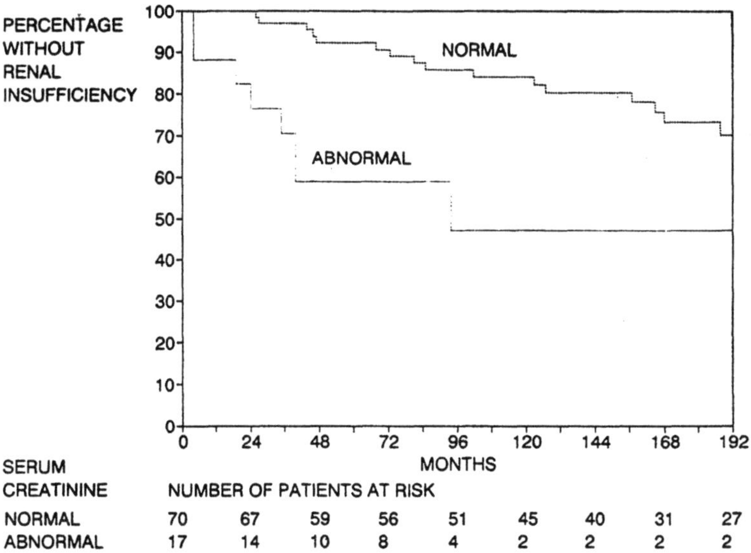

Fig. 2. Life-table of lupus nephritis patients (n = 87) based on the presence of a normal serum creatinine (< 1.5 mgl/100 ml) versus an abnormal creatinine ($P < 0.05$). The outcome is renal insufficiency defined as a serum creatinine persistently greater than 5 mg/100 ml. Additional information on the patients is provided in [18]

nephritis. Other prognostic markers, such as age and sex, are not modifiable. Recently, a number of studies have identified factors that are less directly linked to the nephritis and are potentially modifiable. These include hypertension, other co-morbid diseases, cholesterol, and smoking.

Hypertension can occur in the absence of advanced renal disease and may occur early in the course of lupus nephritis [7]. A number of studies have linked it to a poor prognosis [13, 14, 31, 44, 49, 58, 80, 87]. Hypertension that does not respond to treatment may be a more useful marker than hypertension at presentation [49, 80]. Co-morbid diseases, principally cardiovascular diseases, have also been associated with death [14, 18] (Fig. 3).

Smoking has been linked to end-stage renal disease [87]. Smoking reduced the time to renal failure to almost 50% of that of non-smokers. The effect of smoking was independent of hypertension. While direct evidence is lacking that control of significantly elevated blood pressure or smoking cessation is of benefit in lupus nephritis, the value of these interventions in the general population is well recognized, and justifies their use in SLE.

Hypercholesterolemia has been associated with an increased risk of death.

Reduction of elevated levels of serum cholesterol has been linked to an improvement in survival [80]. The role of hypercholesterolemia as a marker of poor outcome requires further evaluation.

Response to therapy. The preliminary response of an individual patient's disease to a treatment is a predictor of longer-term responsiveness that is commonly used by experienced clinicians. A number of recent studies have evaluated this marker. Levey et al. [44] studied patients with severe nephritis who were participating in a clinical trial. Patients with an abnormal serum creatinine whose test returned to normal within

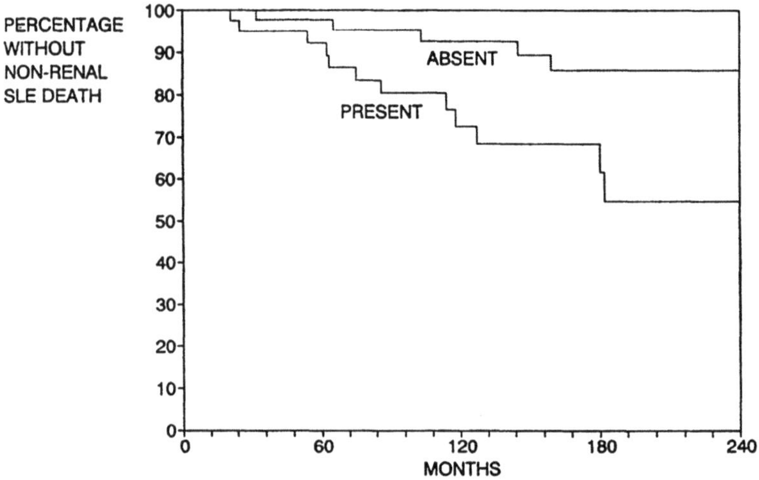

COMORBIDITY	NUMBER OF PATIENTS AT RISK				
ABSENT	44	40	36	21	5
PRESENT	43	32	18	10	3

Fig. 3. Life-table depiction of lupus nephritis patients (n = 87) based on the level of co-morbid disease ($P < 0.05$). Level 0 = absence of co-morbid disease, and levels 1 or 2 = presence of definite co-morbid disease. The outcome is death not attributable to renal involvement (n = 17). Of the 43 patients with a co-morbid disease, 36 (84%) had hypertension, coronary aftery disease or peripheral vascular disease. The patients are described further [18]. Reprinted with permission of Arthritis and Rheumatism

48 weeks of initiating therapy had a much lower likelihood of subsequent renal failure than those whose test remained abnormal. Among patients with less severe nephritis than those studied by Levey, improvement in 24-h urinary protein excretion by 1 year [24] or over the course of the disease [1, 80], or normalization of urinary sediment [80] or serum complement [41], have been associated with better preservation of renal function and improved patient survival.

Short-term prognosis

A small number of studies have evaluated the short-term (from 9 months to 2 years) prognosis of lupus nephritis in general [15, 89], diffuse proliferative lupus nephritis [48], and severe proliferative lupus nephritis [36]. The findings are not dissimilar to the findings for the long-term prognosis, but are perhaps more consistent.

With the exception of the study of severe nephritis, an abnormal serum creatinine was a universal predictor of poorer renal function [15, 48, 89]; increasing age, higher urinary protein excretion, lower serum albumin, hypertension, and co-morbid diseases (principally hypertension, cardiovascular disease, and diabetes mellitus) also predicted poorer renal status [15, 89]. It is not certain whether tests of immunological activity, such as serum complement and anti-dsDNA antibodies, predict short-term outcome.

Renal biopsy

There has been controversy over the role and timing of a renal biopsy in patients with lupus nephritis. A number of studies found that renal biopsy did not add new predictive information over and above that provided by clinical predictors such as serum creatinine and proteinuria (reviewed in [14]). However, in the main these studies considered the World Health Organiztion (WHO) classification of renal biopsy and not the newer classification systems discussed below.

The vast majority of studies that have evaluated the prognostic importance of renal biopsy have done so for long-term outcomes.

WHO classification. The WHO class (Table 1) was *the* biopsy marker two decades ago. However, it is a less consistent predictor today, probably because improved therapy has made proliferative nephritis (class III or IV) a less ominous finding. Nonetheless, proliferative lesions, especially diffuse lesions, continue to bode a poor prognosis even in recent studies [3, 6, 12, 31, 41, 42, 49, 52]. Focal segmental lesions in which more than 50% of the glomeruli are involved carry a prognosis similar to that of diffuse lesions, while lesser involvement carries a better prognosis [70]. The WHO class is also useful in identifying patients with disease confined to the mesangium as this group has a good prognosis.

Table 1. World Health Organization classification of patterns of renal injury in lupus nephritis

Class I	Normal
Class II	Mesangial nephritis
Class III	Focal and segmental proliferative nephritis
Class IV	Diffuse proliferative nephritis
Class V	Membranous nephritis

Activity and chronicity indices. The WHO classification omits information that is intuitively of value in assessing a renal biopsy for prognosis. The WHO class does not assess the activity of the inflammation, the extent of chronic irreversible changes in the glomerulus, or the extent of disease in the vessels and tubulointerstitial region. It cannot assess change over time in these aspects of a renal biopsy. The concept of assessing the activity and chronic changes in a renal biopsy is more than 30 years old, but has attracted considerable attention over the past decade. The National Institutes of Health (NIH) scoring system (Table 2), derived from earlier versions, is commonly used [3].

The activity and chronicity indices derive from a general model of SLE in which the activity of the disorder will, if not controlled by therapy, cause irreversible chronic changes or damage [45]. In the setting of lupus nephritis, damage to the kidney, to other organs as a result of inflammatory disease elsewhere, or as an adverse effect of treatment, may result in organ failure or patient death. There is empirical evidence that this model is correct for lupus nephritis [5, 30].

While a study restricted to severe nephritis [44] and another with particularly long follow-up [1] have not found the chronicity index to predict long-term outcomes, this has in general not been the case. The NIH chronicity index, or a related variant, has been associated with both progressive renal disease [3, 16, 14, 41, 42, 55, 69, 81] and mortality, [14, 18, 41, 42, 52, 55] (Fig. 4). The absence of chronic changes bodes a particularly good prognosis. Among the components of the chronicity index,

Table 2. National Institutes of Health version of a renal pathology scoring system for assessing activity and chronicity

Activity index	Chronicity index
Glomerular abnormalities	
1. Cellular proliferation	1. Glomerular sclerosis
2. Fibrinoid necrosis, karyorrhexis	2. Fibrous crescents
3. Cellular crescents	
4. Hyaline thrombi, wire loops	
5. Leukocyte infiltration	
Tubulointerstitial abnormalities	
1. Mononuclear-cell infiltrate	1. Interstitial fibrosis
	2. Tubular atrophy

Each variable is scored 0–3+. Fibrinoid necrosis and cellular crescents are weighted by a factor of 2. Maximum score of activity index is 24, and that of chronicity index is 12. Reprinted from [3] with permission of the American Journal of Medicine

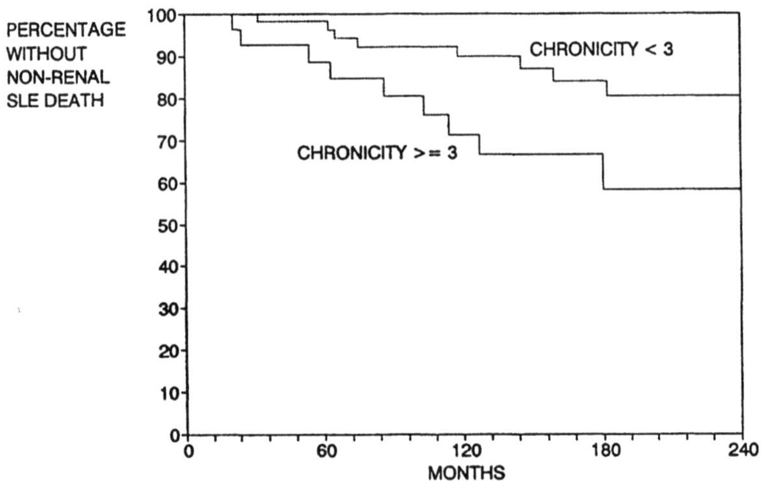

NUMBER OF PATIENTS AT RISK

CHRONICITY < 3	57	50	39	23	7
CHRONICITY >= 3	30	22	15	8	1

Fig. 4. Life-table depiction of lupus nephritis patients ($n = 87$) based on the level of the semi-quantitative chronicity index at the time of first renal biopsy ($P < 0.05$). The outcome is death that was not attributable to renal involvement. Of the 17 deaths, 12 were due to vascular disease (myocardial infarction or stroke), 3 to vasculitis and 2 to infection. The patients are described further in [18]

glomerular sclerosis and tubulointerstitial damage appear to be particularly important in determining the prognosis.

Because the activity index measures a potentially reversible phenomenon, one might expect the activity index to be a less consistent predictor of long-term outcome than the chronicity index. However, to the extent that the activity of the renal lesion is not controlled by therapy, it serves as a marker for subsequent irreversible damage. A number of studies have noted that a high score for the activity index predicts the development of progressive renal disease [3, 4, 6, 14, 42, 48, 49, 55, 61] and mortality [14, 42, 52] (Fig. 5).

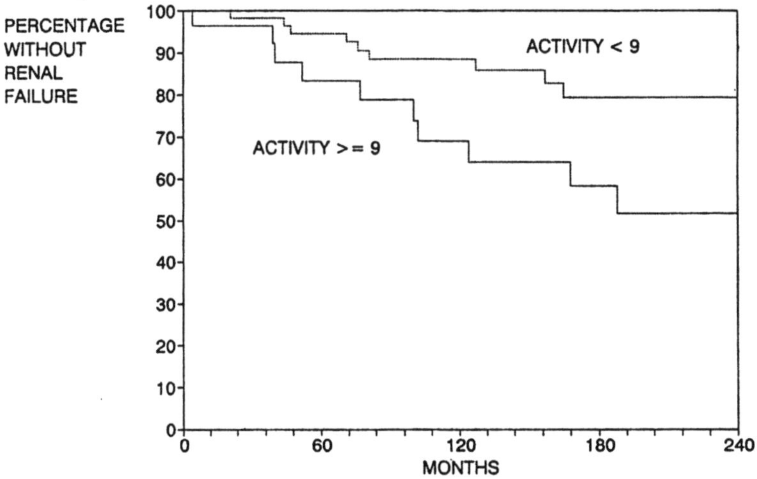

NUMBER OF PATIENTS AT RISK

ACTIVITY < 9	64	50	34	19	4
ACTIVITY >= 9	23	19	14	10	4

Fig. 5. Life-table depiction of lupus nephritis patients (n = 87) based on the level of the semi-quantitative activity index at the time of first renal biopsy ($P < 0.05$). The outcome is renal failure (n = 19) defined as the need for dialysis or renal transplantation. The patients are described further in [18]

Although a number of studies have found the assessment of the activity and chronicity indices to be reproducible, a recent study in a non-referral setting reported only moderate reproducibility [88]. A scoring atlas needs to be developed as this would likely enhance the reliability and comparability of these assessments.

Tubulointerstitial involvement. This has been noted to be a major determinant of prognosis for both end-stage renal disease and fatality in lupus nephritis and in glomerulonephritis in general [4, 14, 18, 42, 54, 93] (Fig. 6). While the changes in the tubulointerstitium were thought previously to be secondary to the glomerular changes, this is no longer the sole explanation. Tubulointerstitial changes in lupus nephritis may be one of the more important histological predictors of long-term renal function.

Electron-dense deposits. Early studies of ultrastructural abnormalities found that subendothelial electron-dense deposits, particularly massive amounts of these deposits, were associated with progressive renal disease. Recent studies have generally not confirmed this for the long-term outcome (reviewed in [14, 15]). However, ultrastructural variables are of predictive value in short-term prognosis (see below). Our own work suggests that these variables are of particular value in assessing a renal biopsy after therapy has been initiated (a repeat biopsy) [17].

Serial renal biopsies. Studies of repeat renal biopsies in patients with lupus nephritis report transformation in WHO class in approximately half of the cases. About one third of those with diffuse proliferative nephritis no longer have this lesion on a second biopsy. A similar proportion of those without a diffuse proliferative pattern initially, will be found to have developed it. No predictors of transformation among WHO classes of biopsy have been identified consistently [17].

Repeat biopsies have demonstrated that with treatment the activity index tends to decline (i.e., improve), while the chronicity index and the extent of tubulointerstitial

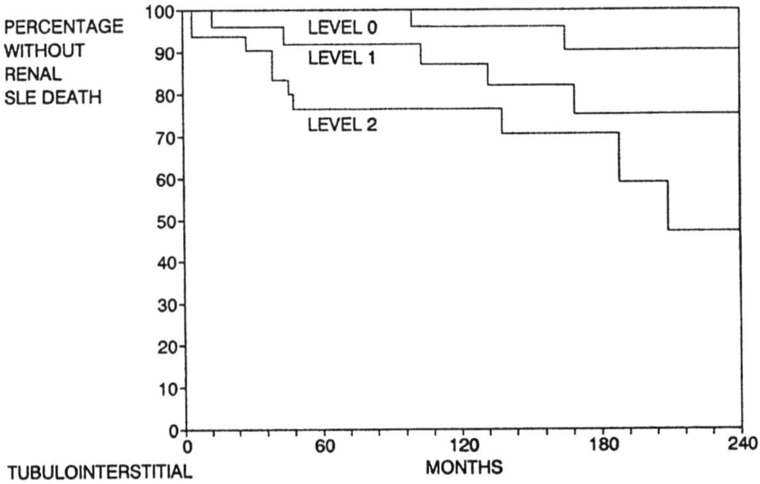

TUBULOINTERSTITIAL DEPOSITS	NUMBER OF PATIENTS AT RISK				
LEVEL 0	30	28	22	14	3
LEVEL 1	25	22	17	10	4
LEVEL 2	32	22	15	7	1

Fig. 6. Life-table depiction of lupus nephritis patients (n = 87) based on the level of a tubulointerstitial index at the time of first renal biopsy ($P < 0.05$). Level 0 = absence of significant damage, and level 2 = marked tubulointerstitial damage. The outcome is death due to involvement (n = 17). The index is described in [14] and additional data on the patients are detailed [18]

involvement stabilizes or deteriorates [5, 12, 17, 42, 55, 65, 69, 78]. Subendothelial and mesangial electron-dense deposits decrease and subepithelial deposits tend to increase between biopsies [17].

Improvement in the amount of subendothelial deposits between biopsies correlated with the between biopsy improvement in both serum creatinine and urinary protein excretion. Furthermore, an improvement in subendothelial or mesangial deposits between the two biopsies were the two strongest predictors of long-term preservation of renal function and patient survival [17].

Renal biopsy and short-term prognosis. Biopsy findings that have predicted a poorer short-term outcome include the presence of proliferative nephritis by WHO class [15, 89], a higher activity index [48, 89], evidence of chronicity or tubulointerstitial damage [15, 48, 89] and the presence of subendothelial deposits [15, 89].

The role of renal biopsy. There is considerable evidence that renal biopsy confirms the prognostic information that is available from clinical and laboratory markers. The role for a renal biopsy as a confirmatory test may be sufficient for many physicians and their patients to justify a renal biopsy. This is likely for a number of reasons. Firstly, while clinicians with considerable experience specifically in the management of lupus nephritis are expert at predicting both short-term and long-term outcome without recourse to renal biopsy data [16], this may not be true for all physicians [90]. Secondly, performing a renal biopsy frequently galvanizes an appropriate decision on treatment. In fact, one study suggests that early treatment particularly with immunosuppressive drugs, had significant long-term benefits for both avoiding renal failure and prolonging patient survival [19]. Given that delay in instituting treatment may increase the risks of end-stage renal disease and death, and that all treatments carry signifcant risks of toxicity, the confirmatory evidence from a renal biopsy may be essential to coming promptly to an appropriate therapeutic decision. Finally, biopsy variables may predict over longer observation periods than clinical markers [18].

Some authors have suggested that confirmatory information alone is not sufficient to justify the risks of renal biopsy. Accordingly, these investigators have demanded that a renal biopsy add predictive information over and above that obtained from the predictions of clinicians or statistically generated clinical models. For short-term prediction, the activity index and subendothelial deposits have each been shown to add significant information to computer generated models based on clinical and laboratory markers in at least two studies [15, 48, 89]. For long-term outcome, the chronicity index has contributed significant additional information to that obtained from clinical models, in three recent studies [3, 51, 55]. In a similar manner, a tubulointerstitial index added signifcantly to the long-term predictions by experienced clinicians [16]. Thus, using this more stringent criterion for evaluating renal biopsy, there is some support for performing renal biopsies in lupus nephritis.

All of these data focus on the prognostic value of a renal biopsy in groups of lupus patients. It has not been possible to demonstrate that information from renal biopsy improves the accuracy of a prediction for an individual patient [14, 15]. Admittedly, this standard is difficult to meet and would be met by few diagnostic procedures that are available today.

Dialysis and renal transplantation

Considerable effort is devoted to avoiding the development of end-stage renal disease. Unfortunately, it occurs all too frequently. At 5, 10, and 20 years, a recent long-term study reported that end-stage renal disease had occurred in 9%, 17% and 30%, respectively, of lupus nephritis patients [18] (Fig. 1).

For SLE patients undergoing dialysis, a number of reports noted a high death rate, especially in the early months after initiating dialysis. However, recent studies have suggested that SLE patients do as well as non-SLE patients on dialysis. Hemodialysis and continuous ambulatory peritoneal dialysis were equally well tolerated. While lupus disease activity was not abolished by dialysis, it did appear to diminish after dialysis was started compared to the activity present in the pre-dialysis period [8, 56].

Two decades ago lupus nephritis was considered a contraindication for renal transplantation. Current data suggest that patient survival, and graft survival and function, are no different for lupus nephritis patients than for those with other non-diabetic causes of end-stage renal disease. For lupus nephritis, the duration of dialysis and the level of disease activity prior to transplantation does not appear to influence the outcome. Recurrence of the nephritis in the transplant is uncommon, especially in those treated with cyclosporin [29, 57].

Neuropsychiatric lupus

Neuropsychiatric lupus is preferred to the term CNS lupus because more than the central nervous system is involved. Neuropsychiatric lupus is a major cause of morbidity and fatality in SLE in most studies [27, 34, 39, 67, 76], but not all [72, 86].

Unfortunately, despite its importance, study of this aspect of SLE has been limited by a number of issues, some of which remain unresolved.

Neuropsychiatric lupus can present in a large variety of ways and classification has proven difficult. A simple scheme is to separate neuropsychiatric events into diffuse and focal disorders. Diffuse disease includes generalized seizures, organic brain syndrome, psychosis, major affective disorders and cognitive dysfunction. Focal disease includes stroke, transient ischemic attacks, amaurosis fugax, cranial and peripheral neuropathies, chorea, transverse myelitis and aseptic meningitis. Other classifications exist [11].

The absence of an external standard, such as tissue biopsy in cutaneous or renal lupus, has made it difficult to confirm a diagnosis in an individual patient. It has also limited acceptance of any one classification system, a step that might facilitate progress in determining prognosis and evaluating pathogenesis. Furthermore, it is frequently difficult to distinguish neuropsychiatric lupus from the identical disorders which may arise from lupus treatment (e.g. steroid psychosis, infection) or co-morbid diseases (e.g., hypertension, atherosclerosis) [92].

Cognitive impairment is well recognized by clinicians as a common complaint in SLE. Recently, scientific studies have greatly increased our knowledge about cognitive impairment and its assessment (reviewed in [11]). However, the need for batteries of psychologic tests, uncertainty as to which tests should be included in a standard assessment, uncertainty as to how to interpret the results of the tests, and uncertainty as to the clinical implications of the mild abnormalities which are present in a large number of SLE patients, has limited the use of these instruments to the research setting.

A study of 354 lupus patients with neuropsychiatric involvement noted that survival is significantly reduced for patients with focal involvement compared to those with diffuse neuropsychiatric lupus [39]. This large study did not provide data on individual subsets within the focal group. Other recent studies suggest that stroke is associated with a particularly poor outcome [20. 23. 72]. Strokes have been linked to previous evidence of systemic thrombosis (e.g. deep venous thrombosis), elevated partial thromboplastin time, spontaneous abortion, age over 60 years, and cardiac valvular disease. Strokes tend to occur in the first 5 years after diagnosis and the risk of recurrence is high. Clearly, large multi-center studies will be needed if progress is to be made in the prognosis of neuropsychiatric lupus.

Conclusions

In SLE, morbidity is universal and fatality is significant. One cannot learn too much about the prognostic markers for this disorder. The identification by means of renal biopsy of subclasses of lupus nephritis spurred the development of new treatment regimens that have improved outcomes. While proliferative nephritis remains a marker of serious renal involvement, the newer indices that attempt to quantify the activity and chronicity of the renal lesion, as well as greater awareness of the importance of tubulointerstitial involvement and improvement in the amount of subendothelial electron-dense deposits with therapy, will likely permit further fine-tuning of the treatment of individual patients with lupus nephritis.

Neuropsychiatric involvement in SLE is another major determinant of financial costs, morbidity and death. Unfortunately, our knowledge of the prognostic markers for this more heterogeneous group of manifestations is less advanced than for lupus renal involvement. Additional studies are needed urgently to determine the factors that predict the subsequent development of the different forms of neuropsychiatric lupus. The determinants will likely differ among the various forms of neuropsychiatric lupus, thereby permitting different preventative or treatment regimens to be developed.

The role of social factors, particularly socioeconomic status, has attracted attention in the United States. The lessons are likely applicable elsewhere. Additional studies to identify social factors that can be modified may bring tangible benefits to SLE patients in this decade.

Although not universally accepted, it does appear that as more SLE patients survive the acute disease, there is an inordinately high risk of developing vascular diseases, including coronary artery disease, stroke and peripheral vascular disease. As with neuropsychiatric lupus, the determinants may differ depending on the specific vascular disease. Better knowledge of these determinants will permit a further improvement in the overall prognosis for patients with SLE.

Acknowledgement. The constructive critique of the manuscript by Drs. Jean-Luc Senecal and Paul Fortin is gratefully acknowledged, as is the help of Drs. John Hayslett, Michael Kashgarian, Lawrence Joseph, and Michael Abrahamowicz, and Mr. Carey Levinton and Mr. Todd MacKenzie in our collaborative studies on the prognosis of SLE. Ms. Barbara Cont provided expert secretarial assistance. Supported by grants from the Arthritis Society of Canada (number 85009) and the Alpha Omicron Pi Foundation.

References

1. Appel GB, Cohen DJ, Pirani CL, Meltzer JI, Estes D (1987) Long-term follow-up of patients with lupus nephritis. Am J Med 83:877
2. Asherson RA (1992) The catastrophic antiphospholipid syndrome. J Rheumatol 19:508
3. Austin III HA, Muenz LR, Joyce KM, Antonovych TA, Kullick ME, Klippel JH, Decker JL, Balow JE (1983) Prognostic factors in lupus nephritis. Am J Med 75:382
4. Austin III HA, Muenz LR, Joyce KM Antonovych TT, Balow JE (1984) Diffuse proliferative lupus nephritis: identification of specific pathologic features affecting renal outcome. Kidney Int 25:689
5. Balow JE, Austin III HA, Muenz LR, Joyce KM Antonovych TT, Klippel JH, Sternberg AD, Plotz PH, Decker JL (1984) Effect of treatment on the evolution of renal abnormalities in lupus nephritis. N Engl J Med 311:49
6. Banfi G, Mazzucco G, Di Belgiojoso GB, Bosisio MB, Stratta P, Confaloniere R, Ferrario F, Imbasciati E, Monga G (1985) Morphological parameters in lupus nephritis: their relevance for classification and relationship with clinical and histological findings and outcome. Q J Med 55:153
7. Budman DR, Sternberg AD (1976) Hypertension and renal disease in systemic lupus erythematosus. Arch Intern Med 36:1003
8. Cheigh JS, Kim R, Stenzel KR, Tapia L, Sullivan JF, Stubenbord W, Riggio RR, Rubin AL (1990) Systemic lupus erythematosus in patients with end-stage renal disease: long-term follow-up on the prognosis of patients and the evolution of lupus activity. Am J Kidney Dis 16:189
9. Clarke AE, Bloch DA, Danoff DS, Esdaile JM (1995) Decreasing costs and improving outcomes in SLE. J Rheumatol 22 (in press)
10. Clarke AE, Esdaile JM, Bloch DA, Lacaille D, Danoff DS, Fries JF (1993) A Canadian study of the total medical costs for patients with systemic lupus erythematosus and the predictors of costs. Arthritis Rheum 36:1548
11. Denburg SD, Denburg JA, Carbotte RM, Fisk JD, Hanly JG (1993) Cognitive deficits in systemic lupus erythematosus. Rheum Dis Clinic North Am 19:81
12. Derksen RHWM, Hené RJ, Kater L (1992) The long-term clinical outcome of 56 patients with biopsy-proven lupus nephritis followed at a single canter. Lupus 1:97

13. Edworthy SM, Bloch DA, McShane DJ, Segal MR, Fries JF (1989) A "State Model" of renal function in systemic lupus erythematosus: its value in the prediction of outcome in 292 patients. J Rheumatol 16:29
14. Esdaile JM, Levinton C, Federgreen W, Hayslett JP, Kashgarian M (1989) The clinical and renal biopsy predictors of long-term outcome in lupus nephritis: a study of 87 patients and review of the literature. Q J Med 72:779
15. Esdaile JM, Federgreen W, Quintal R, Suissa S, Hayslett JP, Kashgarian M (1991) Predictors of one year outcome in lupus nephritis. Q J Med 81:907
16. Esdaile JN, MacKenzie T, Barré P, Danoff D, Osterland CK, Somerville P, Quintal H, Kashgarian M, Suissa S (1992) Can experienced clinicians predict the outcome of lupus nephritis? Lupus 205:244
17. Esdaile JM, Joseph L, MacKenzie T, Kashgarian M, Hayslett JP (1993) The pathogenesis and prognosis of lupus nephritis: information from repeat renal biopsy. Semin Arthritis Rheum 23:135
18. Esdaile JM, Abrahamowicz M, MacKenzie T, Hayslett JP, Kashgarian M (1994) The time-dependence of long-term prediction in lupus nephritis. Arthritis Rheum 37:359
19. Esdaile JM, Joseph L, MacKenzie T, Kashgarian M, Hayslett JP (1995) The benefit of early treatment with immunosuppressive agents in lupus nephritis. J Rheumatol (in press)
20. Eustace S, Hutchinson M, Bresnihan B (1991) Acute cerebrovascular episodes in systemic lupus erythematosus. Q J Med 81:739
21. Finn D, Allen P, Hoffstein P, Goldman D, Petri M (1993) Economic costs of systemic lupus erythematosus (SLE): a five year prospective study (abstract). Arthritis Rheum 36 [Supp]:S192
22. Font J, Cervera R, Navarro M, Pallares L, Lopez-Soto A, Vivancos J, Ingelmo M (1992) Systemic lupus erythematosus in men: clinical and immunological characteristics. Am Rheum Dis 51:1050
23. Futrell N, Millikan C (1989) Frequency, etiology, and prevention of stroke in patients with systemic lupus erythematosus. Stroke 20:583
24. Fraenkel L, MacKenzie T, Joseph L, Kashgarian M, Hayslett JP, Esdaile JM (1992) Response to therapy as a predictor of outcome in lupus nephritis (abstract). Arthritis Rheum 35:S180.
25. Ganczarczyk L, Urowitz MB, Gladman DD (1989) "Latent lupus". J Rheumatol 16:475
26. Ginzler EM, Shorn K (1988) Outcome and prognosis in systemic lupus erythematosus. Rheum Dis Clinic North Am 14:57
27. Ginzler EM, Diamond HS, Weiner M, Schlesinger M, Fries JF, Wasner C, Medsger Jr TA, Ziegler G, Klippel JR, Hadler NM, Albert DA, Hess EV, Spencer-Green G, Grayzel A, Worth D, Hahn BH, Barnett EV (1982) A multicenter study of outcome in systemic lupus erythematosus. I. Entry variables as predictors of prognosis. Arthritis Rheum 25:601
28. Gladman DD, Urowitz MB (1987) Morbidity in systemic lupus erythematosus. J Rheumatol 14 [Suppl 13]:223
29. Goss JA, Cole BR, Jendrisak MD, McCullough CS, So SKS, Windus DW, Hanto DW (1991) Renal transplantation for systemic lupus erythematosus and recurrent lupus nephritis: a single-center experience and a review of the literature. Transplantation 52:805
30. Goulet J-R, MacKenzie T, Levinton C, Hayslett JP, Ciampi A, Esdaile JM (1993) The longterm prognosis of lupus nephritis: the impact of disease activity. J Rheumatol 20:59
31. Gruppo Italiano per lo studio della nefrite lupica (GISNEL) (1992) Lupus nephritis: prognostic factors and probability of maintaining life-supporting renal function 10 years after the diagnosis. Am J Kidney Dis 19:473
32. Harris EN (1994) Antiphospholipid antibodies and the antiphospholipid syndrome. Springer Semin Immunopathol 16:223
33. Hochberg MC, Boyd RE, Ahearn JM, Arnett FC, Bias WB, Provost TT, Stevens NW (1985) Systemic lupus erythematosus: a review of clinico-laboratory features and immunogenetic markers in 150 patients with emphasis on demographic subsets. Medicine 64:285
34. Jonsson H, Nived O, Sturfelt G (1989) Outcome in systemic lupus erythematosus: a prospective study of patients from a defined population. Medicine 68:141
35. Kaplan D, Ginzler EN, Feldman J (1991) Arthritis and nephritis in patients with systemic lupus erythematosus. J Rheumatol 18:223
36. Kasinath BS, Neilson EG, Hebert L, Schwartz MM, Lewis EJ, and the Lupus Nephritis Collaborative Study Group (1986) Short-term prognosis of severe proliferative lupus nephritis. Am J Kidney Dis 8:239
37. Kaslow RA (1982) High rate of death caused by systemic lupus eraematosus among U.S. residents of Asian descent. Arthritis Rheum 25:414

38. Kaufman LD, Gomez-Remo JJ, Heinicke MH, Gorevic PD (1989) Male lupus: retrospective analysis of the clinical and laboratory features of 52 patients, with a review of the literature. Semin Arthritis Rheum 18:189
39. Kovacs JA, Urowitz NW, Gladman DD (1993) Dilemmas in neuropsychiatric lupus. Rheum Dis Clinic North Am 19:795
40. Lacaille D, Clarke AE, Bloch DA, Danoff D, Esdaile JM (1994) The impact of disease activity, treatment and disease severity on short-term costs of systemic lupus erythematosus. J Rheumatol 421:(in press)
41. Laitman RS, Glicklich D, Sablay LB, Grayzel Al, Barland P, Bank (1989) Effect of long-term normalization of serum complement levels on the course of lupus nephritis. Am J Med 87:132
42. Leaker B, Fairley KF, Dowling J. Kincaid-Smith P (1987) Lupus nephritis: clinical and pathological correlation. Q J Med 62:163
43. Lee HS, Spargo BH (1985) A renal biopsy study of lupus nephritis in the United States and Korea. Am J Kidney Dis 5:24
44. Levey AS, Lan S-P, Corwin BL, Kasinath BS, Lachin J. Neilson EG, Hunsicker LG, Lewis EJ and the Lupus Nephritis Collaborative Study Group (1992) Progression and remission of renal disease in the lupus nephritis collaborative study: results of treatment with prednisone and short-term oral cyclophosphamide. Ann Intern Med 116:114
45. Liang MH, Stern S, Esdaile JM (1988) Towards an operational definition of SLE activity for clinical research. In: Klippel JH(Ed), Systemic Lupus Erythematosus. Rheum Dis Clin North Am 14:57
46. Liang MR, Partridge AJ, Daltroy LR Straaton KV, Galper SH, Holman HR (1991) Strategies for reducing excess morbidity and mortality in blacks with systemic lupus erythematosus. Arthritis Rheum 34:1187
47. Lockshin MD (1994) Lupus pregnancies and neonatal lupus. Springer Semin Immunopathol 16:247
48. Magil AB, Puterman ML, Ballon HS, Chan V, Lirenman DS, Rae A, Sutton RAL (1988) Prognostic factors in diffuse proliferative lupus glomerulonephritis. Kidney Int 34:511
49. McCurdy DK, Lehman TJA, Bemstein B, Hanson V, King KK, Nadorra R, Landing BH (1992) Lupus nephritis: prognostic factors in children. Pediatrics 89:240
50. McDonald, J Stewart J, Urowitz MB, Gladman DD (1992) Peripheral vascular disease in patients with systemic lupus erythematosus. Ann Rheum Dis 51:56
51. McLaughlin J. Bombardier C, Gladman D, Urowitz MB, Farewell V, Chang C-H, Cole E, Ritchie S, Churg J (1988) Kidney biopsy in systemic lupus erithematosus. III. Multivariate survival analyses of biopsy results (abstract). Arthritis Rheum 31 [Supp]:S28
52. McLaughlin J. Gladman DD, Urowitz MB, Bombardier C, Farewell VT, Cole E (1991) Kidney biopsy in systemic lupus erythematosus. II. Survival analyses according to biopsy results. Arthritis Rheum 34:1268
53. Miller MH, Urowitz MB, Gladman DD, Killinger DW (1983) Systemic lupus erythematosus in males. Medicine 62:327
54. Nath KA (1992) Tubulointerstitial changes as a major determinant in the progression of renal dammage. Am J Kidney Dis 20:1
55. Nossent HC, Henzen-Logmans SC, Vroom TM, Berden JHM, Swaak TJG (1990) Contribution of renal biopsy data in predicting outcome in lupus nephritis. Arthritis Rheum 33:970
56. Nossent HC,. Swaak TJG, Berden JHM, for the Dutch Working Party on SLE (1990) Systemic lupus erythematosus: analysis of disease activity in 55 patients with end-stage renal failure treated with hemodialysis or contmuous ambulatory peritoneal dialysis. Am J Med 89:169
57. Nossent HC, Swaak TJG, Berden JHM and the Dutch working party on systemic lupus erythematosus (1991) Systemic lupus erythematosus after renal transplantation: patient and graft survival and disease activity. Ann Intern Med 114:183
58. Ostrov BE, Min W, Eichenfield AR Goldsmith DP, Kaplan B, Athreya BH (1989) Hypertension in children with systemic lupus erythematosus. Semin Arthritis Rheum 19:90
59. Panush RS, Greer JM, Morshedian KK (1993) What is lupus? What is not lupus? Rheum Dis Clinic North AM 19:223
60. Petri M, Genovese M. (1992) Incidence of and risk factors for hospitalizations in systemic lupus erythematosus: a prospective study of the Hopkins lupus cohort. J Rheumatol 19:1559
61. Petri M, Bockenstedt L, Colman J, Whiting-O'Keefe Q, Fitz G, Sebastian A, Hellmann D (1988) Serial assessment of glomerular filtration rate in lupus nephropathy. Kidney Int 34:832

62. Petri M, Perez-Guttmann S, Longenecker JC, Hochberg M (1991) Morbidity of systemic lupus erythematosus: role of race and socioeconomic status. Am J Med 91:345
63. Petri M, Pence D, Bone LR, Hochberg MC (1992) Coronary artery disease risk factors in the John Hopkins lupus cohort: prevalence, recognition by patients, and preventative practices. Medicine 71:291
64. Petri M, Perez-Gutthann S, Pence D, Hochberg MC (1992) Risk factors for coronary artery disease in patients with systemic lupus erythematosus. Am J Med 93:513
65. Pillemer SR, Austin III HA, Tsokos GC, Balow JE (1988) Lupus nephritis: association between serology and biopsy measures. J Rheumatol 15:284
66. Pistiner M, Wallace DJ, Nessim S, Metzger AL, Klinenberg JR (1991) Lupus erythematosus in the 1980s: a survey of 570 patients. Semin Arthritis Rheum 21:55
67. Reveille JD, Bartolucci A, Alarcon GS (1990) Prognosis in systemic lupus erythematosus: negative impact of increasing age at onset black race, and thrombocytopenia, as well as causes of death. Arthritis Rheum 33:37
68. Rubin LA, Urowitz MB, Gladman DD (1985) Mortality in systemic lupus erythematosus: the bimodal pattern revisited. Q J Med 55:87
69. Rush PJ, Baumal R, Shore A, Balfe JW, Schreiber M (1986) Correlation of renal histology with outcome in cffildren with lupus nephritis. Kidney Int 29:1066
70. Schwartz MM, Kawala KS, Corwin HL, Lewis EJ (1987) The prognosis of segmental glomerulonephritis in systemic lupus erythematosus. Kidney Int 32:274
71. Seleznick MJ, Fries JF (1991) Variables associated with decreased survival in systemic lupus erythematosus. Semin Arthritis Rheum 21:73
72. Sibley JT, Olszynski WP, Decoteau WE, Sundaram MB (1992) The incidence and prognosis of central nervous system disease in systemic lupus erythematosus. J Rheumatol 19:47
73. Sontheimer RD (1989) Subacute cutaneous lupus erythematosus: a decade's perspective. Med Clinic North AM 73:1073
74. Sthoeger ZM, Geltner D, Rider A, Bentwich Z. (1987) Systemic lupus erythematosus in 49 Israeli males: a retrospective study. Clin Exp Rheumatol 5:233
75. Sturfelt G, Eskilsson J, Nived O, Truedsson L, Valind S (1992) Cardiovascular disease in systemic lupus erythematosus: a study of 75 patients from a defined population. Medicine 71:216
76. Swaak AJG, Nossent JC, Bronsveld W, Van Rooyen A, Nieuwenhuys EJ, Theuns L, Smeenk RJT (1989) Systemic lupus erythematosus. I. Outcome and survival: Dutch experience with 110 patients studied prospectively. Ann Rheum Dis 8:447
77. Swaak AJG, Nossent JC, Smeenk RJT (1991) Prognostic factors in systemic lupus erythematosus. Rheumatol Int 11:127
78. Tateno S, Hiki Y, Hamaguchi K, Tsuchida R Shigematsu R Kobayashi Y (1991) Study of lupus nephritis in males. Q J Med M 81:103
79. Turner-Stokes L, Jones M, Addison I, Mansell NM, Isenberg DA (1989) Does rheumatoid factor protect lupus patients from the developement of nephritis? Ann Rheum Dis 48:14
80. Wallace DJ, Podell TE, Weiner JM Cox MB, Klinenberg JR, Forouzesh S, Dubois EL (1982) Lupus nephritis: experience with 230 patients in a private practice from 1950 to 1980. Am J Med 72:209
81. Wallace DJ, Goldfinger D, Savage G, Nichols S, Goodman D, Fichman M, Stewart M, Klinenberg JR (1988) Predictive value of clinical laboratory, pathologic, and treatment variables in steroid/immunosuppressive resistant lupus nephritis. J Clin Apheresis 4:30
82. Wallace DJ, Pistiner M, Nessim S, Metzger A, Klineberg JR (1992) Cutaneous lupus erythematosus without systemic lupus erythematosus: clinical and laboratory features. Semin Arthritis Rheum 21:221
83. Ward MM, Studenski S (1990) Clinical manifestations of systemic lupus erythematosus: identification of racial and socioeconomic influences. Arch Intern Med 150:849
84. Ward MM, Studenski S (1990) Age associated clinical manifestations of systemic lupus erythematosus: a multivariate regression analysis. J Rheumatol 17:476
85. Ward MM, Studenski S (1990) Systemic lupus erythematosus in men: a multivariate analysis of gender differences in clinical manifestations. J Rheumatol 17:220
86. Ward MM, Studenski S (1991) The time course of acute psychiatric episodes in systemic lupus erythematosus. J Rheumatol 18:535
87. Ward MM, Studenski S (1992) Clinical prognostic factors in lupus nephritis: the importance of hypertension and smoking. Arch Intern Med 152:2082

88. Wernick RM, Smith DL, Houghton DC, Phillips DS, Booth JL, Runcker DN, Johnson DS, Brown KK, Gaboury CL (1993) Reliability of histologic scoring for lupus nephritis: a community-based evaluation. Ann Intern Med 119:805
89. Whiting-O'Keefe, Henke JE, Shearn MA, Hopper J Jr, Biava CG, Epstein WV (1982) The information content from renal biopsy in systemic lupus erythematosus. Ann Intern Med 96:718
90. Whiting-O'Keefe, Henke JE, Shearn MA, Hopper J Jr, Epstein WV (1982) Recognition of information in renal biopsies of patients with lupus nephritis. Ann Intern Med 96:723
91. Wilson HA, Hamilton ME, Spyker DA, Brunner CM, O'Brien WM, Davis IV JS, Winfield JB (1981) Age influences the clinical and serologic expression of systemic lupus erythematosus. Arthritis Rheum 24:1230
92. Wong KL, Woo EKW, Yu YL, Wong RWS (1991) Neurological manifestations of systemic lupus erythematosus: a prospective study. Q J Med 81:857
93. Yamamoto T, Nagase M, Hishida A, Honda N (1993) Interstitial inflammatory and chronic tubulointerstitial lesions in lupus nephritis: comparison with those in IgA nephropathy. Lupus 2:26

MIX
Papier aus verantwortungsvollen Quellen
Paper from responsible sources
FSC® C105338

If you have any concerns about our products,
you can contact us on
ProductSafety@springernature.com

In case Publisher is established outside the EU,
the EU authorized representative is:
Springer Nature Customer Service Center GmbH
Europaplatz 3, 69115 Heidelberg, Germany

Printed by Libri Plureos GmbH
in Hamburg, Germany